CLINICAL NURSING PRACTICE:
The Promotion and Management
of Continence

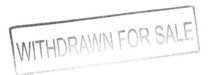

CLINICAL NURSING PRACTICE: The Promotion and Management of Continence

Brenda H. Roe BSc(Hons), MSc, PhD, RGN
Editor

Lecturer in Nursing, University of Liverpool,
Honorary Continence Advisor, Crewe Health
Authority.

Prentice Hall
New York London Toronto Sydney Tokyo

First published 1994 by
Prentice Hall International (UK) Limited
Campus 400, Maylands Avenue
Hemel Hempstead
Hertfordshire, HP2 7EZ
A division of
Simon & Schuster International Group

Typeset in 10/12pt Times
by Mathematical Composition Setters Ltd, Salisbury, Wiltshire

Printed and bound in Great Britain by Redwood Books, Trowbridge, Wilts

British Library Cataloguing in Publication Data

Clinical nursing practice: the promotion and
management of continence.
I. Roe, Brenda H.
616.60071

ISBN 0-13-138207-1

3 4 5   96 95

To J.C. Brocklehurst

Contents

x

List of figures and tables

Figures

Tables

Foreword

Nurses have always dealt with patients' urinary incontinence. Cleaning up others, changing garments or bedding from wet to dry are basic nursing activities. Our long role in providing comfort relates in part to help with toileting needs and attentive response to wetting. In our tradition we have rightly valued the kindly acceptance of another's need at this most personal level. But over the past twenty years nursing has grown in knowledge and understanding. While kindness and comfort remain central values, the importance of systematic patient need assessment, thoughtful care planning, attentive care implementation, and examination of patient outcome in response to care have focused our energies in an increasingly helpful way. This book presents what we need to know about urinary and faecal incontinence in order to provide quality care.

Some years ago I was asked to assist in an education programme for a busy hospital unit which had many elderly patients and a great deal of incontinence. I asked the staff what patient problems they wanted to discuss. They listed many but never mentioned incontinence. When I brought this to their attention, they explained that incontinence wasn't a problem in that they had a solution (adult diapers). They further explained that since incontinence was inevitable and irreversible, they would rather focus on real issues, that is, problems upon which they could truly impact. Those nurses needed this book. Adult diapers, while sometimes helpful in wetting management, are not a solution to incontinence. Loss of urine control with age is neither inevitable nor irreversible. Incontinence is a real issue and nurses can truly make an impact.

Nurses need knowledge in order to act effectively. Most have received little information about incontinence in their basic education programme. This book addresses the knowledge gap in urinary incontinence. It continues a tradition of outstanding British contributions to this clinical problem area from expert authors representing several collaborative disciplines. A useful and needed book, I welcome it into the world of nursing.

Thelma J. Wells, Ph.D., RN, FAAN, FRCN
Professor of Nursing
University of Rochester
Rochester, New York, USA

Preface

Promotion of continence and management of incontinence is an important aspect of nursing practice. Within the last decade, more than 300 specialist continence advisers have been appointed throughout the United Kingdom, following the recommendations of Dame Phyllis Friend, then Chief Nursing Officer at the Department of Health (CNO) (SNC) (77/1) and the Action on Incontinence Working Group (1983). It is a developing speciality with an increasing international profile supported by a number of professional organisations; the International Continence Society (ICS), Association of Continence Advisors (ACA), the Royal College of Nursing of the United Kingdom (RCN) and the British Association of Continence Carers (BACC). There is recognition of the importance of nursing practice for the promotion and management of continence not only by clinical nurse specialists but also by the nursing profession. It is every nurse's responsibility to base clinical practice upon sound research evidence.

The aim of this book is to present contribution chapters by individuals who are specialists within this field, who have undertaken unique research or who have a critical command of the research into incontinence. Each chapter presents their subject along with a critical review of the literature and research evidence from which clinical nursing practice should be based. Recommendations for practice are made and areas for further research identified.

The book is intended for a wide audience, clinically and geographically. It is hoped that not only clinical nurse specialists will find it of benefit but also qualified and student nurses, nurse educationalists and managers, physiotherapists and researchers in the field of incontinence.

In Chapter 1, Ann Mohide reviews recent studies dealing with the prevalence of urinary incontinence, highlighting the need for clear definitions and the difficulty of comparing studies due to different methodological approaches. She also briefly describes the social and psychological effects of urinary incontinence as experienced by sufferers. Francine Cheater in Chapter 2 presents the causes and types of urinary incontinence necessary for deciding upon the most appropriate clinical management. This is further supported by Hilary Duffin in Chapter 3 who deals with the assessment of incontinence using a variety of techniques, such as interview, physical examination, use of bladder charts (frequency/volume, continence) to establish baseline micturition patterns and non-invasive techniques to obtain clinical specimens. Finally, the use of urodynamic investigations for the accurate diagnosis of urinary incontinence are described. This chapter also deals with the difficulties of obtaining accurate and reliable clinical information. Detailed assessment of incontinence is necessary for planning appropriate practice for the promotion of continence or management of incontinence. All positive attempts to promote continence should be endeavoured. Chapters 4 and 5 deal with the promotion of continence using bladder re-education or pelvic floor muscle re-education. In Chapter 4, Anne Kennedy presents behavioural approaches using bladder re-education programmes such as bladder training, habit retraining, timed and prompted voiding, along with indications for the types of incontinence and clients they are most suitable for. Jo Laycock in Chapter 5 goes on to deal with clinical practices for the re-education of pelvic floor muscles, using exercise, electrical stimulation and biofeedback. She not only describes the techniques used in the various research studies but also details the importance of accurate assessment of the pelvic floor muscles by nurses and physiotherapists.

Where promotion of continence cannot be achieved then effective management of incontinence is required. Chapters 6, 7 and 8 deal with the management of incontinence using a variety of incontinence aids and appliances, intermittent self-catheterisation and the use of an indwelling urethral catheter. Alan Cottenden in Chapter 6 provides a comprehensive critical review of the research appertaining to containment aids, such as disposable and reusable pads and bedpads, penile sheaths and urinals. Despite there being a rapidly changing product market, by reviewing the research evidence over a number of years key recommendations can be made for the selection and purchase of incontinence aids and the clinical decisions regarding suitability for clients. In Chapter 7, Ann Winder describes the technique of intermittent self-catheterisation along with the practical aspects of selection of catheters and the ordering and disposal of supplies. She also deals with urinary tract infections and the reuse of catheters. A definition and comprehensive review of research relating to catheter care is presented in Chapter 8 by Brenda Roe. Recommendations for clinical practice and further research relate to the selection of catheters and urine drainage bags, catheterisation, meatal cleansing and the emptying, changing and reuse of drainage bags. Also included are bladder instillations and catheter removal with discussion of clamping catheters and the use of catheter valves.

In Chapter 9, James Barrett presents a definitive account of faecal incontinence, its prevalence, aetiology and practical management. Kath Baker and Brenda Roe in Chapter 10 describe the initiatives and strategies for the promotion of continence and management of incontinence by setting up a Continence Advisory Service. They deal not only with the practical aspects but also consideration of clinical practice, education, management and research. Finally, in Chapter 11, teaching patients and carers about their continence, its promotion or management, is covered. Brenda Roe presents a critical review of the literature appertaining to patient education and incontinence and discusses the role of the nurse versus nurse specialist for continence teaching. A variety of methods and approaches are suggested for the teaching of patients and carers in relation to continence.

It is hoped that this book will not only draw together the expertise and research evidence from which clinical practice for the promotion and management of continence should be based, but also contribute to the further development of nursing and this speciality in particular. Clinical nursing practice for continence is a developing field with further research initiatives required. However, there is already a tremendous body of knowledge that needs to be consolidated and used as the basis for our nursing practice, with the ultimate aim that clients' continence is promoted, their incontinence effectively managed and their suffering alleviated.

I am grateful to Professor Thelma Wells for writing the Foreword. She is not only a nurse specialist, teacher and researcher in the field of continence, but also continues to be an inspiration to us all. This book has been a team effort with all authors making valuable contributions that reflect their expertise, commitment and perseverance. I am also grateful to Prentice Hall International and Mike Cash in particular for allowing the seeds of an idea to grow.

Brenda H. Roe, 1991

Reference

Action on Incontinence Working Group (1983), King's Fund Project. Paper 43. King's Fund Centre, London.

Acknowledgements

We should like to thank Vivien Rooney for carrying out the literature search for Chapter 4, Bladder re-education for the promotion of continence.

We would also like to acknowledge the following sources for giving their permission to reproduce in full or to adapt the diagrams, photographs and tables included in the book.

Chapter 1:
Table 1.1 reproduced with the kind permission of W.B. Saunders, Philadelphia from E.A. Mohide (1986), 'The prevalence and scope of urinary incontinence', *Clinics in Geriatric Medicine*, 2(4): 639–55.

Chapter 5:
Figures 5.1 and 5.2 adapted with the kind permission of J.B. Lippincott Company, Philadelphia.

Figure 5.3 with permission of Doncast, Caterham, Surrey.

Figures 5.4, 5.10, 5.12 with kind permission of Nomeq Healthcare and Rehabilitation Equipment, Redditch, Worcestershire.

Figure 5.5 with permission of Colgate Medical Ltd, Windsor.

Figure 5.6 from *Physiotherapy* (1987), 73(7): 372, with kind permission of *Physiotherapy*, The Journal of the Chartered Society of Physiotherapy.

Figures 5.7 and 5.12 with permission of St Luke's Hospital Medical Illustration Department, Bradford.

Figures 5.8 and 5.9 with the kind permission of Dr Giovanni de Domenico, School of Physiotherapy, Dalhousie University, Nova Scotia, Canada.

Finally we should like to thank Ann Thomson and Sarah Robinson for allowing us to read Sleep, J. (1991), 'Perineal care: a series of five randomised controlled trials', in Robinson, S. and Thomson, A.M. (eds), *Midwives, Research and Childbirth*, vol. 2, London: Chapman and Hall, before it was published.

Contributors

Kathleen E.M. Baker, RGN, RCNT
Projects Manager, formerly District Continence Adviser, Crewe Health Authority, UK.

James A. Barrett, MD, MRCP
Consultant Physician in Geriatric Medicine Rehabilitation, Clatterbridge Hospital, Wirral, Part-time Clinical Lecturer, Department of Geriatric Medicine, University of Liverpool, UK.

Francine M. Cheater, MA (Hons), PhD, RGN
Lecturer in Nursing, Queen Margaret College, Edinburgh, UK.

Alan M. Cottenden, MA, PhD, MBES, MIM CEng
Research Bioengineer, Incontinence Advisory Service, St Pancras' Hospital, London, UK.

Hilary Duffin, RGN, FETC
Clinical Nurse Specialist, Continence Clinic, Leicester General Hospital, Leicester, UK.

Anne P. Kennedy, BSc (Hons), PhD, RGN
Research Nurse, South Manchester Health Authority, Manchester, UK.

Josephine Laycock, MCSP, SRP
Superintendent Physiotherapist, Department of Urotherapy, Bradford Royal Infirmary, Bradford, UK.

E. Ann Mohide, BScN, MHSc, MSc
Associate Professor of School of Nursing, McMaster University, Hamilton, Ontario, Canada.

Brenda H. Roe, BSc (Hons), MSc, PhD, RGN
Lecturer in Nursing, University of Liverpool, Honorary Continence Adviser, Crewe Health Authority, UK.

Ann Winder, RGN
District Continence Adviser, Ham Green Hospital, Pill, Bristol, UK.

1 The prevalence of urinary incontinence

E. ANN MOHIDE

Introduction

The burden of urinary incontinence is considerable, not only on the physical, psychological and social well-being of those who suffer with it but also for their carers and for health care services. How many people suffer from urinary incontinence, who are they and where are they? In this chapter the prevalence of urinary incontinence in community and institutional settings is reviewed together with the implications for those who suffer with it. Empirical studies and literature reviews are presented as well as consideration of the conceptual issues and methodological difficulties when studying urinary incontinence.

Definition of urinary incontinence

The International Continence Society Committee on Standardisation of Terminology (ICSCST) has contributed a standard definition of urinary incontinence that is as clear and succinct as is currently possible. The Committee defines urinary incontinence as 'the involuntary loss of urine which is objectively demonstrable and a social or hygiene problem' (Anderson *et al.*, 1988, p. 17). Further to this, involuntary urine loss through channels other than the urethra is termed extraurethral incontinence (ibid.). The ICSCST points out that involuntary loss can be a symptom, a sign and a condition (Anderson *et al.*, 1988). A subjective report of involuntary loss constitutes a symptom and the objective demonstration of involuntary urine loss denotes incontinence as a sign, while urodynamic studies are required to define urinary incontinence as a condition. Despite the stipulation that the term urinary incontinence requires an objective demonstration, it still involves a judgement about whether the extent of involuntary urine loss is a social or hygiene problem (involuntary urine loss might not be a clinically important issue if the social and/or hygiene aspect was not satisfied). Related to this, the 1988 Consensus Conference on Urinary Incontinence in Adults (Office of Medical Applications of Research, 1989) added the strong qualifier 'so severe as to have social and/or hygienic consequences' (p. 2685) to the definition of incontinence. The qualifier 'so severe' implies that there is a threshold where involuntary loss becomes a clinical problem.

The operational definitions of urinary incontinence used in the surveys cited in Table 1.1 are quite varied and, no doubt, this accounts for some of the variation in estimates of prevalence. Last (1988) defined prevalence as 'the number of instances of a given disease or other condition in a given population at a designated time'. It is a ratio expressing the total number of individuals having the condition at a particular time or during a particular period in the numerator, and the total population at risk of having the attribute or disease at that time or midway through the period of time in question. Most of what is known about the magnitude of this condition is based on prevalence data.

While the ICSCST (Anderson *et al.*, 1988) definition probably minimises the extent of over-reporting by restricting the definition to include only those cases where the problem is viewed to be a social or hygiene problem, it has not been used by all investigators (Table 1.1). In an attempt to avoid overinflating the figures, Feneley *et al.* (1979) and Thomas *et al.* (1980) set a minimum frequency of involuntary urine loss over a specified time period. This probably served to identify clinically important cases and to decrease the likelihood that an individual with a short-term episode of involuntary loss, for instance during an acute illness, would be classified as being incontinent. In contrast, Wolin's (1969) expansive definition of 'ever' experiencing involuntary loss resulted in a very high prevalence estimate. The manner in which the question about involuntary urine loss is asked may bias the results. As an example, the question 'How often do you have difficulty holding your urine until you get to the toilet?' assesses 'difficulty' as opposed to actual involuntary loss (Herzog *et al.*, 1990; Herzog and Fultz, 1990).

Variation in prevalence may also be related to the patterns or types of incontinence considered in the study. For example, Milne *et al.* (1972) examined urge and stress incontinence, while Wolin (1969) and Yarnell *et al.* (1981) only included stress incontinence. In addition to differences in prevalence explained by pattern or type of incontinence, failure to include less obvious forms of involuntary loss can result in underestimation. For instance, both urethral and external catheters (penile sheaths) are used frequently as a management strategy for incontinence in long-term institutions. While Ouslander *et al.* (1982) included subjects with catheters (excluding cases of hypotonic bladder and obstruction), Jewett *et al.* (1981) did not, and underestimated the prevalence considerably (35 per cent as opposed to 58 per cent). Similarly, the US Department of Health Education and Welfare (1975) survey of nursing homes reported that 55 per cent of residents were incontinent, although it was higher (61 per cent) after taking catheters into account. Sullivan and Lindsay (1984) probably skewed the incontinence figures for males relative to females by classifying subjects with penile sheaths as incontinent and subjects with urethal catheters as continent. Only two community-based studies, Feneley *et al.* (1979) and Mohide *et al.* (1988), incorporated usage of catheters (urethral and external), and extraurethral continence appliances into the definition of incontinence. In a study of incontinence among patients receiving organised home health services, Mohide *et al.* (1988) found that 25 per cent of those classified as incontinent were using an appliance, catheter or

Table 1.1 Description of urinary incontinence prevalence studies

Survey	Study sample	Setting	Definition of incontinence	Data source	Data collection	Overall prevalence (%)
Studies in community settings						
Wolin, 1969	Nulliparous unmarried females aged 17–25; N = 4,211	17 nursing schools in the New York City area and 6 in Denver, Colorado, USA	Stress incontinence was defined as the accidental passing of urine on laughing, coughing, sneezing, or excitement not related to the desire to void.	Subjects	Written questionnaire administered by the investigator, response rate not given	51
Vetter *et al.*, 1981	Random sample of those ≥70 years; N = 1,280	2 large general practices in South Wales	'Do you ever wet yourself if you are unable to get to the lavatory as soon as you need to, or when you are asleep at night, or if you cough or sneeze?' If answered yes, questions followed about frequency and amount.	Subjects	Interviewed using a standardised questionnaire; type of interviewer not identified; response rate 95%	14

(Continued)

Table 1.1 Continued

Survey	Study sample	Setting	Definition of incontinence	Data source	Data collection	Overall prevalence (%)
Diokno et al., 1986	Random sample of ≥60 years, August, 1983 to July, 1984; N = 1,955	Households in Washtenaw County, Michigan, USA	'Any respondent who reported losing urine of any volume with a minimum frequency of 6 days within the last 12 months.' Those who lost urine on less than 6 occasions were examined for a fit with the types of incontinence, e.g. stress. If there was a fit, the respondent was classified as incontinent.	Subjects	Face-to-face interview in the home; response rate 65%	30
Holst and Wilson, 1988	Random sample of women ≥18 years; N = 851	Dunedin, New Zealand	Not specified; subjects responded to a presence/absence question examining a 12 month period. If incontinent, frequency, severity and social implications were examined.	Subjects	Standardised telephone interview; response rate 76%	31
Jolleys, 1988	Census survey of all women, ≥25 years and those taking oral contraceptives <21	A rural general practice in Leicestershire, England	Patients were asked whether they experienced leakage of urine on	Subjects	Postal survey with one follow-up reminder, response rate 89%	41

Reference	Population	Setting	Definition	Informants	Method	No.
	years, registered with the practice 1 May 1987; N = 833		coughing, laughing, exercise, lifting, climbing stairs, a full bladder, or other occasions. Frequency of occurrence was categorised.			
Mohide *et al.*, 1988	All patients ≥16 years receiving organised home health care; N = 2,850	A large urban area, Hamilton, in southern Ontario, Canada	Involuntary loss of urine that was a social or hygienic problem and was objectively demonstrable. Included use or urethral, extraurethral and external catheters, intermittent catheterisation, and incontinence that would occur if a toileting routine was not implemented.	Subjects, family, and home health care staff (including family physicians and homemakers)	Standardised written continence assessment form completed by the primary home health care professional (88% nurses); response rate 97%	22

Studies including subjects from both community and institutional settings

Reference	Population	Setting	Definition	Informants	Method	No.
Brocklehurst *et al.*, 1968	All patients ≥65 years; N = 557	1 general practice in a London suburb; England; N = 7,000	'Does urine ever come away unexpectedly or without your being able to stop it and you get wet? Does this only happen when you cough, laugh or move?'	Subjects	Questionnaire administered by a nurse; response rate 85%	20

(Continued)

Table 1.1 Continued

Survey	Study sample	Setting	Definition of incontinence	Data source	Data collection	Overall prevalence (%)
Milne et al., 1972	Random sample of those ≥62–90 years; N = 487	Elderly people living in a defined area of Edinburgh, Scotland; N = 27,000	'Do you lose control of your bladder if unable to go to the lavatory as soon as you need to pass urine?' 'Does your urine come away if you cough or sneeze?'	Subjects, and when mentally impaired, staff	Questionnaire; does not state who administered the questionnaire; no response rate given	34
Feneley et al., 1979 1. Recognised incontinence	All those known to health, social and welfare agencies; total active caseloads not provided; N of incontinent = 368	In a British community; N = 37,000	Involuntary excretion or leakage of urine and/or faeces in inappropriate places and at inappropriate times. The threshold consisted of dribbling incontinence, or two or more episodes of incontinence in the previous month. Included the use of catheters and appliances.	General practitioners, community nurses, and staff in health, social and welfare agencies	Asked to report cases to investigators; did not specify about the use of any standardised questionnaire or response form; no follow up procedures were reported; response rate not given	1
2. Unrecognized incontinence	≥5 years of age; N = 6,510	One group practice; N = 7,000	Same as above.	Subjects and parents of subjects aged 5–15 years	Postal survey with two follow up reminders; response rate 93%	5
Yarnell and St Leger, 1979	Women and men ≥65 years in 1975; N = 368	All medical practices in a South Wales town; N = 27,696	'Was there any leakage of urine in the previous 12 months?' If answered	Subjects, and when mentally unreliable, the next-of-kin or	Questionnaire administered by first author in each subject's place of	14

Reference	Sample	Location; N	Definition / questions	Respondent	Methods / response rate	Prevalence
(continued from previous page)			yes, questions followed about frequency and time of day.		residence; response rate 98%	15–64 years <1; ≥65 years 2
Thomas *et al.*, 1980, 1. Recognised incontinence	All those ≥15 years known to health and social agencies; total number not provided for active caseloads; N of incontinent = 1,944	In the London boroughs and health districts of Brent and Harrow, England; N = 359,000	'Regular' incontinence was involuntary excretion or leakage of urine in inappropriate places or at inappropriate times – twice or more a month regardless of the quantity of urine lost. Incontinence occurring less than twice a month was termed 'occasional'.	Health and social agency workers	Did not specify about the use of any standardised questionnaire; no follow up procedures were reported; response rate not given	15–64 years <1; ≥65 years 2
2. Unrecognised incontinence	All patients ≥5 years; N = 17,694	~12 general practices in 5 British communities; N = 22,430	Same as above	Subjects and parents of subjects aged 5–15 years	Mail survey sent out to patients by their physicians; up to two reminders were sent at 3-week intervals; response rate 87%	15–64 years 16; ≥65 years 22
Yarnell *et al.*, 1981	A random sample of women ≥17 years; N = 1,022	A light-industrial town in South Wales; N = 38,000	'Do you ever have to rush to the toilet to pass water? If you have to rush to the toilet, do you ever lose any water before reaching the toilet?' 'Do you lose urine at any other time, for example, when you cough, laugh, or sneeze, etc.?'	Subjects	Interviewed by a nurse using a standardised questionnaire; response rate 90%; complete data available on 1,000 of 1,022 subjects for the purpose of analyses	45

(Continued)

Table 1.1 Continued

Survey	Study sample	Setting	Definition of incontinence	Data source	Data collection	Overall prevalence (%)
Campbell et al., 1985	Random stratified sample of those ≥65 years; N = 559	Gisborne, New Zealand	'Do you have any trouble controlling your water?' If answered no, then asked 'Do you ever wet yourself or do you always get to the toilet on time?'	Subjects and, when an accurate history was not possible, an individual most closely associated with the subject	Questionnaire administered by a physician; response rate 95%	10
Koyano et al., 1986	Subsample (N = 2,567) of a random sample of those ≥65 years; N = 3,906	Over 25% of elderly population in Koganei City, a residential district of Metropolitan Tokyo, Japan	Not specified; subjects responded in one of three categories: incontinent, occasionally incontinent, never incontinent	Subjects	Postal survey, no details provided; response rate where data on continence status and disability were completed 66%	3
Elving et al., 1989	Age stratified random sample of females aged 30–59; N = 2,631	6% of the female population aged 30–59 in the municipality of Aarhus, Denmark	Involuntary urine loss ever experienced in adult life and in 1987. Included a question about whether the urine loss was a social or hygienic problem.	Subjects	Postal survey with two follow up reminders; 85% response rate	10, for 1987
Molander et al., 1990	Random sample of females aged 65–85 years; N = 4,206	10% of the female population of Goteborg, Sweden	Not specified.	Subjects	Postal survey with one follow up reminder; 70% response rate	Current 17 at some time in adult life 23

(Continued)

Studies in long-term care institutional settings

Isaacs and Walkey, 1964	All patients; N = 552	A geriatric hospital in Glasgow, Scotland; 85% of patients were ≥65 years and 51% had been in hospital over 1 year	Bed wet on rising or one 'accident' during the day, incontinence more than once, doubly incontinent.	Not stated	'Enquiries' were made but no information about the data collection was provided	43
US Department of Health, Education and Welfare, Public Health Service, 1975	15 randomly selected nursing home residents in each of 288 nursing homes; N = 4,320	US nursing homes in the Medicare/Medicaid programme; total nursing home population = 283,915	Involuntary loss of urine at least occasionally.	Nursing home staff	Standardised written assessment form used; response rate not given	55
Jewett et al., 1981	All ≥65 years admitted over a 13-month period; N = 277	An urban long-term care hospital with 321 chronic care beds, 75% geriatric care; Ontario, Canada	Involuntary loss of urine that was a social or hygienic problem and was objectively demonstrated.	Subjects, subjects' family and hospital staff	Standardised questionnaire administered by a research nurse; response rate not given	38
Ouslander et al., 1982	All patients ≥65 years; N = 842	Seven US nursing homes: four proprietary, too non-profit and a Veterans Administration nursing home care unit	Any uncontrolled leakage of urine regardless of the amount or frequency. Included the use of catheters except in cases of hypotonic bladder or obstruction.	Nursing home nurses	Verbal report from nurses with follow up verification using patient, staff and family interviews, as well as the review of each health record; response rate not given	50

Table 1.1 Continued

Survey	Study sample	Setting	Definition of incontinence	Data source	Data collection	Overall prevalence (%)
Fernie et al., 1983	All patients ⩾65 years admitted over a 21-month period; N = 437	An urban long-term care hospital with 321 chronic care beds, 75% geriatric care, Ontario, Canada	Involuntary loss of urine that was a social or hygienic problem and was objectively demonstrated.	Subjects, subjects' family and hospital staff	Standardised questionnaire administered by a research nurse; response rate not given	38
Ouslander and Fowler, 1985	All patients; N = 7,853	90 US Veterans Administration nursing home care units	Any involuntary leakage of urine, regardless of frequency and amount. Included the use of catheters.	Nursing home nursing supervisors	Standardised mail questionnaire; response rate 94%	41
Tobin and Brocklehurst, 1986	Permanent long-term care residents; N = 1,189	30 Local Authority Residential Homes in Greater Manchester, England	'Involuntary loss of urine on one or more occasions per week.' Frequent incontinence was one or more occasions per day and intermittent was less than once per day.	Residential home staff	Face-to-face interview; no details or response rate provided about the interview	Frequent 25 Intermittent 7
Studies in acute-care hospitals						
Sullivan and Lindsay, 1984	All patients ⩾65 years admitted over a 6-week period; N = 315 completed a hospital stay during the study period	A 730-bed acute-care teaching hospital in Charlottesville, Virginia, USA	Any inappropriate loss of urine regardless of amount and frequency. Included the use of condom catheters but	Nursing staff	Daily verbal report to one of the investigators; response rate not given	19

Sier *et al.*, 1987	Census survey of patients ≥65 years admitted during a 14-week period; N = 363	Three general medical wards, 2 surgical wards and 1 medical intensive care unit at UCLA Medical Centre, Los Angeles, California, USA	excluded the use of urethral or suprapubic catheters. Non-catheterised patients who had one or more episodes of incontinence during the hospitalisation.	Hospital nursing staff	Predeveloped and pretested Incontinence Monitoring Record completed twice every eight hours per patient by the nursing staff after receiving inservice training; response rate not given	35
Sudbury and Mohide, 1990	One day census survey of all admitted patients ≥65 years; N = 230	622-bed acute-care teaching hospital in active treatment beds in Hamilton, Ontario, Canada	Involuntary urine loss was objectively demonstrated. Patients with catheters were classified as incontinent except where there were medical indications.	Medical record and hospital nursing staff	A predeveloped and pretested standardised pre-coded form was used by nurse research assistants to abstract the medical records and interview the nursing staff; response rate 100%	20

intermittent catheterisation. With the exception of Mohide *et al*. (1988), studies of older adults have not identified study subjects who would be incontinent if they did not have reliable assistance for using the toilet, as incontinent.

Measurement of urinary incontinence

The measurement of urinary incontinence in research investigations is fraught with problems. The measurement attributes of research instruments used in surveys have not been examined in depth (Mohide, 1986; Herzog and Fultz, 1990). Both reliability and validity are required measurement attributes in order to come as close as possible to the 'true' ascertainment of incontinence. Yet, most studies do not elaborate on instrument development issues. Herzog and Fultz (1990) provide examples of such instrument development and testing.

The quantification of involuntary urine loss is difficult to establish when comprehensive clinical examinations and urodynamic tests are not included as part of the study. In fact, Table 1.1 illustrates that most prevalence studies have not validated self-reported involuntary urine loss. This is an important point where self-reports are the only source of data. Molander *et al*. (1990) conducted clinical assessments on 300 of the 677 subjects reporting that they experienced involuntary urine loss. In 4.6 per cent of the cases this could not be validated objectively.

As mentioned earlier, individuals assessing the involuntary loss of urine, whether they are patients, informal caregivers or health professionals, are likely to have varying points of view about what extent of involuntary urine loss constitutes a problem. Careful examination of an investigator's operational definition of urinary incontinence is warranted, since the inclusion of infrequent urine loss in scant amounts would serve to inflate the prevalence (Mohide, 1986) above what would be deemed to be clinically important. As an example, Thomas *et al*. (1980) found that few subjects experiencing minimal involuntary urine loss considered that they had a problem. Inclusion of these subjects would inflate the figures beyond what is clinically important.

Other issues influencing prevalence estimates

Different methods used in studies (Mohide, 1986; Thiede, 1989; Herzog and Fultz 1990) have contributed to the variations in prevalence. For example, some investigators did not determine the extent to which the non-respondents were similar to the respondents. If the response rate is not high and the respondents differ from the non-respondents, then the results will not reflect the truth in the population to which the results are being inferred. As another factor, differences in the study samples, for example sex, age, type of setting (long-term care institution versus community living), influence the prevalence figures.

Under-reporting is such an important issue that it deserves some detailed discussion.

It is most problematic in studies where information about involuntary urine loss is based entirely on self-reports. Some subjects do not volunteer information about involuntary urine loss (Holst and Wilson, 1988; Jolleys, 1988; Molander *et al.*, 1990) even when the individual feels that it is a social or hygiene problem. This may be due to the shame, the fallibility of memory or other reasons. Because urinary incontinence is not life-threatening, not solely associated with life-threatening disease, not painful, not necessarily a functional impairment, and not impossible to manage without medical intervention, it can be a 'hidden' condition among individuals living in the community. Thomas *et al.* (1980) found that only 10 out of 34 patients with moderate to severe incontinence were receiving health and social services for the incontinence. Yarnell *et al.* (1981) also found under-reporting on the part of some subjects; and in Wolin's (1969) study, none of the subjects who were interviewed had sought medical attention because they were either ashamed or did not perceive the incontinent episodes as abnormal. In cases where health professionals provide data about incontinence, under-reporting can occur as a result of failure to assess continence status. In two studies of nursing home residents (Ouslander *et al.*, 1982; Ribeiro and Smith, 1985), urinary incontinence was recorded as a problem by physicians in less than 15 per cent of the identified cases of incontinence. Both Feneley *et al.* (1979) and Thomas *et al.* (1980) attempted to differentiate between the prevalence of recognised incontinence (i.e. cases of incontinence that were known to health or social agency workers) and unrecognised incontinence (i.e. incontinence case-finding by means of a postal survey to the subjects). Both groups of investigators reported much lower figures for recognised incontinence, compared with those for unrecognised incontinence. They concluded that there was significant underestimation of urinary incontinence by health and social agency workers. In summary, the issue of under-reporting by subjects and clinicians probably swamps the influence of over-reporting in prevalence studies.

The burden of illness

The burden of illness of a condition can be examined in terms of the magnitude of the problem (prevalence and incidence), the associated morbidity and mortality, the impact of the condition on individuals other than the patient, and the costs.

Whether for the purposes of planning health services or conducting research, it is important to know the extent to which the burden of illness is avoidable as opposed to unavoidable (Tugwell *et al.* 1985). Avoidable burden describes disability, symptoms, or mortality that can be reduced by preventive action or treatment that is known to be effective. Alternatively, unavoidable burden describes the magnitude of illness for which there is no known effective prevention or treatment. The former is of principal interest to clinicians, while researchers focus on the latter.

Examination of the prevalence data in Table 1.1 illustrates the wide range of the estimates ($<1-55$ per cent). Some of this variation, due to differences in study populations, is reduced when the studies are categorised according to study setting (Table 1.2); however, the range of estimates is still wide within the types of settings.

Table 1.2 Range in prevalence of urinary incontinence according to survey settings[1]

Study setting	Number of studies	Range in prevalence (%)
Community	6	14–51
Community and institution	10	<1–45
Long-term care institution	7	38–55
Acute care institution	3	19–35

1. See Table 1.1 for survey descriptions.

A number of conceptual and methodological explanations for the variation have been explored.

As can be seen from Table 1.2, the smallest range of figures are found in studies of the acute and long-term institutional settings. The high prevalence of incontinence in long-term institutions is probably a reflection of the extent of physical disability and impaired functional ability related to urinary incontinence (Isaacs and Walkey, 1964; Milne, 1976; Jewett *et al.*, 1981; Ouslander *et al.*, 1982). Because there are several objective sources of data available in these institutions, as opposed to self-reports alone, the prevalence data are probably more accurate than in studies where multiple data sources such as written documentation, reports of health professionals, or results of clinical examinations are not available (Mohide, 1986). The prevalence of urinary incontinence in long-term care institutions probably can be safely estimated at 50 per cent or more. In countries such as Canada, where long-term care institutions are almost always the last home, rather than a convalescent facility, the prevalence may be much higher.

Incontinence in acute care institutions has not been studied sufficiently; however, the three available studies (Sullivan and Lindsay 1984; Sier *et al.*, 1987; Sudbury and Mohide, 1990) indicate that it is a problem for at least 20 per cent of elderly patients admitted to hospital. Further study is required to determine the extent to which the incontinence is related to iatrogenic causes, such as inappropriate drug use and use of restraints.

Although all community-based studies do not demonstrate a consistent gradient of increasing prevalence with increasing age, the Consensus Conference on Urinary Incontinence in Adults (Office of Medical Applications of Research, 1989) included age, with gender (female) and parity as established risk factors. Less rigorous evidence suggests that the following factors might also be risk factors: urinary tract infection, menopause, genitourinary surgery, lack of postpartum exercise, chronic illness and various medications (ibid.) The estimate for community dwelling older adults was placed by the Conference experts and participants as 15–30 per cent, with 20–25 per cent of incontinent individuals being classified as having severe incontinence.

Over the past five years, some incidence data have provided valuable information about its development and prognosis. Incidence describes 'the number of new cases of a disease in a defined population within a specified period of time' (Last, 1988). In a study examining episodes of urinary incontinence during adult life Elving *et al.* (1989) found the cumulative incidence reported by subjects up to age 59 to be 30 per cent and Herzog and Fultz (1990) found one-year incidence rates of 20 per cent for older women and 10 per cent for older men.

Although urinary incontinence is not a life-threatening disease, there are significant adverse social, psychological and biological sequelae associated with it. Thiede (1989) provides an overview of major categories of problems encountered by patients with urinary incontinence summarised in Table 1.3. The scientific evidence for the physical problems has not been well-documented but clinical experience indicates that two problems are skin irritation and discomfort. Incontinence has been shown to be weakly associated with depression, negative affect and low life satisfaction (Herzog *et al.*, 1988). Up until the late 1980s, measurement instruments to assess the specific psychological and social problems of incontinence were not available. Recently several condition-specific instruments have now been developed and tested (Wyman *et al.*, 1987; Yu and Kaltreider, 1987; Yu *et al.*, 1989).

Urinary incontinence can be burdensome for family caregivers (Norton, 1982; Noelker, 1983: Mohide *et al.*, 1988; Ouslander *et al.*, 1990) and predispose a person to long-term institutionalisation. In a study that examined the reasons for long-term institutionalisation, 44 per cent of the family members reported that urinary incontinence was a significant factor in the decision to institutionalise their relative (Johnson and Werner 1982). Smallegan (1985) found that incontinence was a precipitating cause of admission to nursing homes for 89 per cent of elderly subjects who received a substantial amount of care at home. Even within institutions, caregivers can be stressed by caring for people who are incontinent (Yu and Kaltreider, 1987).

Ouslander *et al.* (1982) and Hu (1986, 1990) have estimated the economic costs of urinary incontinence. In the United States, a conservative estimate of the direct costs alone of caring for incontinent people in the community is $7 billion annually, and the comparable figure for direct incontinence care costs in the US nursing homes is $3.3 billion (Office of Medical Applications of Research, 1989). Figures for the United Kingdom are not so readily available, although it has been reported that some £57 million were spent in the community on disposable incontinence products for 1989–90 (Roe, personal communication, independent industrial source).

Table 1.3 Problems experienced by patients with urinary incontinence

Odours and smells
Restricted diet
Discomfort
Restricted physical exercise
Impaired sexual life
Emotional problems
Limited social activities
Inability to perform housework
Unemployment
Increased financial costs

Summary

In summary there are several basic messages suggested by the data presented in this chapter. The first is quite obvious: despite the wide variation in magnitude of estimates, urinary incontinence is common, particularly in women and older adults. The second message is that we are obtaining evidence of significant problems accompanying incontinence, whether considered from the patient, family or health care system perspective. The third message is particularly important for clinicians: there is a great deal of under-reporting, and in light of the fact that much of the burden is avoidable through appropriate treatment, identifying people who are incontinent and making an accurate diagnosis is important, especially for front-line health professionals (Freer, 1990). Finally, further research is required, not on prevalence (except in the case of acute care hospitals), but rather to detect high risk groups, examine risk factors, improve treatment and most importantly to prevent its occurrence. Without this research, we will not reduce the unavoidable burden of urinary incontinence.

References

Anderson, J. (Chairman), Abrams, P., Blaivas, J.G. and Stanton, S.L. (1988), 'The standardization of terminology of lower urinary tract function', *Scandinavian Journal of Urology and Nephrology, Supplementation*, 114: 5–19.

Brocklehurst, J.C., Dillane, J.B. and Griffiths, L. (1968), 'The prevalence and symptomatology of urinary infection in an aged population', *Gerontologia Clinica*, 10: 242–53.

Brocklehurst, J.C., Andrews, K., Richards, B. and Laycock, P.J. (1985), 'Incidence and correlates of incontinence in stroke patients', *Journal of the American Geriatrics Society*, 33(8): 540–2.

Campbell, A.J., Reinken, J. and McCosh, L. (1985), 'Incontinence in the elderly: prevalence and prognosis', *Age and Ageing*, 14: 65–70.

Diokno, A.C., Brock, B.M., Brown, M.B. and Herzog, A.R. (1986), 'Prevalence of urinary incontinence and other urological symptoms in the noninstitutionalized elderly', *The Journal of Urology*, 136: 1022–5.

Elving, L.B., Foldspang, A., Lam, G.W. and Mommsen, S. (1989), 'Descriptive epidemiology of urinary incontinence in 3,100 women age 30–59', *Scandinavian Journal of Urology and Nephrology Supplementum*, 125: 37–43.

Feneley, R.C.L., Shepherd, A.M., Powell, P.H. and Blannin, J. (1979), 'Urinary incontinence: prevalence and needs', *British Journal of Urology*, 51: 493–6.

Fernie, G.R., Jewett, M.A.S., Autry, D., Holliday, P.J. and Zorzitto, M.L. (1983), 'Prevalence of geriatric urinary dysfunction in a chronic care hospital', *Canadian Medical Association Journal*, 128: 1085–6.

Freer, C.B. (1990), 'Screening the elderly', *British Medical Journal*, 300: 1447–8.

Herzog, A.R., Diokno, A.C., Brown, M.B., Normolle, D.P. and Brock, B.M. (1990), 'Two-year incidence, remission and change patterns of urinary incontinence in noninstitutionalized older adults', *Journal of Gerontology*, 45(2): M67–74.

Herzog, A.R. and Fultz, N.H. (1990), 'Prevalence and incidence of urinary incontinence in community-dwelling populations', *Journal of the American Geriatrics Society*, 38: 273–81.

Herzog, A.R., Fultz, N.H., Brock, B.M., Brown, M.B. and Diokno, A.C. (1988), 'Urinary incontinence and psychological distress among older adults', *Psychology and Aging*, 3(2): 115–21.

Holst, K. and Wilson, P.D. (1988), 'The prevalence of female urinary incontinence and reasons for not seeking treatment', *New Zealand Medical Journal*, 101: 756, 758.

Hu, Teh-wei (1986), 'The economic impact of urinary incontinence', *Clinics in Geriatric Medicine*, 2(4): 673–87.

Hu, Teh-wei. (1990), 'Impact of urinary incontinence on health-care costs', *Journal of the American Geriatrics Society*, 38: 292–5.

Isaacs, B. and Walkey, F.A. (1964), 'A survey of incontinence in elderly hospital patients', *Gerontologia Clinica*, 6: 367–76.

Jeter, K.F. and Wagner, D.B. (1990) 'Incontinence in the American home: a survey of 36,500 people', *Journal of the American Geriatrics Society*, 38: 379–83.

Jewett, M.A.S., Fernie, G.R., Holliday, P.J. and Pim, M.E. (1981), 'Urinary dysfunction in a geriatric long-term care population: prevalence and patterns', *Journal of the American Geriatrics Society*, 29(5): 211–14.

Johnson, M.J. and Werner, C. (1982), 'We had no choice: a study of familial guilt feelings surrounding nursing home care', *Journal of Gerontological Nursing*, 8(11): 641–5, 654.

Jolleys, J.V. (1988), 'Reported prevalence of urinary incontinence in women in a general practice', *British Medical Journal*, 296: 1300–2.

Kirshen, A.J. (1983), 'Urinary incontinence in the elderly: a review', *Clinical and Investigative Medicine*, 6(4): 331–9.

Koopman-Boyden, P.G. and Wells, L.F. (1979), 'The problems arising from supporting the elderly at home', *New Zealand Medical Journal*, 89: 265–8.

Koyano, W., Shibata, H., Haga, H. and Suyama, Y. (1986), 'Prevalence and outcome of low ADL and incontinence among the elderly: five years follow-up in a Japanese urban community', *Archives of Gerontology and Geriatrics*, 5: 197–206.

Last, J.M. (ed.) (1988), *A dictionary of epidemiology*, New York: Oxford University Press.

Milne, J.S. (1976), 'Prevalence of incontinence in the elderly age groups', in Willington, F.L. (ed.), *Incontinence in the elderly*, London: Academic Press.

Milne, J.S., Williamson, J., Maule, M.M. and Wallace, E.T. (1972), 'Urinary symptoms in older people', *Modern Geriatrics*, 198–212.

Mohide, E.A. (1986), 'The prevalence and scope of urinary incontinence', *Clinics in Geriatric Medicine*, 2(4): 639–55.

Mohide, E.A., Pringle, D.M., Robertson, D. and Chambers, L.W. (1988), 'Prevalence of urinary incontinence in patients receiving home care services', *Canadian Medical Association Journal*, 139: 953–6.

Molander, U., Milsom, I., Ekelund, P. and Mellström, D. (1990), 'An epidemiological study of urinary incontinence and related urogenital symptoms in elderly women', *Maturitas*, 12: 51–60.

Noelker, L. (1983), 'Incontinence in aged cared for by family', *Gerontology*, 23 (special issue): 258.

Norton, C. (1982), 'The effects of urinary incontinence in women', *International Rehabilitation Medicine*, 4(1): 9–14.

Norton, P.A. (1990), 'Prevalence and social impact of urinary incontinence in women', *Clinical Obstetrics and Gynecology*, 33(2): 295–7.

Office of Medical Applications of Research (1989), Consensus Conference, 'Urinary incontinence in adults', *Journal of the American Medical Association*, 261(18): 2685–90.

Ouslander, J.G. (1989), 'Urinary incontinence: out of the closet', *Journal of the American Medical Association*, 261(18): 2695–6.

Ouslander, J.G. (1990), 'Urinary incontinence in nursing homes', *Journal of the American Geriatrics Society*, 38: 289–91.

Ouslander, J.G. and Fowler, E. (1985), 'Management of urinary incontinence in veterans administration nursing homes', *Journal of the American Geriatrics Society*, 33(1): 33–40.

Ouslander, J.G. and Kane, R.L. (1984), 'The cost of urinary incontinence in nursing homes', *Medical Care*, 22(1): 69–79.

Ouslander, J.G., Kane, R.L. and Abrass, I.B. (1982), 'Urinary incontinence in elderly nursing home patients', *Journal of the American Medical Association*, 248(10): 1194–8.

Ouslander, J.G., Zarit, S.H., Orr, N.K. and Muira, S.A. (1990), 'Incontinence among elderly community-dwelling dementia patients: characteristics, management and impact on caregivers', *Journal of the American Geriatrics Society*, 38: 440–5.

Ribeiro, B.J. and Smith, S.R. (1985), 'Evaluation of urinary catheterization and urinary incontinence in a general nursing home population', *Journal of the American Geriatrics Society*, 33(7): 479–81.

Sier, H., Ouslander, J. and Orzeck, S. (1987), 'Urinary incontinence among geriatric patients in an acute-care hospital', *Journal of the American Geriatrics Society*, 257(13): 1767–71.

Smallegan, M. (1985), 'There was nothing else to do: needs for care before nursing home admission', *Journal of the American Geriatrics Society*, 25(4): 364–9.

Sudbury, F. and Mohide, E.A. (1990), 'Prevalence and factors associated with urinary incontinence in elderly patients in an acute-care hospital'. Submitted for publication.

Sullivan, D.H. and Lindsay, R.W. (1984), 'Urinary incontinence in the geriatric population of an acute care hospital', *Journal of the American Geriatrics Society*, 32(9): 646–50.

Thiede, H.A. (1989), 'The prevalence of urogynecologic disorders', *Obstetrics and Gynecology Clinics of North America*, 16(4): 709–16.

Thomas, T.M. (1986), 'The prevalence and health service implications of incontinence', in Mandelstam, D. (ed.), *Incontinence and Its Management* (2nd edn), London: Croom Helm.

Thomas, T.M., Plymat, K.R., Blannin, J. and Meade, T.W. (1980), 'Prevalence of urinary incontinence', *British Medical Journal*, 281: 1243–6.

Tobin, G.W. and Brocklehurst, J.C. (1986), 'The management of urinary incontinence in local authority residential homes for the elderly', *Age and Ageing*, 15: 292–8.

Tugwell, P., Bennett, K.J., Sackett, D.L. and Haynes, R.B. (1985), 'The measurement iterative loop: a framework for the critical appraisal of need, benefits and costs of health interventions', *Journal of Chronic Diseases*, 38(4): 339–51.

US Department of Health, Education, and Welfare, Public Health Service, Office of Nursing Home Affairs (1975), 'Long term care facility improvement study' (PHS publication No. 588459), Washington, D.C.

Vetter, N.J., Jones, D.A. and Victor, C.R. (1981), 'Urinary incontinence in the elderly at home', *The Lancet*, 1275–7.

Wells, T. (1984), 'Social and psychological implications of incontinence', in Brocklehurst, J.C. (ed.), *Urology in elderly*, Edinburgh: Churchill Livingstone.

Williams, M.E. (1983), 'A critical evaluation of the assessment technology for urinary continence in older persons', *Journal of the American Geriatrics Society*, 31(11): 657–64.

Wolin, L.H. (1969), 'Stress incontinence in young, healthy nulliparous female subjects', *Journal of Urology*, 101: 545–9.

Wyman, J.F., Harkins, S.H., Choi, S.C., Taylor, J.R. and Fantl, A. (1987), 'Psychosocial impact of urinary incontinence in women', *Obstetrics and Gynecology*, 70(3): 378–81.

Wyman, J.F., Harkins, S.W. and Fantl, J.A. (1990), 'Psychosocial impact of urinary incontinence in the community-dwelling population', *Journal of the American Geriatrics Society*, (32): 282–8.

Yarnell, J.W.G. and St Leger, A.S. (1979), 'The prevalence, severity and factors associated with urinary incontinence in a random sample of the elderly', *Age and Ageing*, (8): 81–5.

Yarnell, J.W.G., Voyle, G.J., Richards, C.J. and Stephenson, T.P. (1981), 'The prevalence and severity of urinary incontinence in women', *Journal of Epidemiology and Community Health*, 35: 71–4.

Yu, L.C. (1987), 'Incontinence stress index: measuring psychological impact', *Journal of Gerontological Nursing*, 13(7), 18–25.

Yu, L.C. and Kaltreider, D.L. (1987), 'Stressed nurses dealing with incontinent patients', *Journal of Gerontological Nursing*, 13(1): 27–30.

Yu, L.C., Kaltreider, D.L., Hu, T., Igou, J.F. and Craighead, W.E. (1989), 'The ISQ-P tool: measuring stress with incontinence', *Journal of Gerontological Nursing*, 15(2): 9–15.

2 The aetiology of urinary incontinence

FRANCINE M. CHEATER

Introduction

Urinary incontinence – the consequence of a breakdown in eliminatory function – can occur in childhood, adulthood and old age. Alternatively, continence is a skill which some people may never have acquired. Incontinence is a common health problem with not only physical, but profound psychological and social implications for the sufferer, the sufferer's family and carers.

The nurse has a key role in the prevention of incontinence and the restoration of continence. Where this is not a viable goal of care, the nurse is instrumental in helping the patient, and the patient's family and carers where relevant, to cope effectively with the physical, psychological, social and economic consequences of the problem. If nurses are to fulfil this role they need firstly, to know how the bladder functions normally, and secondly to have a thorough knowledge of the various ways in which it may become impaired. It is through understanding the mechanisms which maintain normal bladder function, and how these might be adversely affected by illness, injury, therapy or psycho-social factors, which enable nurses to recognise continence problems. Then in response to these problems nurses are able to carry out systematic assessments and appropriate and informed interventions.

The aim of this chapter is to provide nurses with up-to-date, and where possible, research-based information about the main causes of incontinence. It begins by attempting to define normal bladder function. This is followed by a brief overview of the structure of the lower urinary tract and the process of micturition. The way in which continence is acquired is then described. The remainder of the chapter presents a review of the literature concerning the major causes of urinary incontinence. Throughout this chapter the word 'incontinence' refers specifically to urinary incontinence unless otherwise stated.

Normal bladder function

The definition of normal bladder function is problematic since the limits of what constitutes 'normality' are wide. Any attempt at definition is constrained by a lack of sufficient research-based evidence obtained from healthy individuals in the population at large. Micturition does not conform to a uniform pattern, but exhibits a wide variation between individuals. Research has shown that patterns of micturition alter with age. Nocturia, for example, defined as being woken at night by the need to micturate, has been reported to increase with age (Brocklehurst et al., 1971; Abrams et al., 1983; Hale et al., 1986). Thus age, as well as other factors, needs to be considered when attempting to define normal variations in bladder function.

In most adults, the bladder will hold a maximum of 400–600 ml of urine at capacity (Abrams et al., 1983; Stephenson and Wein, 1984; Brocklehurst, 1985), although many individuals micturate before this volume is reached. In a cystometric study (that is, the method by which pressure/volume measurements of the bladder are made), of ten healthy female subjects, Ulmsten et al. (1977) found that the first desire to void was experienced at approximately 300 ml bladder volume.

The distribution of diurnal voiding frequency in 3,276 patients (age range 5–84 years) attending the Clinical Investigations Unit in Bristol has been reported by Abrams et al. (1983). These patients attended the clinic for investigations of bladder dysfunction, so it should be remembered that these findings may not be representative of the general population. The range of voids per day (day being defined as rising from bed to falling asleep at night) was wide and found to be from 1 to 20 with a mean frequency of 8 times a day. There was little difference in frequency of voiding with age and sex.

In Sweden, Larsson and Victor (1986) studied the frequency of micturition in 141 'normal' healthy female volunteers with a mean age of 43.6 years (range 19–81 years). The mean frequency per 24 hours was found to be 5.9 (range 3–11 times); a slightly lower rate than reported in Abrams et al.'s (1983) study. Similarly, no age-related changes in the frequency of micturition were demonstrated. Abrams et al. (1983) suggested that 'normal' diurnal frequency of micturition was probably between 4 and 8 times per day.

A very broad definition of normal bladder function has been offered by Feneley (1986) who stated that it is the ability to store and void urine at will in suitable places and convenient times. Norton (1986) identified the importance of the additional skill of 'anticipatory voiding', that is, the ability to empty the bladder in the absence of any sensation of the need to do so (for example before going on a long journey).

Normal bladder function is further defined as the ability to remain continent if micturition has been delayed, during exercise, coughing or standing up, or during sleep (Stanton, 1978; Norton, 1986). On completion of voiding, significant residual urine (the volume of urine remaining in the bladder immediately after the completion of micturition), defined by Stanton (1978) as being less than 50 ml, should not be present in the bladder. However, in the elderly, in whom bladder emptying may be less efficient (Brocklehurst and Dillane, 1966a; Eastwood, 1979), a higher limit of up to 100 ml may be accepted as normal.

Further research is needed to better define the limits of acceptable variation in bladder function in healthy individuals across all ages. Nevertheless, it is wise to heed Abrams et al. (1983). They suggested that bladder function is considered within the context of what is perceived as 'normal' by the patient, but this may not necessarily be what the health carer considers to be 'normal'.

The lower urinary tract: structure and function

The lower urinary tract is composed of the bladder and the urethra (Fig. 2.1). The principal functions of the bladder are storage and evacuation of urine (Bradley and Scott, 1978). Urine is conveyed from the kidneys via the ureters, which enter the bladder obliquely (Lich *et al.*, 1978; Boyarsky *et al.*, 1979; Gosling and Chilton, 1984). The bladder consists of the detrusor and trigone muscles (Fig. 2.1) (Woodburne, 1961; Tanagho *et al.*, 1968). The detrusor muscle forms the smooth muscle of the body of the bladder and consists of a meshwork of interlacing fibres mounted upon the trigone muscle of the bladder (Powell, 1983; Gosling and Chilton, 1984). The trigone is the triangular area between the two ureteric orifices and the bladder neck (Crane *et al.*, 1978). The capacity for urine storage is assured by elasticity of the detrusor muscle which allows the bladder to stretch to accommodate urine with minimal increase in pressure (Bradley and Scott, 1978; Mundy, 1984; Diokno, 1988).

It was traditionally believed that the bladder neck was held closed by an 'internal sphincter' (Kohlraush, 1854). Today, most regard this concept as untenable since no internal sphincter has ever been actually demonstrated (Woodburne, 1961; Crane *et al.*, 1978; Mundy, 1984). Instead, the accumulation of circular or oblique muscle

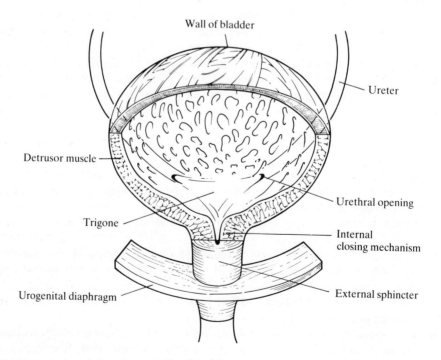

Fig. 2.1 Cross-section of the urinary bladder (female).

fibres passing from the bladder into the urethra may rather be thought of as an opening mechanism rather than a sphincter.

The urethra serves as a channel for urine (and products of the reproductive system in males) and extends from the bladder to the external surface of the body at the meatus (Lich *et al.*, 1978, Tanagho 1978). Adequate compression of the mucosal folds of the urethra provide a watertight closure for maintaining continence (Feneley, 1986). The external urethral sphincter allows voluntary closure of the urethra (Woodburne, 1961) and is thought to function to interrupt voiding (Peterson *et al.*, 1962; Turner-Warwick, 1968; Wheatley, 1983).

The chief support of the bladder is the pelvic floor (Lich *et al.*, 1978). The pelvic floor muscles form a hammock comprising the levator ani, which subdivides into the pubococcygeus and ileococcygeus, and the coccygeus (Chilton, 1984) through which the urethra, vagina in females, and the rectum pass (Sampselle *et al.*, 1989). Any increase in abdominal pressure from a cough or sneeze, for example, is transmitted equally to both the bladder and the urethra so the intraurethral pressure remains greater than the bladder pressure (Lapides, 1982), thus maintaining continence.

The nerves supplying the bladder consist of both sympathetic and parasympathetic components (Gosling and Chilton, 1984). Research by Denny-Brown and Robertson (1933) showed that the bladder and the urethra were reciprocally innervated, relaxation of the urethra occurring with contractions of the bladder and with relaxation of the bladder the urethra resumes its normal tone. In the bladder wall itself there are stretch receptors which relay information about the state of the bladder via both the parasympathetic sensory nerves and the pudendal nerve centrally to the brain (Feneley, 1986).

Bladder control has long been thought to be via a sacral micturition reflex through the parasympathetic nerves to a centre in the second, third and fourth sacral segments of the spinal cord (Fig. 2.2) (Denny-Brown and Robertson, 1933). The sacral micturition centre, however, is modulated by the inhibitory (preventing micturition) and facilitatory (initiating micturition) influence of specific areas of the brain (Fig. 2.2) (Bradley, 1976). Parts of the frontal lobe (Andrew and Nathan, 1964), among other areas of the brain, have been identified as important in the control of micturition (Bradley and Scott, 1978). Feneley (1986) maintains that the main influence of the brain is to suppress bladder (detrusor) contractions thereby inhibiting micturition.

Bladder function may be thought of in terms of cycles of filling and emptying (Yeates, 1976; Powell, 1983). Urine production by the kidneys is continuous and the bladder normally fills at an average rate of approximately 1 ml per minute (Mundy, 1984). Throughout the filling phase, continence is maintained so long as the pressure within the bladder is lower than the urethral pressure (Powell, 1983; Wein, 1986). At approximately 200–300 ml capacity (Ulmsten *et al.*, 1977; Brocklehurst, 1978b; Powell, 1983) an awareness of distension and a mild desire to void is normally experienced. Sensory impulses from the bladder reach the second, third and fourth sacral segments of the spinal cord and travel to micturition centres in the brain (Hald, 1975). If the time or the place is not suitable for micturition, there follows a phase of postponement during which elimination is suppressed by conscious inhibitory

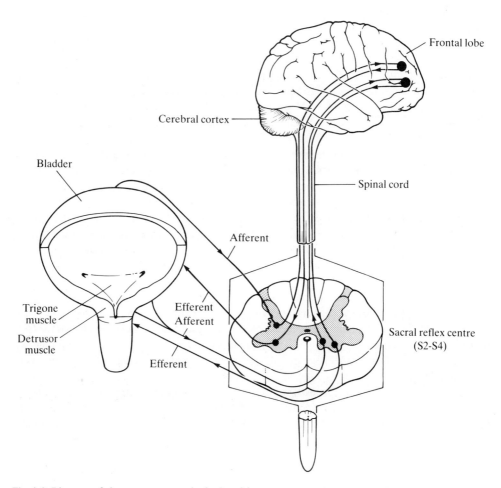

Frontal lobe

Cerebral cortex

Spinal cord

Bladder

Afferent

Trigone
muscle

Efferent
Afferent

Detrusor
muscle

Sacral reflex centre
(S2-S4)

Efferent

Fig. 2.2 Diagram of the nervous control of micturition.

impulses from the frontal lobe (Andrew and Nathan, 1964). When a suitable place for micturition has been selected, the inhibitory impulses from the brain are removed, the sustained contraction of the detrusor muscle raises the bladder pressure which overcomes the resistance of the urethra and voiding occurs (Wein, 1986).

Voiding is a complex process and begins by relaxation of the voluntary muscles of the pelvic floor (Harrison, 1983). As a result, the bladder neck descends, and when a certain critical point is reached, the bladder neck opens (Vincent, 1966). Contraction of the trigone muscle opens the bladder outlet further and the detrusor contracts, further opening the bladder outlet and increasing bladder pressure. This is accompanied by relaxation of the external sphincter (Brocklehurst, 1978a).

Acquisition of continence

The acquisition of continence is a complex skill which occurs early in childhood. The issue of whether continence is learned or developed spontaneously as a process of natural maturation, or is the result of an interaction between the two, has been reviewed by Smith and Smith (1987). Findings were inconclusive and the authors thought it likely that maturation and learning were both necessary.

In the normal infant, the incomplete development of the central nervous system results in an automatic spinal reflex for both bladder and bowel (Millard, 1979). As a consequence the infant's bladder (and bowel) empties involuntarily anywhere and at any time (Brocklehurst, 1967).

It is usual for a child in his or her first year to begin to acquire appropriate urination behaviour under parental instruction (Willington, 1975a). This is normally achieved by the process of toilet ('potty') training. Newson and Newson (1963) found that 83 per cent of mothers in England had started toilet training before the infant was 12 months old. The range of skills needed to acquire continence are considerable and are thought to only progress according to the stage of development of the child's central nervous system (Willington, 1975a).

At about two years of age, with full development of the cerebral cortex, conscious inhibition appears (Willington, 1975a). As physical maturation continues sensations of bladder fullness and imminent voiding are perceived by the infant and the ability briefly to inhibit micturition is acquired (Muellner 1960; Brocklehurst, 1967). Bladder capacity increases and successful toileting develops gradually with practice (Willington, 1975a). By the age of five or six years, 80–90 per cent of children have both day and night bladder control (Brazelton, 1962; Newson and Newson, 1968). Continence becomes subconscious and automatic in most circumstances (Brocklehurst, 1967).

Causes of incontinence

There are a variety of causes and types of incontinence and this has led to a number of attempts at classification of the problem (Borrs and Cormarr, 1971; Gibbon, 1976; Krane and Sirosky, 1979; Wein, 1981). Each classification has its shortcomings: some are very complex and all are limited to specific clinical specialties, and they have rarely accounted for causes other than those of physiological origin. Psychological, environmental and social factors may also play an important part in determining continence, or lack of it, in many individuals. Incontinence is also a symptom which, particularly in the elderly, can be multifactorial; the cause being two or more inter-related factors. For example, incontinence is a symptom commonly associated with the occurrence of a stroke (Milne, 1976; Brocklehurst, 1984b; Green, 1986; Barer, 1989). A stroke may cause impaired mobility, perceptual problems or communication dysfunction together with one or more specific physiological bladder disturbances, such as detrusor instability, any one or all of which may predispose a patient to incontinence. Thus where incontinence is perceived solely in terms of impaired bladder function, important aspects of the problem may be easily overlooked.

Norton (1986) utilised a simple scheme for considering the main causes of incontinence which were classified into three broad categories: physiological bladder dysfunction, factors affecting the individual's ability to cope with bladder function, and factors directly influencing bladder functioning. She stressed that these categories were intimately related and often overlapped. This scheme would seem to be particularly appropriate to nursing, allowing sufficient scope and flexibility to encompass physiological, functional, environmental, psychological and social dimensions which nurses need to consider if they are to adequately assess, plan and carry out interventions to help patients achieve continence or to better manage incontinence. An overview of the main causes of incontinence is presented according to Norton's classification in Fig. 2.3. Any discussion of causes of incontinence is hampered by wide differences in terminology; so, where possible, terms adopted by the International Continence Society are used.

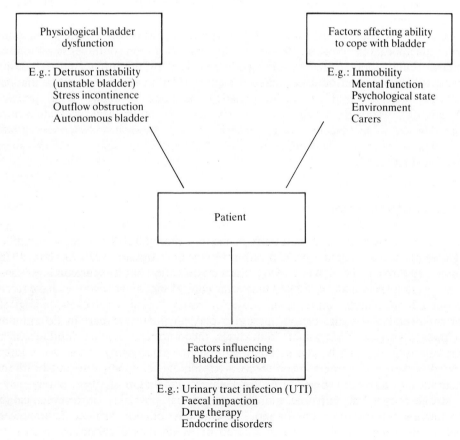

Fig. 2.3 Causes and predisposing factors of urinary incontinence.

Physiological bladder dysfunction

Physiological bladder dysfunction may be classified into four main types: detrusor instability, genuine stress incontinence, outflow obstruction, and autonomous bladder (Fig. 2.3) (Norton, 1986).

Detrusor instability

Normally the bladder contracts during voluntary voiding and at no other time, this controlled behaviour being referred to as 'stable' (Turner-Warwick, 1984). Detrusor instability ('unstable bladder') is the term used to describe the objectively demonstrated contraction of the detrusor (by means of cystometry) occurring either spontaneously or on provocation (for example, on coughing or jumping up and down), during bladder filling, or while the patient is attempting to inhibit micturition (Bates *et al.*, 1975). Individuals with this condition normally experience symptoms of urgency (a strong desire to void) persistent frequency, and nocturia, and where the detrusor contraction is sufficient, urge incontinence (a strong desire to void with involuntary loss of urine) and nocturnal enuresis (incontinence at night time) (Farrar *et al.*, 1975; Cantor and Bates, 1980; Overstall *et al.*, 1980; Abrams *et al.*, 1983; Fernie *et al.*, 1983; Pannill, 1987). Patients with this condition frequently complain of very short or no warning of the need to micturate, and may be incontinent of urine before reaching, or on the way to, the toilet (Diokno, 1988). Studies by Cantor and Bates (1980) and Farrar *et al.* (1975) found that nocturia and urge incontinence were symptoms which positively correlated with a urodynamic diagnosis of detrusor instability. Residual volumes in excess of 100 ml are common (Brocklehurst and Dillane, 1966a; Eastwood, 1979) and bladder capacity is reduced (Fleigner and Glenning, 1979; Castleden *et al.*, 1981).

Detrusor instability is claimed to be the most common cause of incontinence in the elderly (Brocklehurst and Dillane, 1966b; Gleason *et al.*, 1974; Eastwood, 1979; Field, 1979; Castleden and Duffin, 1981; Fossberg *et al.*, 1981; Hilton and Stanton, 1981; Williams and Pannill, 1982; Farrar, 1984). Between 39 per cent and 75 per cent of elderly patients have been reported as having the condition (Brocklehurst and Dillane, 1966b; Castleden *et al.*, 1981; Hilton and Stanton, 1981; Eastwood and Warrell, 1984; Ouslander *et al.*, 1986). It should be remembered, however, that patients in the studies mentioned above were attending urodynamic clinics or were hospital inpatients and may not, therefore, be representative of the general population.

Detrusor instability may arise with loss of the normally inhibiting impulses from the micturition centre in the brain. As discussed earlier, these impulses normally modulate activity in the sacral reflex arc which controls micturition. Loss of these inhibitory impulses leads to inappropriate activation of the sacral reflex arc and the bladder begins to contract before micturition is voluntarily initiated, so causing incontinence (Brocklehurst, 1978a; Johnson, 1980; Overstall *et al.*, 1980).

The underlying causes of detrusor instability are varied. Sensory input from the bladder may be increased in intensity (sensory urgency), for example as a result of local causes such as acute urinary tract infection, stones, faecal impaction or prostatic enlargement (Brocklehurst, 1978b; Wheatley, 1983). In the elderly, neurological causes are common, for example strokes, Alzheimer's disease and Parkinson's disease, while incomplete spinal cord lesions and brain tumours may also cause detrusor instability (Brocklehurst and Dillane, 1966b; Williams and Pannill, 1982; Wheatley, 1983). It has also been suggested that age-related brain changes in general might cause the majority of elderly people to suffer from some degree of detrusor instability (Brocklehurst, 1984b), although this does not necessarily result in incontinence.

'Idiopathic' detrusor instability occurs in the absence of detectable pathology (Brocklehurst, 1984a). It is thought that emotional or psychological problems can manifest as urological symptoms (Newman, 1962; Margolis, 1965; Willington, 1975c; Abrams et al., 1983; Brocklehurst, 1985) and that idiopathic detrusor instability may in some cases be psychosomatic in origin (Frewen, 1972). The successful treatment of detrusor instability with placebo therapy or hypnotherapy tends to support this view (Frewen, 1978; Freeman and Baxby, 1982). Yarnell et al. (1981) found that neuroticism was associated with symptoms of urge and combined urge and stress incontinence in females. The extent to which this can be implicated in causation of incontinence, however, is unknown as neuroticism might well have arisen as a consequence of being incontinent.

Results from urodynamic investigation have shown that patients with detrusor instability often experience warning of impending micturition simultaneously or only a few seconds before urine appears in the urethra (Castleden and Duffin, 1981). In these circumstances, it is easy to see why frequent toileting, or nearby positioning of commodes or bottles may not alleviate the situation. Castleden and Duffin (1981) claimed that toileting would be unsuccessful in patients with unstable detrusor contractions at volumes less than 150 ml, thus highlighting the importance of first trying to estimate the patient's bladder capacity.

Genuine stress incontinence
Genuine stress incontinence is defined as involuntary loss of urine when the bladder pressure exceeds the maximum urethal pressure but in the absence of detrusor activity (Bates et al., 1975). 'Stress incontinence' is a symptom which is the patient's statement of involuntary urine loss and a sign which denotes the observation of involuntary urine loss from the urethra immediately upon an increase in abdominal pressure (ibid.).

In patients so affected, small amounts of urine loss usually occur immediately with the onset of physical exertion or coughing (Pannill, 1987). Studies by Glezerman et al. (1986) and Farrar et al. (1975) have demonstrated that small volumes of urine loss related to physical activity were positively correlated with stress incontinence. It is important that genuine stress incontinence is distinguished from detrusor instability, however, as a movement or a cough may cause involuntary urine loss in both situations (Brocklehurst, 1978a; Norton, 1986), in the latter condition acting as a stimulus to a detrusor contraction. This often necessitates the patient having to undergo urodynamic investigations in order to differentiate between the two causes of incontinence (Hilton and Stanton, 1981). Diokno et al. (1986) reported that 'mixed' incontinence, that is, symptoms of stress and urge incontinence, is common among elderly women.

Stress incontinence is rare in males; it can arise as a complication following prostatic surgery or occur in chronic retention (Abrams *et al.*, 1983; Brocklehurst, 1984b). Stress incontinence, however, is common in women and Stanton (1984) suggests this might be due to a fundamental anatomical weakness in the female partly associated with the evolutionary change from horizontal to vertical position. In the vertical position, the urethra leaves the bladder at the point of maximal gravitational force and lacks the buttressing support of the symphysis.

The prevalence of stress incontinence is difficult to determine due to its variable level of tolerance and definition. Community-based studies relying upon subjective reporting of symptoms have indicated that approximately 50 per cent of young, healthy nulliparous women experienced some degree of stress incontinence (Nemir and Middleton, 1954; Wolin, 1969). Fifty-seven per cent of women aged 45–64 years have been found to experience stress incontinence (Brocklehurst *et al.*, 1972) while in elderly females (65 years or older) between 12 per cent and 17 per cent were identified as having the symptom (Brocklehurst *et al.*, 1971; Yarnell *et al.*, 1981).

Results obtained from urodynamic studies of elderly women vary widely. Interpretations of studies are limited by highly selected samples as well as lack of comparative data for continent women. Of 263 consecutive admissions of patients 65 years and older to a urology clinic in the United States, 16 per cent of the females and 2 per cent of the males were shown to have genuine stress incontinence following urodynamic investigation (Ouslander *et al.*, 1986). This is a prevalence comparable to that for elderly women as discussed above. Of 75 elderly women consecutively investigated at a continence clinic in the United Kingdom, however, none were shown to have stress incontinence following urodynamic investigation (Castleden *et al.*, 1981). In contrast, a study in the United States by Diokno *et al.* (1987) of 200 elderly women consecutively attending an outpatient clinic showed that 77 per cent had genuine stress incontinence.

Stress incontinence is usually associated with bladder outlet incompetence because of weakness of the supporting pelvic muscles (Brocklehurst, 1978a; Wheatley, 1983). The bladder should be situated within the abdominal cavity to allow equal transmission of any increase in abdominal pressure (Stanton, 1984). The intra-abdominal location of the bladder, adequate urethral support beneath the pubic bone, and the angle of the pelvic floor to the urethra have been shown to be important determinants of the bladder outlet resistance (Wheatley, 1983). If the pelvic tissue relaxes, the effects of gravity pull the organs downward (Sampselle *et al.*, 1989). An alteration in the anatomical relationship between the bladder and the urethra and their muscular supports can then result in stress incontinence (Stanton, 1984).

Pregnancy, childbirth, obesity, the menopause, and conditions associated with impaired innervation of the pelvic floor have been implicated as causal factors (Hodgkinson, 1970; Thomas *et al.*, 1980; Yarnell *et al.*, 1981; Wheatley, 1983; Snooks *et al.*, 1984; Stanton, 1986). A study of the factors associated with incontinence by Yarnell *et al.* (1981) did not establish any relationship between stress incontinence and perineal damage during childbirth and it was suggested that parity was a far more important aetiological factor. Hodgkinson (1970), however, maintained that there was no correlation with number of vaginal deliveries and either the occurrence or severity of stress incontinence. More recently, electrophysiological investigation of pelvic floor innervation in women postnatally, by Snooks *et al.* (1984), indicated that nerve damage, rather than overstretched muscles, may be the cause of incontinence.

Stress incontinence may be associated with urogenital prolapse in females, for example cystocoele or rectocoele (Abrams *et al.*, 1983; Robinson, 1984a; Leach and Yip, 1986). A study by Ouslander *et al.* (1986) however, found that of 32 elderly females examined, 13 showed evidence of prolapse but remained continent. The investigators concluded that prolapse was not a major causal factor of stress incontinence.

Inadequate levels of oestrogen in postmenopausal women may lead to atrophy of muscles, ligaments and fascia involved with bladder outlet control (Stanton, 1984) and so predispose to stress incontinence. The association of oestrogen deficiency and incontinence is discussed further in the section on endocrine disorders. Obesity, chronic cough and habitual straining at stool are factors which are thought to aggravate the problem (Parks *et al.*, 1966; Norton, 1986).

Outflow obstruction
The obstruction of outflow of urine during voiding may be caused by, among other factors, prostatic enlargement, bladder neck hypertrophy, urethral stenosis or stricture, and chronic constipation (Abrams *et al.*, 1983; Brocklehurst, 1984b; Turner-Warwick, 1984). Abrams *et al.* (1983) suggested that outflow obstruction may also be caused by psychological or emotional factors which can lead to inhibition of urethral relaxation.

Outflow obstruction is associated with hesitancy, poor urinary stream, and postmicturition dribble (Brocklehurst, 1984b; Turner-Warwick, 1984). A slow stream and difficulty in starting micturition have been shown to be associated with proven outflow obstruction following urodynamic investigation (Abrams and Feneley, 1978). Other symptoms such as nocturia, frequency, urge micturition and urgency incontinence are also commonly associated with obstruction, most often as a result of unstable detrusor contractions (Turner-Warwick, 1984). Turner-Warwick estimated that 75–80 per cent of males with outflow obstruction had secondary symptoms of frequency, urgency and nocturia. Of 318 males aged between 45–85 years attending a urodynamic clinic, 17 per cent had obstruction alone while 40 per cent were diagnosed as having obstruction and detrusor instability (Abrams *et al.*, 1983). Overstall *et al.* (1980) reported a higher proportion with both outflow obstruction and detrusor instability; 80 per cent of elderly men attending a urodynamic clinic having both conditions.

In severe cases, the detrusor contraction is unsustained and leaves a residual volume of urine which gradually builds up, the bladder becomes progressively distended and in some patients leads to overflow incontinence (Abrams *et al.*, 1983; Brocklehurst, 1984b). The bladder is emptied by frequent voiding of small amounts, and at the same time urine may be dribbling constantly (Diokno, 1988). The most common cause of outflow obstruction is prostatic enlargement (Yeates, 1976; Abrams *et al.*, 1983) which increases with age in men over the age of 55 years (Abrams *et al.*, 1983). Bladder outflow obstruction is rare in females; of 2,124 females who attended a urodynamic clinic, 3.7 per cent were so diagnosed (ibid.).

Autonomous bladder
In the autonomous bladder, the detrusor muscle is underactive and fails to provide a sustained or adequate voiding contraction during micturition (Norton, 1986). The condition is usually caused by damage to the peripheral nerves to the bladder or by damage to the lower spinal cord. The sensation of bladder filling may be absent or reduced (Robinson, 1984a); the bladder often increases in capacity and large residual volumes of urine (500–2,000 ml) may accumulate and result in overflow incontinence (Castleden et al., 1981; Mundy and Blaivas, 1984). Diabetic neuropathy, particularly in middle or old age, pelvic injuries, lesions of the cauda equina, multiple sclerosis and herpes zoster are some of the causes (Brocklehurst, 1978a; Wheatley, 1983; Mundy and Blaivas, 1984).

Factors affecting ability to cope with bladder

The precise role of factors such as impaired mobility, diminished mental awareness or environmental limitations, as predisposing or causal factors of incontinence is relatively unknown. The association between impaired mobility and incontinence, for example, may be connected with poor physical health, mental impairment, inaccessible toilets and lack of carers, factors which may cumulatively predispose towards the problem.

A number of institutional and community surveys of elderly people were concerned with the relationship between incontinence and such factors. Comparisons between studies, however, are hindered by different methods of data collection, widely varying and sometimes inadequately described patient samples and, in some cases, lack of data about continent individuals with which to compare findings.

Mobility problems and related factors
Physical restrictions which impede access to the toilet are likely to induce incontinence, either directly or in association with other factors such as detrusor instability or diuretic therapy (Isaacs and Walkey, 1964; Field, 1979; Millard, 1979; Williams and Pannill, 1982; Brocklehurst, 1984a; Kennedy, 1984; Robinson, 1984a; Green, 1986). A number of studies of elderly institutionalised patients have reported a relationship between level of mobility and continence status (Isaacs and Walkey, 1964; Ouslander et al., 1982; Fernie et al., 1983; McCormick et al., 1985; Sier et al., 1987). Similar findings have been reported in studies of elderly people living in the community (Vetter et al., 1981; Vehkalahti and Kivelda, 1985; Resnick et al., 1986).

In contrast to these studies, Castleden et al. (1981) did not find any relationship between level of mobility and incontinence in a study of 100 elderly people consecutively assessed in a continence clinic. They concluded that mobility was not an important factor in the causation of incontinence in the elderly. It should be noted, however, that their sample was highly selected; all patients were attending a continence clinic and the majority were mobile.

In addition to limited mobility, associated factors such as poor manual dexterity, impaired eyesight, and unsuitable clothing and footwear are frequently cited as adversely affecting an individual's functional ability for independent toileting (Millard, 1979; Whitehead *et al.*, 1984; Norton, 1986).

Mental state

The association between impaired mental function and incontinence is well-documented (Isaacs and Walkey, 1964; Brocklehurst and Dillane, 1966b; Arie *et al.*, 1976; Ouslander *et al.*, 1982; Campbell *et al.*, 1985; Berrios, 1986; Sier *et al.*, 1987). In contrast, Castleden *et al.* (1981), in the study previously mentioned, found little relationship between mental test scores and incontinence. Differences between the findings of Castleden *et al.*'s study and those mentioned above are again, likely to be the result of biases in sample selection. The sample in Castleden *et al.*'s study comprised patients attending a continence clinic, the majority of whom were mobile, whereas in most of the other studies, mentioned above, samples comprised hospital or nursing home inpatients in whom physical and mental impairment was likely to be common.

Mental impairment associated with dementia and cerebrovascular disease has been shown to be positively correlated with incontinence, the severity of the incontinence being related to degree of mental impairment (Brocklehurst and Dillane, 1966b; Borrie *et al.*, 1985; Brocklehurst *et al.*, 1985; Campbell *et al.*, 1985; Berrios, 1986; Barer, 1989). Vetter *et al.* (1981) found that clinical anxiety and depression were also much more common in incontinent than continent people living in the community. As previously discussed, it is difficult to know whether anxiety and depression are secondary to incontinence or whether they are factors in its causation. In addition, it is unclear from the study by Vetter *et al.* (1981) whether anxiety or depression existed independently or coexisted, or resulted from other mental impairment such as dementia or cerebrovascular disease.

Conditions causing impaired mental functioning may have a direct effect on bladder function by damage to micturition centres in the brain. This damage is normally due to Alzheimer's disease, vascular dementia or a stroke (Brocklehurst and Dillane, 1966b; Arie *et al.*, 1976; Campbell *et al.*, 1985; Berrios, 1986). The cognitive impairment and disinhibition found in these conditions may also indirectly affect continence as a result of inability to remember or locate the toilet, lack of appreciation of impending need to empty the bladder or of the social need to do so (Brocklehurst, 1984a; Robinson, 1984a; Norton 1986).

Psychological state

The influence of psychological factors upon bladder function is well-documented although their precise role in the causation of incontinence is unclear (Schwartz and Stanton, 1950; Newman, 1962; Margolis, 1965; Willington, 1969; Sutherland, 1971; Stone and Judge, 1978; Frewen, 1979; Abrams *et al.*, 1983; Wells, 1984; Scott, 1985; Ory *et al.*, 1986). Sutherland (1971) stressed that without an adequate consideration of psychological aspects, neither the understanding of incontinence nor its treatment are complete. Wells (1984) warned, however, against prematurely attributing incontinence to an emotional disorder in the absence of consideration of other causal mechanisms. Specific symptoms such as urinary retention (Margolis, 1965; Abrams *et al.*, 1983) and urge or urge incontinence (Frewen, 1972; 1979) have been attributed, in some circumstances, to be psychosomatic in origin. Frewen (1979) claimed that 80 per cent of female patients with symptoms of urge incontinence attending gynaecology outpatient clinics belonged to this group, though further data to substantiate this surprisingly high figure have not been reported.

While a considerable amount has been written about the role of psychological factors in the causation of incontinence, little systematic research has been carried out in this area, thus information remains largely anecdotal.

Newman (1962) suggested that incontinence was a symptom of emotional breakdown in elderly institutionalised people. It is frequently claimed that incontinence in an elderly person may arise as a consequence of a sudden life crisis such as a bereavement. An elderly patient newly admitted to hospital may become disoriented in unfamiliar surroundings which can lead to difficulties with locating the toilet and consequent incontinence. Scott (1985) and Sutherland (1971) considered that incontinence was, in some cases, the result of patients' psychological coping reactions, or of defence mechanisms which may manifest in regressive, overly dependent, rebellious or attention-seeking behaviour.

Willington (1969) attributed the cause of psychologically induced incontinence to a loss of learned conditioned reflexes. He indicated the importance of negative stimuli such as lack of privacy or uncomfortable toileting positions, which exert a strong inhibitory effect on voiding behaviour, and positive stimuli, such as appropriate staff attitudes and the use of suitable clothing which help maintain continence.

Environmental factors

The physical design, layout and facilities afforded by the environment, in both community and institutional settings, are considered to be important determinants of continence or incontinence (Millard, 1979; Hu, 1982; Williams and Pannill, 1982; Brink and Wells, 1986). Thus, bed and chair height (including the angle of the seat), the proximity to mobility aids, the provision of a working call bell system, and the location and accessibility of toilet facilities, among other factors, have been identified (Calder, 1976; Hu, 1982; Brink and Wells, 1986).

A Scottish Home and Health Department report (1970) recommended that toilets be no more than 12 m from oriented, continent elderly individuals. The rationale upon which this recommendation was based is not, however, made explicit. Interestingly, Vehkalhti and Kivelda (1985), and Vetter *et al.* (1981), in surveys of the elderly living in the community, found no relationship between incontinence and location of toilet. In institutions, the recommended toilet to patient ratio is 1 : 6 or 1 : 4 in wards in which patients are more dependent (Chamberlain and Stowe, 1982). An investigation of 246 long-stay wards for the elderly by Norton (1967) showed that 68 per cent of the toilets were unsatisfactory in size and design. Wells (1975), in an investigation of 13 care of the elderly wards, found that 83 per cent of the toilets were too small for a wheelchair, only one ward had the recommended number of toilets and 43 per cent of the patients' beds were further than 12 m from the toilet. More recently, Chamberlain and Stowe (1982) assessed the bathroom and toilet facilities of 21 surgical and medical wards. They found the ratio of toilets to patients highly variable ranging from 1 : 4 to 1 : 16.

Of 65 toilets inspected, 14 (22 per cent) had room for a wheelchair and an attendant with the door closed, and only two wards had raised toilet seats.

The effects of improving the physical environment have received little systematic research. There remains a considerable need to carry out studies to establish the extent to which incontinence can be accounted for by general environmental changes. Chanfreau-Rona et al. (1984) made simple environmental adaptations to the ward environment to increase the sensory cues to enable elderly female psychiatric patients to visit the toilet. No measurable improvement of continence was observed after a 2-week period. It is doubtful, however, whether this was a sufficient length of time to allow for any changes in behaviour to occur.

Several other studies undertaken in care of the elderly settings have reported a reduction in the level of incontinence as a consequence of environmental adaptations (Lepine et al., 1979; King, 1980; Mandelstam and Tuck, 1986).

Anecdotal evidence describing the move of a group of elderly patients from a hospital ward to bungalow accommodation has highlighted beneficial changes in both their mental and physical functioning, which included 'a great reduction in incontinence' (Adams, 1979; Davies, 1979; Northwood, 1979).

The effect of the 'social' environment as an important determinant of incontinence has also been highlighted (Dunn and Strang, 1970; Isaacs, 1976; Norton, 1986). It is often claimed that improving the social environment, for example through the introduction of activity programmes and social events, has resulted in less incontinence in care of the elderly wards. Goat (1988) reported a reduction in the level of incontinence in 12 patients in a long-stay care of the elderly ward following the introduction of a nurse therapist who provided ward-based activities and outings. More carefully designed studies to evaluate the precise benefits of such interventions are now needed.

Carers

It is frequently claimed that carers' low expectations and negative attitudes may be responsible for causing or exacerbating incontinence (Schwartz and Stanton, 1950; Willington, 1969; Arie et al., 1976; Calder, 1976; Isaacs, 1976; Tarrier and Larner, 1983; Miller, 1985a; Miller, 1985b; Mitteness, 1987). This was vividly portrayed in a published letter in the Nursing Times written by a 22-year-old man who was admitted to hospital for investigations of 'mild' urinary incontinence:

> I was taken into a treatment room by a young male nurse who explained that they were going to try some incontinence aids, and he gave me a pair of plastic pants . . .
> When I felt the need to urinate and attempted to find the toilet, an auxiliary nurse escorted me back to my chair and said in a loud voice, 'It's ok, you've waterproof pants on' . . .
> After four days in that place I had 'progressed' to wearing adult all-in-one diapers . . . and was readily wetting myself instead of using the toilet . . .
> After seven days I had regressed to being totally dependent on aids . . .
> I went into hospital, a good looking 22-year-old with self respect and

confidence. I am now totally incontinent of urine and rely on baby's underwear.

(Cullodine, 1987)

Observational studies investigating the nursing care of elderly people in hospital (Norton *et al.*, 1962; Wells, 1975; Baker, 1978; Wright, 1984) found that nurses focused on soiling rather than measures to encourage continence and that many nursing practices, such as the routine use of incontinence aids, frequently encouraged incontinence. The routine giving of care may be less demanding on staff than the encouragement of self-care. Isaacs (1976) and Baker (1978) suggested that attending to individual patient requests for toileting does not readily fit into the ward routine, while the cleaning and changing of incontinent patients can occur at a time which is convenient to the nursing staff.

Ory *et al.* (1986) claimed that carers commonly sublimate their negative feelings towards patients with incontinence by overindulgence and 'excessive' caring; a strategy which is unlikely to promote self-care. Sutherland (1971) suggested that many nursing procedures related to caring for patients with incontinence might actually encourage patient dependency.

Evidence to suggest that patient dependency can be nurse-induced has been reported by Miller (1985a). She carried out a study to compare two different styles of nursing care, traditional task-oriented nursing and individualised nursing care. She found that where traditional task allocation nursing was carried out, patients were significantly more physically dependent (which included incontinence) than patients in wards which individualised nursing care took place. Similar, although anecdotal findings, have been reported by Savage and Widdowson (1974a, 1974b) in a psychiatric ward for elderly patients. Changes in work pattern from a rigid routine to more flexible individualised nursing was reported to produce a decrease in episodes of incontinence. Thus, the way in which nursing care is organised may be an important determinant in the causation of incontinence in the ward environment.

Despite apparent changes in attitudes towards incontinence in recent years there is evidence to suggest that common misconceptions persist. For example incontinence is still viewed by some carers (and patients) as a normal, inevitable part of ageing (Mitteness, 1987; Herzog and Fultz, 1988; Cheater, 1990). Cheater (1990) found that nurses working in acute medical and care of the elderly wards appeared to have a very limited appreciation of their own potential for initiating rehabilitative care in response to patient's continence problems. Many nurses tended to view their role as restricted primarily to the provision of incontinence aids.

Attitudes such as those described above, are important to consider, since they may result in health professionals, relatives and patients themselves subscribing to the notion that little can be done to alleviate the problem.

The difficulties of changing staff attitudes towards incontinence in a male psychiatric ward have been highlighted by Bridgewater and Christie (1974). They described the staff as paternal, affectionate but defeatist. A new implemented toileting programme was poorly accepted; staff resented the change and were anxious that the workload would be increased as a result of the new procedure.

Further research is needed to examine in more detail nurses' and other health professionals' attitudes towards incontinence, and in particular, to ascertain their effect on patient care.

Factors influencing bladder function

Urinary tract infection

Acute urinary tract infection is frequently cited as causing or predisposing to transient urinary incontinence (Helps, 1977; Brocklehurst, 1978a; Norton, 1986; Ouslander, 1986). An acute infection is thought to sensitise the stretch receptors in the bladder and, in an elderly person, present as incontinence associated with urgency, frequency and dysuria (painful micturition) (Brocklehurst, 1978a; Ouslander, 1986; Diokno, 1988). The precise role of urinary tract infection as a causal factor of incontinence, however, remains uncertain (Brocklehurst *et al.*, 1968; Ouslander, 1986; Abrutyn *et al.*, 1988), particularly in the elderly where asymptomatic bacteriuria (i.e. 10^5 or more colony forming units per millilitre of urine) is common (Sourander, 1966, Walkey *et al.*, 1967; Brocklehurst *et al.*, 1968; Akhtar *et al.*, 1972; Brocklehurst *et al.*, 1977). A study by Sourander (1966) reported an association between bacteriuria and incontinence but Brocklehurst *et al.* (1968) and Yarnell *et al.* (1981) found no such relationship.

Brocklehurst (1984b) maintained that chronic bacteriuria in many elderly people is probably secondary to residual urine associated with bladder dysfunction, and treatment of the infection will not affect incontinence which is likely to recur. Despite the lack of data to support a clear association with incontinence, most clinicians consider it important to try and eradicate a urinary tract infection, where present, in those patients with urinary incontinence.

People who suffer from incontinence may restrict their fluid intake. Norton *et al.* (1988) found that 70 per cent of the 60 incontinent women in their sample practised fluid restriction. Low fluid intake is thought to predispose towards urinary tract infection (and constipation), and concentrated urine itself may irritate the bladder causing sensory urgency and frequency (Norton, 1986). Spangler *et al.* (1984) reported that when they tested the specific gravity of urine specimens of 16 incontinent elderly nursing home residents, four patients were found to be dehydrated.

Faecal impaction

Willington (1980) claimed that the most common cause of incontinence in the elderly was chronic constipation. Elderly people are known to be particularly prone to constipation, and consequent faecal impaction. Constipation in the elderly may arise from increased colonic transit time, drug therapy such as analgesics, diuretics and anticholinergics, reduced mobility (Avery-Jones and Godding, 1973; Tallis and Norton, 1985) and low fluid intake (Norton, 1986). A study by King (1979) found that 26 per cent of incontinent psychiatric inpatients had faecal impaction and 19 per cent chronic constipation.

Incontinence caused by an impacted rectum may be characterised by voiding of small amounts, constant dribbling of urine and faecal incontinence (Diokno, 1988). The precise mechanisms by which constipation may lead to incontinence of urine have not, however, been examined. It is postulated that chronic constipation or faecal impaction may cause urinary incontinence by compressing the bladder and urethra leading to outflow obstruction, retention of urine and overflow (Brocklehurst, 1985; Tallis and Norton, 1985; Diokno, 1988; Wells, 1988). Abdominal and rectal distension is also thought to precipitate detrusor instability in some circumstances (Tallis and Norton, 1985). Evidence from a study by O'Reagan *et al.* (1985) indicated that chronic constipation can cause unstable detrusor contractions. Investigations of 47 children with chronic constipation, recurrent urinary tract infection and enuresis and/or faecal incontinence showed that all had unstable bladder contractions following urodynamic investigation. Elimination of constipation resulted in cessation of urinary tract infection, enuresis and faecal incontinence in the majority of individuals. The authors postulated that compression of the bladder due to the faecal pressure might trigger unstable detrusor contractions. It has also been suggested that faecal loading may stretch the pelvic floor muscles and precipitate stress incontinence (Parks *et al.*, 1966).

Drug therapy
Many different types of drugs have been reported to affect bladder function adversely (Brocklehurst, 1978a; Perkash, 1982; Williams and Pannill, 1982; Paillard and Resnick, 1984; Shimp, 1988).

As polypharmacy is common in the elderly, they may be particularly prone to drug induced incontinence (Green, 1986; Shimp, 1988). A recent study by Keister and Creason (1989) of 84 elderly incontinent females in nursing homes found that 70 per cent were taking a drug having the potential to cause urinary incontinence. However, evidence is contradictory. Yarnell and St Leger (1979) in a study of a random sample of 388 elderly people living in the community found increased drug use was positively correlated to prevalence of incontinence although they did not specify the nature of the drugs used. In contrast, a study of 437 elderly patients admitted to a long-term care hospital found that incontinent patients were receiving slightly fewer diuretic and sedative drugs than those who were continent (Jewett *et al.*, 1981). A study of 363 elderly patients admitted to medical and surgical wards by Sier *et al.* (1987) found no difference between continent and incontinent individuals in the use of anticholinergic, psychotropic or diuretic drug therapy. A study of elderly, predominantly community dwelling individuals, however, found that incontinence was significantly related to the use of diuretics (Vehkalahti and Kivelda, 1985).

Diuretics, particularly the rapid-acting loop diuretics, are thought to predispose towards frequency, urge and urge incontinence (Willington, 1975b; Brocklehurst, 1984a; Paillard and Resnick, 1984; Ouslander, 1986). Reduction in bladder contractility and retention of urine, with or without overflow incontinence, may be caused by anticholinergic, antidepressant, anti-Parkinsonian, phenothiazine and antihistamine drugs (Brocklehurst, 1978a; Perkash, 1982; Williams and Pannill, 1982).

The use of certain analgesics, for example opiates such as morphine sulphate, may cause bladder sensation to be decreased. Twycross and Lack (1990) claim that the use of morphine in the pain management of patients with terminal cancer can occasionally exacerbate hesitancy of micturition and rarely, may cause urgency incontinence. The use of opiates frequently cause constipation and faecal impaction, which in turn can lead to retention of urine with overflow incontinence (ibid.). The long-term administration of certain cytotoxic agents may produce cumulative effects on the kidney tissue, for example cisplatin can cause oliguria (a diminished capacity to form and pass urine) or renal toxicity (Ames and Kneisl, 1988). Cyclophosphamide, one of the nitrogen mustards, can cause haemorragic cystitis. Cyclophosphamide metabolites in the urine irritate the bladder lining and can cause frequency, urgency or urge incontinence (ibid.).

Beta blockers, such as propanolol, can increase urethral pressure and cause voiding difficulties leading to retention of urine (Perkash, 1982). Progesterone can lower urethral resistance and cause stress incontinence (ibid.). Norton (1986) claimed that diazepam may also lower urethral resistance. Psychotropic, sedative and hypnotic drugs may cause oversedation, confusion and immobility which can reduce an individual's response to micturition cues or ability to get to the toilet (Willington 1975b; Williams and Pannill, 1982; Paillard and Resnick, 1984; Norton, 1986). Castleden and Davies (1987) reported that 55 per cent of hospital patients aged 85 years and over who were given 10 mg of nitrazepam at night were found to be sedated the next day.

Alcohol may also cause frequency, urgency, sedation, confusion and immobility (Paillard and Resnick, 1984; Ouslander, 1986), all of which may predispose to urinary incontinence. Beverages such as coffee, tea and cocoa contain caffeine, a diuretic, which stimulates micturition (Brink, 1988).

Endocrine disorders
The effect of diabetic neuropathy on bladder function has been discussed earlier in this chapter. In the elderly incontinence may be associated with an undiagnosed recent onset of diabetes mellitus. Diabetes mellitus and insipidus may also cause polyuria with consequent effects on bladder function. Incontinence in these situations is usually of the urge type (Diokno, 1988).

Oestrogen deficiency in postmenopausal women causes atrophic changes in the vagina and urethra which may cause or exacerbate incontinence (Robinson, 1984a; Brocklehurst, 1984b). Cardozo et al. (1986) found that the level of circulating oestradiol in postmenopausal women negatively correlated with symptoms of urgency, thus leading them to conclude that oestrogen withdrawal influenced lower urinary tract function.

A study by Robinson (1984b) found that 77 per cent of 219 women attending a continence clinic (mean age 79 years) had atrophic vaginal mucosa when examined, and of these, 81 per cent of the clinical diagnoses were histologically confirmed. She found that a third of the patients who were treated with oestrogen alone, 53 per cent of those on oestrogen and other drugs such as anticholinergic and/or antibiotic therapy, and 44 per cent of those treated without oestrogen, with or without other drug treatment, became dry. She concluded that oestrogen deficiency may contribute to incontinence in the presence of other factors but it was not a major cause of incontinence in its own right.

The effect of ageing on bladder function

While it is generally assumed that bladder function diminishes with increasing age, current knowledge about age changes in the lower urinary tract and the neurological mechanisms controlling micturition is scanty (Brocklehurst, 1984b). Little information concerning bladder functions in 'normal' elderly people is available (Abrams et al., 1983; Brocklehurst, 1984b). A progressive deterioration of renal function and structure has been shown to accompany ageing (Anderson and Brenner, 1987).

Research by Brocklehurst (1985) has shown that bladder epithelium becomes thinner and there is some replacement of smooth urethral muscle by connective tissue associated with ageing. The closing pressure of the urethra has also been shown to diminish in elderly females, which Brocklehurst (1982) has suggested may be related to replacement of urethral tissue. Trabeculation and diverticulae of the bladder, in both sexes, are common (Brocklehurst, 1985; Staskin, 1986). The bladder appears to empty less completely with increasing age and there is a tendency for residual urine volume to increase (Eastwood, 1979). Cystometric studies by Brocklehurst and Dillane (1966a) in 40 elderly, continent females found that bladder capacity and compliance, as well as the ability to postpone voiding were diminished. Post-voiding residual urine was increased to more than 100 ml in 73 per cent, and 42 per cent of the women leaked urine during bladder filling. Similar findings in males have been reported by Eastwood (1979).

Staskin (1986) suggested that fibrotic changes induced by radiotherapy, chronic infection, interstitial disease, chronic overdistension and long-term use of indwelling catheters may be contributory factors which reduce bladder compliance in the elderly. The closing pressure of the urethra has also been shown to diminish in elderly females, which Brocklehurst (1982) has suggested may be related to replacement of the smooth muscle by collagen, as mentioned above. Oestrogen depletion may also affect the urethral closing mechanism, as previously discussed, and may lead to stress incontinence (Brocklehurst, 1982; Staskin, 1986). Benign prostatic hypertrophy is generally considered to be a pathological condition associated with ageing in men (Staskin, 1986).

According to Brocklehurst (1982), the most important age change associated with the control of bladder function is that which occurs within the central nervous system. The long and complex nerve tracts might be affected by what Brocklehurst (1984b) termed 'neuronal fall-out' in the neo-cortex and cerebellum of the brain. This may affect the inhibition of spinal reflex activity, allowing spontaneous bladder contractions to occur causing urgency and diminished bladder capacity, both of which predispose towards incontinence (Brocklehurst, 1982). Whether these alterations in central nervous control reflect true ageing changes or are associated with age-related disease (e.g. Alzheimer's disease, cerebrovascular disease) remains unclear.

As already discussed, there is evidence that the pattern of micturition alters with age. Brocklehurst et al. (1971) and more recently, Hale et al. (1986), among others, have found nocturia to be a very common symptom in elderly men and women living in the community. Nocturia appears to become more common and severe with increasing age (Brocklehurst et al., 1971).

It is important to remember that incontinence is not an inevitable consequence of ageing, indeed the majority of elderly people remain continent all of their lives. Elderly people are, however, more susceptible to incontinence than younger people because of the additional pathological, physiological, pharmacological and psychological factors from which they are at risk. Brocklehurst (1985) suggested that there are factors which lead to inefficient and impaired bladder function with which an elderly person can cope provided his or her environment is undisturbed. There are also a number of precipitating factors (for example, the sudden loss of mobility due to a stroke), however, which may tilt the balance so that the elderly person with impaired bladder control is no longer able to maintain continence. The precise role of many of these factors and the way in which they interact to affect whether an elderly person remains continent or not, has still to be determined.

Summary

Over the last two decades there have been considerable improvements in the assessment and management techniques available for incontinence sufferers. However, research into the causes of incontinence, across all age groups, needs to be further built upon if the provision and the quality of care for people with continence problems is to continue to improve. It is clear from the literature reviewed that while some aspects of the aetiology of incontinence have still to be determined, it is a symptom which has many causes and may result from more than one causal or predisposing factor. The literature identifies not only the role of different types of physiological bladder dysfunction in the causation of incontinence, but also stresses the role of many other important aspects such as environmental, psychological and social factors. A comprehensive assessment of the patient with incontinence, therefore, necessitates the exploration of many areas if the causes of incontinence are to be identified, and appropriate management planned and carried out.

References

Abrams, P.H. and Feneley, R. (1978), 'The significance of the symptoms associated with bladder outflow obstruction', *Urology International*, 33: 171–4.

Abrams, P.H., Feneley, R. and Torrens, M. (1983), *Urodynamics*, Berlin: Springer-Verlag.

Abrutyn, E., Boscia, J.A. and Kaye, D. (1988), 'The treatment of asymptomatic bacteriuria in the elderly', *Journal of the American Geriatrics Society*, 36: 473–5

Adams, J. (1979), 'Features of the bungalow', *Nursing Times*, 75: 1160–1.

Akhtar, A.J., Andrews, G.R., Caird, F.L. and Fallon, R.J. (1972), 'Urinary tract infection in the elderly: population study', *Age and Ageing*, 1: 48–54.

Ames, S.W. and Kneisl, C.R. (1988), *Adult Health Nursing*, California: Addison-Wesley.

Anderson, S. and Brenner, B. (1987), 'The ageing kidney: structure, function, mechanisms and therapeutic implications', *Journal of the American Geriatrics Society*, 35: 590–3.

Andrew, J. and Nathan, P. (1964), 'Lesions of the anterior frontal lobes and disturbance of micturition and defaecation', *Brain*, 87: 233–61.

Arie, T., Clarke, M. and Slattery, Z. (1976), 'Incontinence in geriatric psychiatry', in Willington, F.L. (ed.), *Incontinence in the Elderly*, London: Academic Press, pp. 70–81.

Avery-Jones, F.A. and Godding, E.W. (1973), *Management of Constipation*, Oxford: Blackwell Scientific (2nd edn).

Baker, D.E. (1978), 'Attitudes of nurses to the care of the elderly', PhD thesis, University of Manchester.

Barer, D.H. (1989), 'Continence after stroke: useful predictor or goal of therapy?', *Age and Ageing*, 18: 183–91.

Bates, C.P., Bradley, W.E., Glen, E., Melchior, M., Rowan, D., Stirling, A. and Hald, T. (1975), 'First report of the standardisation of terminology of lower urinary tract function', *Scandinavian Journal of Urology and Nephrology* (1977), 11: 193–6.

Bates, C.P., Bradley, W.E., Glen, F., Melchior, M., Rowan, D., Stirling, A., Sundrin, T., Thomas, D., Torrens, M., Turner-Warwick, R., Zinner, N.R. and Hald, T. (1979), 'Fourth report on the standardisation of terminology of lower urinary tract function', International Continence Society, Manchester, September 1978.

Berrios, G.E. (1986), 'Urinary incontinence and pathophysiology of the elderly with cognitive failure', *Gerontology*, 32: 119–24.

Borrie, M.J., Campbell, A.J. and Caradoc-Davies, T.H. (1985), 'Urinary incontinence following stroke: a prospective study', London: International Continence Society (papers read by title).

Borrs, E. and Cormarr, A. (1971), *Neurological Urology*, Baltimore: University Park Press.

Boyarsky, S., Labay, P., Hanrick, P., Abramson, A. and Boyarsky, L. (1979), *Care of the patient with neurogenic bladder*, Boston: Little Brown.

Bradley, W.E. (1976), 'Neural control of urethral vestical function', *American Journal of Obstetrics and Gynaecology*, 125: 653–66.

Bradley, W.E. and Scott, F.B. (1978), 'Physiology of the urinary bladder', in Harrison, J.H., Gittes, R.F., Perlmutter, A.D., Stamey, T. and Walsh, P.C.W.B. (eds), *Campbell's Urology, Volume 1*, Philadelphia: Saunders Company, pp. 87–118 (4th edn).

Brazelton, T.B. (1962), 'A child orientated approach to toilet training', *Paediatrics*, 29: 121–8.

Bridgewater, J. and Christie, H. (1974), 'Glyme – "A silk purse"', *Nursing Mirror*, 139: 58–61.

Brink, C.A. (1988), 'Evaluation of urinary incontinence', *Topics in Geriatric Rehabilitation*, 3: 21–9.

Brink, C.A. and Wells, T.A. (1986), 'Environmental support for geriatric incontinence', *Clinics in Geriatric Medicine*, 2: 829–39.

Brocklehurst, J.C. (1967), 'Incontinence of urine', *Nursing Times*, 63: 954–6.

Brocklehurst, J.C. (1978a), 'Differential diagnosis of urinary incontinence', *Geriatrics*, April: 36–9.

Brocklehurst, J.C. (1978b), 'The investigation and management of incontinence', in Isaacs, B. (ed.), *Recent advances in geriatric medicine*, Edinburgh: Churchill Livingstone.

Brocklehurst, J.C. (1982), 'The ageing bladder', *Geriatric Medicine*, 12: 11–15.

Brocklehurst, J.C. (1984a), 'Urinary incontinence in the elderly', *The Practitioner*, 228: 275–83.

Brocklehurst, J.C. (1984b), 'Ageing, bladder function and incontinence', in Brocklehurst, J.C. (ed.), *Urology in the Elderly*, Edinburgh: Churchill Livingstone, pp. 1–18.

Brocklehurst, J.C. (1985), 'The genitourinary system – the bladder', in Brocklehurst, J.C. (ed.), *Textbook of Geriatric Medicine and Gerontology*, Edinburgh: Churchill Livingstone, pp. 626–47 (3rd edn).

Brocklehurst, J.C., Andrews, K., Richards, B. and Laycock, P.J. (1985), 'Incidence and correlates of incontinence in stroke patients', *Journal of the American Geriatric Society*, 33: 540–2.

Brocklehurst, J.C., Bee, P., Jones, D. and Palmer, M.K. (1977), 'Bacteriuria in geriatric hospital patients: its correlates and management', *Age and Ageing*, 6: 240–5.

Brocklehurst, J.C. and Dillane, J.B. (1966a), 'Studies of the female bladder in old age: cystometrograms in non-institutional women', *Gerontologia Clinica*, 8: 285–305.

Brocklehurst, J.C. and Dillane, J.B. (1966b), 'Studies of the female bladder in old age II: cystometrograms in 100 incontinent women', *Gerontologia Clinica*, 8: 306–19.

Brocklehurst, J.C., Dillane, J.B., Griffiths, L.L. and Fry, J. (1968), 'The prevalence and symptomatology of urinary infection in an aged population', *Gerontologia Clinica*, 10: 242–53.

Brocklehurst, J.C., Fry, J., Griffiths, L.L. and Karlton, G. (1971), 'Dysuria in old age', *Journal of the American Geriatrics Society*, 197: 582–92.

Brocklehurst, J.C., Fry, J., Griffiths, L. and Karlton, G. (1972), 'Urinary incontinence and symptoms of dysuria in women aged 45–64 years', *Age and Ageing*, 1: 41–7.

Calder, M. (1976), 'The nursing of incontinence', in Willington F.L. (ed.), *Incontinence in the Elderly*, London: Academic Press, pp. 202–9.

Campbell, J.A., Reinken, J. and McCosh, L. (1985), 'Incontinence in the elderly: prevalence and prognosis', *Age and Ageing*, 14: 65–70.

Cantor, T.J. and Bates, C.P. (1980), 'A comparative study of symptoms and objective urodynamic findings in 214 incontinent women', *British Journal Obstetrics and Gynaecology*, 87: 889–92.

Cardozo, L., Versi, E., Tapp, A. and Studd, J. (1986), 'Oestrogens and urgency', Proceedings of the International Continence Society, Boston, Mass, 370–1.

Castleden, C.M. and Davies, K.N. (1987), 'Hypnotics in the elderly', *The Practitioner*, 282: 885–8.

Castleden, C.M. and Duffin, H.M. (1981), 'Guidelines for controlling urinary incontinence without drugs or catheters', *Age and Ageing*, 10: 186–90.

Castleden, C.M., Duffin, H.M. and Asher, M.J. (1981), 'Clinical and urodynamic studies in 100 elderly incontinent patients', *British Medical Journal*, 82: 1103–5.

Chamberlaine, M.A. and Stowe, J. (1982), 'Bathing in hospital', *British Medical Journal*, 284: 1693–4.

Chanfreau-Rona, D., Bellwood, S. and Wylie, B. (1984), 'Assessment of a behavioural programme to treat incontinent patients in psychogeriatric wards', *British Journal of Clinical Psychology*, 23: 273–9.

Cheater, F.M. (1990), 'Urinary incontinence in hospital in-patients: a nursing perspective', PhD thesis, University of Nottingham.

Chilton, C.P. (1984), 'The distal urethral sphincter mechanism and the pelvic floor', in Mundy, A.P., Stephenson, T.P. and Wein, A.J. (eds), *Urodynamics: Principles, Practice and Application*, Edinburgh: Churchill Livingstone, pp. 9–13.

Crane, D., David, B. and Hackler, R. (1978), *Urology in Practice*, Devine, C. and Streckler, J. (eds), Boston: Little Brown.

Cullodine, S. (1987), 'Urinary incontinence – a lesson for nurses' (letter), *Nursing Times*, 83: 14.

Davies, J.E. (1979), 'Effects of the new home on patients and nurses', *Nursing Times*, 75: 1725–6.

Denny-Brown, D. and Robertson, G. (1933), 'On the physiology of micturition', *Brain*, 54: 149–90.

Diokno, A.C. (1988), 'The cause of urinary incontinence', *Topics in Geriatric Rehabilitation*, 3: 13–20.

Diokno, A.C., Brock, B.M., Brown, M.B. and Herzog, R. (1986), 'Prevalence of urinary incontinence and other urological symptoms in the non institutionalised elderly', *Journal of Urology*, 136: 1022–5.

Diokno, A.C., Wells, T.J. and Brink, C.A. (1987), 'Urinary incontinence in elderly women: urodynamic evaluation', *Journal of the American Geriatrics Society*, 35: 940–6.

Dunn, A. and Strand, C. (1970), 'Ward hostess experiment', *Gerontologia Clinica*, 2: 267–74.

Eastwood, H.D.H. (1979), 'Urodynamic studies in the management of urinary incontinence in the elderly', *Age and Ageing*, 8: 41–8.

Eastwood, H.D.H. and Warrell, R. (1984), 'Urinary incontinence in disabled elderly females; Prediction in diagnosis and outcome of management', *Age and Ageing*, 13: 230–334.

Farrar, D.J. (1984), 'Urology in the elderly', in Mundy, A.R., Stephenson, T.P. and Wein, A.J. (eds), *Urodynamics: Principles, Practice and Application*, Edinburgh: Churchill Livingstone, pp. 249–55.

Farrar, D.J., Whiteside, C.G., Osborne, J.L., Turner-Warwick, R.T. (1975), 'A urodynamic analysis of micturition symptoms in the female', *Surgery, Gynaecology and Obstetrics*, 141: 875–81.

Feneley, R.C.L. (1986), 'Normal micturition and its control', in Mandelstam, D. (ed.), *Incontinence and its management*, London: Croom Helm (2nd edn), pp. 16–34.

Fernie, G.R., Jewett, M.A.S., Autry, D., Holliday, P.J. and Zorzitto, M.L. (1983), 'Prevalence of geriatric urinary dysfunction in a chronic care hospital', *Canadian Medical Association Journal*, 128: 1085–6.

Field, M.A. (1979), 'Urinary incontinence in the elderly: an overview', *Journal of Gerontological Nursing*, 5: 12–19.

Fleigner, J.R. and Glenning, P.P. (1979), 'Seven years experience in the evaluation and management of patients with urge incontinence of urine', *Australian and New Zealand Journal of Obstetrics and Gynecology*, 19: 42–4.

Fossberg, E., Sanders, S. and Beisland, H. (1981), 'Urinary incontinence in the elderly: a pilot study', *Scandinavian Journal of Urology and Nephrology*, 60 (supp): 51–3.

Freeman, R.M. and Baxby, K. (1982), 'Hypnotherapy for incontinence caused by the unstable detrusor', *British Medical Journal*, 284: 1831–6.

Frewen, W.K. (1972), 'Urgency incontinence: review of 100 cases', *Journal of Obstetrics and Gynaecology*, 79: 77–9.

Frewen, W.K. (1978), 'An objective assessment of the unstable bladder of psychosomatic origin', *British Journal of Urology*, 50: 246–9.

Frewen, W.K. (1979), 'Role of bladder training in the treatment of unstable bladders in females', Symposium on clinical urodynamics, *Urological Clinics of North America*, 6: 273–7.

Gibbon, N.L. (1976), 'Nomenclature of neurogenic bladder', *Urology*, 8: 423.

Gleason, D.M., Bottaccini, M.R. and Reilly, R.J. (1974), 'Active and passive incontinence: differential diagnosis', *Urology*, 4: 693–701.

Glezerman, M., Glasner, M., Ritover, M., Tauber, E., Barziv, J. and Insler, D. (1986), 'Evaluation of the reliability of the history in females complaining of urinary stress incontinence', *European Journal of Obstetrics and Gynaecological Reproductive Biology*, 21: 159–64.

Goat, S. (1988), 'Incontinence can improve', *Nursing Standard*, 3: 34–5.

Gosling, J.A. and Chilton, C.P. (1984), 'The anatomy of the bladder, urethra and pelvic floor', in Mundy, A.R., Stephenson, T.P. and Wein, A.J. (eds), *Urodynamics. Principles, Practice and Application*, Edinburgh: Churchill Livingstone, pp. 3–9.

Green, M.F. (1986), 'Old people and disorders of continence', in Mandelstam, D. (ed.), *Incontinence and its Management*, London: Croom Helm (2nd edn), pp. 110–34.

Hald, T. (1975), 'Problems of urinary incontinence', in Caldwell, K.P.S. (ed.), *Urinary Incontinence*, London: Sector Publishing, pp. 11–25.

Hale, W.E., Perkins, L.L., May, F.E., Marks, R.G. and Stewart, R.B. (1986), 'Symptom prevalence in the elderly: an evaluation of age, sex, disease and medication use', *Journal of the American Geriatrics Society*, 34: 333–40.

Harrison, S.M. (1983), 'Stress incontinence and the physiotherapist', *Physiotherapist*, 69: 144–7.

Helps, E.P.W. (1977), 'Disorders of the urinary system: urinary incontinence in the elderly', *British Medical Journal*, 2: 754–7.

Herzog, A.R. and Fultz, N.H. (1988), 'Urinary incontinence in the community: prevalence, consequences, management and beliefs', *Topics in Geriatric Rehabilitation*, 2: 1–12.

Hilton, P. and Stanton, S.L. (1981), 'Algorithmic method of assessing urinary incontinence in elderly females', *British Medical Journal*, 282: 940–2.

Hodgkinson, C.P. (1970), 'Stress incontinence', *American Journal of Obstetrics and Gynaecology*, 108: 1141–68.

Hu, S.A. (1982), 'ABC of incontinence', *Nursing Times*, 78: 1194.

Isaacs, B. (1976), 'The preservation of continence', in Willington F.L. (ed.), *Incontinence in the Elderly*, London: Academic Press, pp. 245–51.

Isaacs, B. and Walkey, F.A. (1964), 'A survey of incontinence in elderly hospital patients', *Gerontologia Clinica*, 6: 367–76.

Jewett, M.A.S., Fernie, G.R., Holliday, P.J. and Pim, M.E. (1981), 'Urinary dysfunction in a geriatric long-term population: prevalence and patterns', *Journal of the American Geriatrics Society*, 29: 211–14.

Johnson, J.H. (1980), 'Rehabilitative aspects of neurologic bladder dysfunction', *Nursing Clinics of North America*, 15: 293–307.

Keister, K.J. and Creason, N.S. (1989), 'Medications of elderly institutionalised incontinent females', *Journal of Advanced Nursing*, 14: 980–5.

Kennedy, A.P. (1984), 'Nursing and the incontinent patient', in Brocklehurst, J.C. (ed.), *Urology in the Elderly*, Edinburgh: Churchill Livingstone, pp. 127–43.

King, M.R. (1979), 'A study of incontinence in a psychiatric hospital', *Nursing Times*, 75: 1133–5.

King, M.R. (1980), 'Treatment of incontinence', *Nursing Times*, 76: 1006–10.

Kohlraush, O. (1854), *Zur Anatomie und Physiologie der beckenorgane*, Leipzig: Hirzel.

Krane, R.J. and Sirosky, M.B. (1979), 'Classification of neurourological disorders', in Krane, R.J. and Sirosky, M.B. (eds), *Clinical Urology*, Boston: Little Brown, p. 143.

Lapides, J. (1982), 'Physiology of the bladder and urinary sphincter: relationship to stress incontinence', in *Disorders of the female urethra and urinary incontinence*, Baltimore: Williams and Wilkin, pp. 15–24.

Larsson, G. and Victor, A. (1986), 'A study of the volume-frequency micturition chart in healthy women', Proceedings of the Incontinence Society, third joint meeting, Boston, Mass., pp. 458–60.

Leach, G.E. and Yip, C.M. (1986), 'Urologic and urodynamic evaluation of the elderly population', *Clinics in Geriatric Medicine*, 2: 731–55.

Lepine, A., Renault, R. and Stewart, I. (1979), 'The incidence and management of incontinence in a home for the elderly', *Health and Social Services Journal*, 89: 9–12.

Lich, R., Howerton, L.W. and Amin, M. (1978), 'Anatomy and surgical approach to the urogenital tract in the male', in Harrison, J.H., Ruben, F.G., Perlmutter, A.D., Stamey, T.A. and Walsh, P.C. (eds), *Campbell's Urology, Volume 1* (4th edn), Philadelphia: W.B. Saunders, pp. 3–31.

McCormick, K.A., Engel, B.J., Burgio, L.K. and Burgio, L.D. (1985), 'Comparative characteristics of incontinent patients in outpatient day care and inpatient environments', *Gerontologist* (Supp), 25: 247.

Mandelstam, D. and Tuck, S.M. (1986), 'Continence and nursing management in the elderly'. Proceedings of the International Continence Society, Boston, Mass., pp. 477–8.

Margolis, G.L. (1965), 'A review of the literature on psychogenic urinary retention', *Journal of Urology*, 94: 257–8.

Millard, P.H. (1979), 'The promotion of continence', *Health Trends*, 11: 27–8.

Miller, A. (1985a), 'A study of the dependency of elderly patients in wards using different methods of nursing care', *Age and Ageing*, 14: 132–8.

Miller, A. (1985b), 'Nurse/patient dependency – is it iatrogenic?', *Journal of Advanced Nursing*, 10: 63–9.

Milne, J.S. (1976), 'Prevalence of incontinence in elderly age groups', in Willington, F.L. (ed.), *Incontinence in the elderly*, London: Academic Press, pp. 9–21.

Mitteness, L.S. (1987), 'So what do you expect when you are 85? Urinary incontinence in late life', in Roth, J.A. and Conrad, P. (eds), *Research in the sociology of health care* (vol. 6), Connecticut: Jai Press.

Muellner, S.R. (1960), 'Development of urinary control in children', *Journal American Medical Association*, 171: 1256–61.

Mundy, A.R. (1984), 'Clinical physiology of the bladder, urethra and pelvic floor', in Mundy, A.R., Stephenson, T.P. and Wein, A.J. (eds), *Urodynamics. Principles, practice and application*, Edinburgh: Churchill Livingstone, pp. 14–25.

Mundy, A.R. and Blaivas, J.C. (1984), 'Non-traumatic neurological disorders', in Mundy, A.R., Stephenson, T.P. and Wein, A.J. (eds), *Urodynamics. Principles, practice and application*, Edinburgh: Churchill Livingstone, pp. 278–87.

Nemir, A. and Middleman, R.P. (1954), 'Stress incontinence in young healthy nulliparous female subjects', *American Journal of Obstetrics and Gynaecology*, 68: 1166–8.

Newman, J.L. (1962), 'Old folk in wet beds', *British Medical Journal*, 1: 1824–8.

Newson, J. and Newson, E. (1963), 'Infant care in an urban community', London: George Allen & Unwin.

Newson, J. and Newson, E. (1968), 'Four years old in an urban community', London: George Allen & Unwin.

Northwood, J. (1979), 'The progress of two patients after moving to Ridge Hill', *Nursing Times*, 75: 1769–70.

Norton, C. (1986), *Nursing for continence*. Beaconsfield: Beaconsfield Publishers.

Norton, D. (1967), *Hospitals of the long-stay patient*, Oxford: Pergamon Press.

Norton, D., McClaren, R. and Exton-Smith, A. (1962), 'An investigation into geriatric nursing problems in hospital. London, National Corporation for the care of old people' (reprinted 1976) Edinburgh: Churchill Livingstone.

Norton, P.A., MacDonald, L.D., Sedgwick, P.M. and Stanton, S.L. (1988), 'Distress and delay associated with urinary incontinence, frequency and urgency in women', *British Medical Journal*, 297: 1187–9.

O'Reagan, S.O., Yasbeck, S. and Schick, E. (1985), 'Constipation, bladder instability and urinary tract infection syndrome', *Clinical Nephrology*, 23: 152–4.

Ory, M.G., Wyman, J.F. and Yu, L. (1986), 'Psychosocial factors in urinary incontinence', *Clinics in Geriatric Medicine*, 2: 657–71.

Ouslander, J.G. (1986), 'A diagnostic evaluation of geriatric urinary incontinence', *Clinics in Geriatric Medicine*, 2: 715–27.

Ouslander, J.G., Hepps, K.P., Raz, S. and Su, H.L. (1986), 'Genitourinary dysfunction in a geriatric outpatient population', *Journal of the American Geriatrics Society*, 34: 507–14.

Ouslander, J.G., Kane, R.L. and Abrass, B. (1982), 'Urinary incontinence in elderly nursing home patients', *Journal of American Medical Society*, 248: 1194–8.

Overstall, R.W., Rounce, K. and Palmer, J.K. (1980), 'Experience with an incontinence clinic', *Journal of the American Geriatrics Society*, 28: 534–8.

Paillard, M. and Resnick, N. (1984), 'Natural history of nosocomial urinary incontinence', *Gerontologist*, 24: 212.

Pannill, F.L. (1987), 'Urinary incontinence' (Editorial), *Journal of the American Geriatrics Society*, 35: 880–2.

Parks, A.G., Porter, N.H. and Hardcastle, J.D. (1966), 'Syndrome of the descending perineum', *Proceedings of the Royal Society of Medicine*, 59: 477–82.

Perkash, I. (1982), 'Management of neurogenic dysfunction of the bladder and bowel', in Kotte, F.J., Stillwell, G.K. and Lehman, J.F. (eds), *Krusen's Handbook of Physical Medicine and Rehabilitation*, Philadelphia: W.B. Saunders, pp. 724–45.

Peterson, I., Sterner, I., Selleden, U. and Kollberg, S. (1962), 'Investigation of urethral sphincter in females with simultaneous electromyographic and micturition urethrocystography', *Acta Neurologica Scandinavica*, Supplement 3: 145.

Powell, P.H. (1983), 'Incontinence, function and dysfunction and investigation', *Physiotherapy*, 69: 105–8.

Resnick, N.M., Wetle, T.T., Scherr, P., Branch, L. and Taylor, J. (1986), 'Urinary incontinence in community dwelling elderly: prevalence and correlates'. International Continence Society Meeting, Boston, Mass., pp. 76–8.

Robinson, J.M. (1984a), 'Evaluation of methods for assessment of bladder and urethral function', in Brocklehurst, J.C. (ed.), *Urology in the elderly*, Edinburgh: Churchill Livingstone, pp. 19–54.

Robinson, J.M. (1984b), 'Is oestrogen deficiency related to urinary incontinence?', *Geriatric Medicine*, 14: 173–5.

Sampselle, C.M., Brink, C.A. and Wells, T. (1989), 'Digital measurement of pelvic muscle strength in childbearing women', *Nursing Research*, 38: 134–8.

Savage, B.J. and Widdowson, T. (1974a), 'Revising the use of nursing resources – 1', *Nursing Times*, 71: 1372–4.

Savage, B.J. and Widdowson, T. (1974b), 'Revising the use of nursing resources – 2', *Nursing Times*, 71: 1424–7.

Schwartz, M. and Stanton, A. (1950), 'A social psychological study of incontinence', *Psychiatry*, 13: 399–413.

Scott, J.N. (1985), 'This malodorous malady', *Geriatric Nursing*, 5: 5–10.

Scottish Home and Health Department (1970), *Geriatric Accommodation Report*, Edinburgh.

Shimp, L.A. (1988), 'Influence of drug therapy on urinary incontinence', *Topics in Geriatric Rehabilitation*, 2: 30–41.

Sier, H., Ouslander, J.G. and Orzeck, S. (1987), 'Urinary incontinence among geriatric patients in an acute-care hospital', *Journal American Medical Association*, 257: 1767–71.

Smith, P.S. and Smith, L.J. (1987), 'The role of maturation and learning', in *Continence and Incontinence*, London: Croom Helm, pp. 55–72.

Snooks, S.J., Setchell, M., Swash, M. and Henry, M. (1984), 'Injury to innervation of pelvic floor sphincter musculature in child birth', *Lancet*, 2: 546–50.

Sourander, L.B. (1966), 'Urinary tract infection in the aged: an epidemiological study', *Annales Medicinae Internae Fennaie*, Supplement 45: 56.

Spangeler, B.F., Risley, T.R. and Bilyew, D.D. (1984), 'The management of dehydration and incontinence in non-ambulatory geriatric patients', *Journal Applied Behavioural Analysis*, 17: 397–401.

Stanton, S.L. (1978), 'Preoperative investigation and diagnosis', *Clinical Obstetrics and Gynaecology*, 21: 705–24.

Stanton, S.L. (1984a), 'Sphincter incompetence', in Mundy, A.R., Stephenson, T.P. and Wein, A.J. (eds), *Urodynamics. Principles, Practice and Application*, Edinburgh: Churchill Livingstone, pp. 229–41.

Stanton, S.L. (1984b), 'Gynecological aspects', in Mandelstam, D. (ed.), *Incontinence and Its Management*, London: Croom Helm, pp. 55–75.

Stanton, S.L. (1986), 'Gynecological aspects', in Mandelstam, D. (ed.), *Incontinence and Its Management*, 2nd ed, London: Croom Helm, pp. 55–75.

Staskin, D.R. (1986), 'Age-related physiological and pathological changes affecting lower urinary tract function', *Clinics in Geriatric Medicine*, 2: 701–9.

Stephenson, T.P. and Wein, A.J. (1984), 'The interpretation of urodynamics', in Mundy, A.P., Stephenson, T.P. and Wein, A.J. (eds), *Urodynamics. Principles, Practice and Application*, Edinburgh: Churchill Livingstone, pp. 93–115.

Stone, C.B. and Judge, C.E. (1978), 'Psychogenic aspects of urinary incontinence in females', *Clinical Obstetrics and Gynaecology*, 21: 807–15.

Sutherland, S. (1971), 'Emotional aspects of incontinence in the elderly', *Modern Geriatrics*, May: 270–4.

Tallis, R. and Norton, C. (1985), 'Incontinence in the elderly', *Nursing Times*, 81: 21–4.

Tanagho, E.A. (1978), 'The anatomy and physiology of micturition', *Clinics in Obstetrics and Gynaecology*, 5: 3–26.

Tanagho, E.A., Smith, D. and Myers, F. (1968), 'The trigone: anatomical and physiological considerations in relation to the bladder neck', *Journal of Urology*, 100: 633–9.

Tarrier, N. and Larner, S. (1983), 'The effect of management of social reinforcement on toilet requests on a geriatric ward', *Age and Ageing*, 12: 234–9.

Thomas, S.M., Plymat, K.R., Blannin, J. and Meade, T.W. (1980), 'Prevalence of urinary incontinence', *British Medical Journal*, 281: 1243–6.

Turner-Warwick, R. (1968), 'The repair of urethral structure in membranous urethra', *Journal of Urology*, 100: 303–14.

Turner-Warwick, R. (1984), 'Bladder outflow obstruction in the male', in Mundy, A.R., Stephenson, T.P. and Wein, A.J. (eds), *Urodynamics. Principles, Practice and Application*, Edinburgh: Churchill Livingstone, pp. 183–201.

Twycross, R.G. and Lack, S.S. (1990), *Therapeutics in Terminal Cancer*, Edinburgh: Churchill Livingstone.

Ulmsten, U., Andersson, K.E. and Persson, C.G.A. (1977), 'Diagnostic and therapeutic aspects of urge incontinence in women', *Urology International*, 32: 88–96.

Vehkalahti, I. and Kivelda, S.L. (1985), 'Urinary incontinence and its correlates in very old age', *Gerontology*, 31: 391–6.

Vetter, N.J., Jones, D.A. and Victor, C.R. (1981), 'Urinary incontinence in the elderly at home', *Lancet*, 2: 1275–7.

Vincent, S.A. (1966), 'Postural control of urinary incontinence', *Lancet*, 2: 631–2.

Walkey, F.A., Judge, T.G., Thomson, J. and Sakari, N.B.S. (1967), 'Incidence of urinary tract infection in the elderly', *Scottish Medical Journal*, 12: 411–14.

Wein, A.J. (1981), 'Classification of neurogenic voiding dysfunction', *Journal of Urology*, 125: 605.

Wein, A.J. (1986), 'Physiology of micturition', *Clinics in Geriatric Medicine*, 2: 682–99.

Wells, T. (1975), 'Towards understanding nursing problems in care of the hospitalised elderly', PhD thesis, University of Manchester.

Wells, T. (1984), 'Social and psychological implications of incontinence', in Brocklehurst, J.C. (ed.), *Urology in the Elderly*, Edinburgh: Churchill Livingstone, pp. 107–26.

Wells, T. (1988), 'Additional treatments for urinary incontinence', *Topics in Geriatric Medicine Rehabilitation*, 3: 48–57.

Wheatley, J.K. (1983), 'Causes and treatment of bladder incontinence', *Comprehensive Therapy*, 9: 27–33.

Whitehead, W.E., Burgio, K.L. and Engel, B.T. (1984), 'Behavioural methods in the assessment and treatment of urinary incontinence', in Brocklehurst, J.C. (ed.), *Urology in the Elderly*, Edinburgh: Churchill Livingstone, pp. 74–92.

Williams, M.E. and Pannill, F.C. (1982), 'Urinary incontinence in the elderly: physiology, pathophysiology, diagnosis and treatment', *Annals of Internal Medicine*, 97: 895–907.

Willington, F.L. (1969), 'Problems of urinary incontinence in the aged', *Gerontologia Clinica*, 2: 330–56.

Willington, F.L. (1975a), 'Significance of incompetence of personal sanitary habits', *Nursing Times*, 71: 340–1.

Willington, F.L. (1975b), 'Problems in the aetiology of urinary incontinence', *Nursing Times*, 71: 378–81.

Willington, F.L. (1975c), 'Incontinence, psychological and psychogenic aspects', *Nursing Times*, 71: 378–81.

Willington, F.L. (1980), 'Urinary incontinence: a practical approach', *Geriatrics*, 35: 41–8.

Wolin, L.H. (1969), 'Stress incontinence in young healthy nulliparous female subjects', *Journal of Urology*, 101: 545–9.

Woodburne, R.T. (1961), 'The sphincter mechanisms of urinary bladder and urethra', *Anatomical Medicine*, 141: 11.

Wright, M. (1984), 'Study into problems of incontinence in two long-stay wards for the elderly', Unpublished report undertaken for level III Health Studies Course, University of Sheffield.

Yarnell, J.W.G. and St Leger, A.S. (1979), 'The prevalence, severity and factors associated with urinary incontinence in a random sample of the elderly', *Age and Ageing*, 8: 81–5.

Yarnell, J.W.G., Voyle, G.J., Seetnam, P.M., Milbank, J., Richards, C.J., Stephenson, T.P. (1981), 'Factors associated with urinary incontinence in women', *Journal of Epidemiology and Community Health*, 36: 58–63.

Yeates, W.K. (1976), 'Normal and abnormal bladder function in incontinence of urine', in Willington, F.L. (ed.), *Incontinence in the Elderly*, London: Academic Press, pp. 22–4.

3   Assessment of urinary incontinence
HILARY DUFFIN

Introduction

What is the value of assessment, and how reliable is the information obtained? Does variability depend on such factors as the environment for the interview or the expectations and past experiences of both patient and nurse? Assessment of incontinence is a necessary preliminary step in planning and appropriate intervention and management of presenting problems and the promotion of continence.

This chapter focuses on current methods and approaches in the nursing assessment of patients with urinary incontinence. It presents a general concept of patient assessment, followed by detailed aspects of the information required and how it is selected. Such techniques include interview, observation, physical examination and measurements using frequency/volume charting. The reliability of the information collected is discussed along with recommendations for practice. Finally invasive techniques for the assessment of incontinence which includes urodynamics are described.

Assessment of the patient with urinary incontinence

Assessment is a key factor in individualised nursing. It is defined by Roper *et al.* (1990) as 'collecting information, reviewing the collected information, identifying the patient's problems and identifying the priority of problems. Information', they state, 'is gained through observation, interview, examination, measurement and by tests as appropriate to the individual.' This initial information is used as 'a base-line against which any further information can be compared.' Relatives of the patient or primary carers may also provide a valuable secondary source of information.

The method of assessing patients has been developed over the past 30 years into a systematic approach which consolidates a nurse's observations and interprets the responses (McCain, 1965). Such a systematic approach was described in a study made by Campbell *et al.* (1985) which highlights the method of assessment using interview and physical examination. By responding to appropriate structured questioning, the patient's status in each area is established. Collectively the whole assessment data are used by the nurse to plan management, treatment and goals. A full account of a 'functional health patterns assessment tool' for nursing use was given by Gordon (1982) who advocated a two-phase assessment: firstly history taking and examination, followed by observation and further questions if necessary. However, the nurse should be alert to the possibility of being given misleading information, or making a poor interpretation of the patient's response. In her paper analysing the components of basic nursing care, Henderson (1969) described the skills required by the nurse to make an assessment of the patient's needs. She warned that the nurse must understand that human beings do not necessarily convey the intended meaning in what is spoken, and that understanding of each other can be limited.

Good interviewing skills ensure a better response. The posture of the nurse and verbal interaction can encourage the patient. It may be necessary to repeat a question or change the original wording, to make it more easily understood or more relevant to that patient. Replies may be vague or muddled, so clarification will be needed.

The nursing assessment and interview should be conducted in an atmosphere of peace and privacy where the patient can feel relaxed and safe (Campbell et al., 1985). The patient's own home can provide the ideal location (Norton, 1986), especially if there are difficulties with personal mobility, or obtaining transport to a clinic.

This assessment tool can be retained as a record of the initial situation. It should be filed within the patient's hospital or clinic notes to be used as a reference by nursing staff and other health care professionals, to monitor the progress of that patient (Norton, 1980).

Nursing attitudes

The nurse should try not to hurry the patient or give the impression that the patient is taking up too much time. By showing an attitude of understanding and empathy and genuine warmth of feeling, the interviewing nurse will be fulfilling the criteria for desirable behaviour as described by Brown (1988).

The patient is the main and most important information source (after all it is he or she who has the problem). There may be areas causing particular concern or distress which do not have the same priority to the nurse making the assessment. Experience and in-depth knowledge of incontinence will enable the nurse to be selective in expanding or curtailing subjects broached.

Henderson (1969) called upon the nurse to possess a sensitivity to feelings expressed in non-verbal communication, and to encourage the patients to describe feelings, symptoms or difficulties. The nurse is required to share the patient's interpretation of problems in order to develop their relationship. Brown (1988) also referred to the importance of establishing a relationship of trust between patient and nurse, by the creation of an environment in which the patient is able to confide in the nurse. This will be particularly helpful later on when working towards goals set. He also identified the importance of self-awareness in the nurse conducting the interview: this helps him or her to relate to the needs of others. One example of this which applies especially to the elderly, is a frequent preference to be addressed formally as Mr, Mrs or Miss, rather than by their given name. The nurse should first remember to introduce him or herself, explaining his or her own place within the health care team.

The responses made by the patient to the assessment questions must be recorded exactly as they are expressed to the nurse (Campbell *et al.*, 1985). An assessment form or 'check-list' appropriate to the interview provides a helpful guideline and continuity of practice. The patient's own perception of health will have a major influence on his or her replies to questions. This will also affect participation in the setting of goals, acceptance of nursing management, implementation of treatment, and expectations of outcome (Henderson, 1969; Gordon, 1982; Campbell *et al.*, 1985).

Recent life events, particularly a 'loss experience' may precede the onset of symptoms of incontinence. It is known that a variety of reasons cause patients to overplay their response to questions at interview (Totman, 1987).

Confidentiality

Members of the patient's family may wish to be involved with assessment. Often it is necessary for the nurse to consult relatives, or a member of the care team if the patient is living in residential care accommodation. The presence of another person may inhibit the patient from fully expressing problems and needs. Indeed the patient may have kept certain aspects (or the whole problem) hidden from others. It is therefore essential to ask permission from the patient before consulting anyone else. If discussion does take place with relatives or carers it should be together with the patient (Campbell *et al.*, 1985).

Observations

In addition to noting verbal and non-verbal communication from the patient, observations made by the nurse and other health care professionals make a valuable and essential contribution towards making a nursing assessment. Observations during the interview should include attitude, mood, beliefs, tolerance and coping ability, and a specific examination of mental and physical status, activity and exercise (Gordon, 1982). It will be necessary to know about the patterns of elimination, and sleep at a later date.

Social impact

Between 4 and 10 per cent of elderly people living in the community are said to suffer from a significant degree of urinary incontinence (McGrother *et al.*, 1986). That is to say, the amount of urine lost is such that it interferes with normal everyday life. McGrother *et al.* (1986) also predicted that the numbers of elderly people over 85 years of age would double in the following twenty years, and over 75 year olds increase by one-third. The absolute number of incontinent elderly people will therefore rise considerably in that period. Since studies have shown that the greater proportion of incontinence is associated with ageing and disability (Yarnell and St Leger, 1979; Vetter *et al.*, 1981), future developments in health care will need to include improved services for incontinent people.

It has been argued that urinary incontinence is a common cause of admission to geriatric units (Shuttleworth, 1970; Tattersall, 1985). The recent white paper *Caring for People* (1989) sets out the proposals for developing care and support in the community, rather than in institutions. In particular it targets the elderly, the mentally ill, the handicapped and the disabled. These are arguably the groups most likely to encounter incontinence problems. It is therefore essential that the causes of incontinence are properly diagnosed, and the differing conditions treated and cured so that the increased numbers of elderly people can remain active and independent within the community. If this is done huge improvements in their lifestyle could be achieved. The devastating effect of incontinence with consequent loss of dignity and self-esteem is a disability which can destroy the sufferer's personal relationships and social contacts. The problems and work caused by incontinence to families struggling to cope, is often the extra burden which leads to a breakdown in care and precipitates requests for many elderly people to be admitted into hospital (Tattersall, 1985). It has been shown by McGrother *et al.* (1987a) that elderly people with urinary incontinence in the community were three times more likely to have a low level of social contact (shopping, visiting, etc.) than others living locally.

Psychological aspects

Although not a life-threatening condition, chronic urinary incontinence has been found to be a source of 'appreciable morbidity' (Macaulay *et al.*, 1987), causing depression and anxiety which become incorporated into the patient's lifestyle and personality. These mood changes were found by Macaulay *et al.* (1987) to worsen the very condition by causing urgency, frequency and urge incontinence.

Feelings of anger, shame, depression, fear (of social embarrassment resulting from urine leakage and smell) and concerns about sexual relationships, are all too familiar to the incontinent person (Smith and Smith, 1989). To many sufferers the problems are enormous and appear unresolvable. These feelings cause many patients to deny the presence of incontinence, by preferring instead to focus on other physical symptoms (Hafner *et al.*, 1977). This makes it difficult to assess whether underlying emotional and interpersonal problems are a result of incontinence, or a contributing factor. Frewen (1978) found that such patients were unable to be cured without either adapting themselves, or changing the cause of the stress. A study by Norton *et al.* (1990) showed that 21 women of a total of 105 presenting with urinary incontinence had received psychiatric treatment. It would therefore seem that psychological factors are an extremely important cause (Freeman and Baxby, 1982).

Successful outcome of treating incontinence depends largely on patient participation in fairly simple techniques. Patient motivation to become continent was found by

	FREQUENCY / VOLUME CHART		

JOHN WELLS

consultant DR HARRIS   ward

Go to the toilet when you want to go.
Measure the amount passed each time.

date DEC '90

14th		15th		16th									
time	vol.	time	vol.	time	vol.	time	vol.	time	vol.	time	vol.	time	vol.
4 AM	WET 150	3.15	WET 100	4.30	WET 100								
7.15	200	7.30	WET 150	6.30	150								
9.10	150	8.30	100	8 AM	100								
11 AM	WET 100	11 PM	175	10.30	WET 50								
12.45	125	1 PM	WET 50	11.30	75								
2 PM	100	2 PM	50	12.45	100								
SHOPPING		SLEEPING		3.10	175								
4.50	WET 150	5 PM	WET 100	4.45	100								
6.20	WET 50	7 PM	200	6.30	WET 100								
8.30	175	8.15	125	8.20	200								
9 PM	50	9.30	150	9.45	175								
		11.45	175										

Fig. 3.1 Frequency volume chart.

Consultant:
Ward:
Month: Dec. '90

Name: MRS. M WRIGHT

Go to the toilet ~~every~~ .... ~~hours,~~ WHEN YOU WANT TO ~~whether you want to or not, and whether you are wet or dry.~~

Date: Day:	17 MON		18 TUES		19 WED		20 THURS		21 FRI		22 SAT		23 SUN	
	wet or dry	was urine passed	wet or dry	was urine passed	wet or dry	was urine passed	wet or dry	was urine passed	wet or dry	was urine passed	wet or dry	was urine passed	wet or dry	was urine passed
12 midnight														
1 am														
2 am			W	✓	W	✓			W	✓				
3 am	W	✓					D	✓						
4 am														
5 am			W	✓	W	✓			W	✓				
6 am							W	✓						
7 am	W	✓	D	✓			D	✓	W	✓				
8 am					W	✓			D	✓				
9 am	W	✓			D	✓	D	✓	D	✓				
10 am	D	✓	W	X			W	X	W	X				
11 am									D	✓				
12 noon	D	✓	W	✓										
1 pm					W	✓	W	✓						
2 pm			D	✓										
3 pm	W	✓			D	✓	D	✓	W	✓				
4 pm					D	✓								
5 pm	W	✓	D	✓			D	✓	D	✓				
6 pm	D	✓			D	✓	W	X						
7 pm	W	X	W	✓										
8 pm							D	✓						
9 pm	D	✓	D	✓	W	✓	D	✓						
10 pm									W	✓				
11 pm					D	✓								
X WET	6		5		5		4		6					

Fig. 3.2 Urinary continence chart.

Castleden *et al.* (1984) to be the most significant predictor of cure. This motivation may be difficult to generate when so many patients display negative attitudes of hopelessness and embarrassment as reasons for not consulting their general practitioner for help. Many believe that the doctor will think incontinence trivial, and that it is incurable (McGrother *et al.*, 1987a).

Assessment charts

The information obtained by charting episodes of incontinence, voiding frequency, and urine volumes, complements the assessment interview and physical examination. It is unnecessary for charts to be kept for long periods; a week at the most is usually adequate (Lofting, 1990) and where possible the details should be entered on to the chart by the patient (Castleden and Ekelund, 1989).

Types of chart
The frequency volume chart (Fig. 3.1) requires the patient to enter a record of the usual micturition pattern. Times of voiding, volumes of urine, and episodes of wetness are recorded. This then provides a baseline for possibly implementing a regular toileting regime to ensure urine is passed before incontinence occurs, or to regain bladder control if frequency is the major problem (Blannin, 1987). This type of chart often clarifies details of symptoms described by the patient at interview. Normal micturition patterns have been found by Boedker *et al.* (1989) to be unaffected by ageing.

The diary chart (Fig. 3.2) does not require urine volumes to be measured. A record is made of the times of micturition together with whether the patient is 'wet' or 'dry' at that time. Episodes of incontinence between visits to the toilet are also noted. Again where possible the patient should complete the chart, since this can have beneficial effects on motivating participation in treatment and management. This chart can also be used as a 'preliminary check' described by Clay (1978). The patient is asked to pass urine regularly every two hours. Entries are made in the same manner as for the diary chart. Assessment is then made in the light of this regular regime of voiding, and adjustment to the timing is subsequently made until continence is achieved.

Assessment interview

Every nurse is familiar with the process of gathering data from patient or client (McFarlane and Castledine, 1984). In order to be able to use these data it is necessary to know what elements to select so that the information will be relevant. It is also desirable that the nurse is aware of the best way to obtain that information (Chalmers, 1990). Every nurse has a personal concept of what are priority questions. Since these will vary it is appropriate to have an assessment tool or 'check list' that standardises the procedure within a unit or area. Using an assessment form also ensures that information gathered can be safely kept together, so that decisions about nursing intervention can be made (Fig. 3.3).

Name: Date
Address:

                                               Consultant:
                        Tel:
D.O.B.   M/F   Ref. by:

Onset:

Duration:

Presenting problems:

Warning of incontinence?

How long can you hold on after you feel the desire to pass urine?

Urgency?

Do you know when urine is leaking?

Are you wet all the time?

Urinary tract infection?

Dysuria?

Do you leak a little when you laugh, cough or sneeze?

Made worse by?

Can you interrupt the stream?

Is the stream of urine good?

Do you have to strain to pass water?

Post micturition dribble?

Complete emptying?

Fig. 3.3 Urinary incontinence assessment form.

Toileting
Frequency   Day: Night: | Urine test

Incontinence:
Frequency   Day: Night:

No. of changes
of pad/clothes   Day: Night:

Fluid intake: Number of cups per 24 hours
        (Tea, Coffee, Alcohol?)

Diet:
(Added salt?)

History:
Medical

Surgical

Obstetric/Gynaecological

Urological

Social history:

Smoking:

Attitude to problem:

Is the incontinence affecting relationship/sexuality?

Fig. 3.3 (*Continued*)

Mobility:

Dexterity:

Aids in use:

Mental score (1–10):

Medication:

Allergies:

On examination:

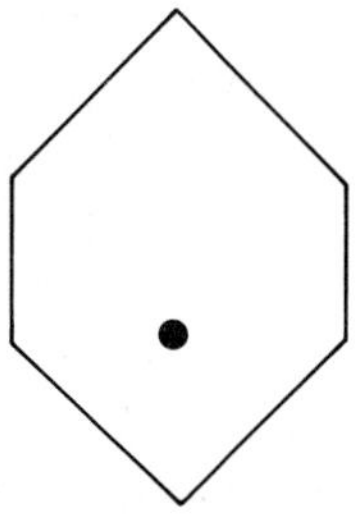

Eyesight:

Hearing:

Bowel pattern:

Rectal examination:

Skin condition: Healthy
                Red
                Excoriated

Vaginal assessment

Vaginitis:
Other:

Pelvic floor assessment
Squeeze felt on p.v.?

BP – Lying:
     Standing:

Fig. 3.3 (*Continued*)

Clinical Diagnosis

Management plan:

Bladder retraining   Pads:

Pelvic floor exercises

Self-catheterisation

Refer to continence adviser   Appliances:

Refer to urodynamics   Other:
(for Cystometry)

Cystometry
Initial residual (after voiding)   Urethral pressure:

Vol 1st desire: Urethral length:

Vol 1st spasm: pressure: Post incontinence residual:

Vol capacity: pressure   Max flow rate

Diagnosis:

Treatment:

Fig. 3.3 (*Continued*)

Research has shown that nurses lack skills in communicating with their patients (Faulkner, 1987), and that there is a great difference between skills required for professional interaction, and those used socially (Faulkner, 1988). Because urinary incontinence is such a socially unacceptable condition (Watson and Royle, 1987), sufferers often find difficulty in answering personal questions, especially those which touch on aspects that are upsetting or embarrassing. Passing urine is something we normally do in private. When control is lost urine is passed without warning, often in public. It is therefore important that the assessment interview is conducted in an atmosphere of privacy. Patients are usually more willing to discuss their problems with the nurse who shows an attitude of tact and empathy (Norton, 1980).

It is important that rather than simply noting data on the form, the nurse considers each symptom or problem carefully and report relevant points to appropriate members of the health care team (Resnick, 1990). Recognition that incontinence is present is an important step towards regaining continence (Foster, 1989). However, it may be some time before the sufferer is able to admit this to another person.

When making an assessment of incontinence the nurse should allow time for the patient to express feelings about the main presenting problems. This information may come not from the patient, but from the primary carer. It is important to clarify that any special terminology which is used by patient or nurse is properly understood. Patients usually use terms to describe bladder and bowel functions which are not medical, so the nurse should always remember that patients are unlikely to be familiar with such medical terms as 'enuresis' (Watson and Royle, 1987).

The word incontinent means 'wanting in self restraint' (*Oxford English Dictionary*, 1964), this definition being placed before 'being able to hold something in – urine etc'. Many elderly people may recall that this term was used to describe women of loose moral behaviour, so to use it in reference to some elderly patients is therefore offensive. To speak of 'difficulties in holding your water' is generally more acceptable and more easily admitted to (Norton, 1986).

Going through the assessment form

The cause of incontinence is often established by relating the onset to specific life events. Emotions, interpersonal problems as described by Hafner *et al.* (1977), stressful situations such as moving into residential accommodation, bereavement (Kennedy, 1988), anxiety, depression and interpersonal difficulties (Macaulay *et al.*, 1987) are all contributing factors and occur in all age groups (Frewen, 1983; Castleden *et al.*, 1984).

Childbirth can be the precipitating event for many women with stress incontinence following delivery of large babies, long labours and multigravidae (Norton, 1986). Swash (1988) demonstrated damage of pelvic nerves and thus pelvic floor dysfunction following a difficult labour with forceps delivery and multiple births as contributing factors.

Neurological diseases such as Parkinson's disease (Mundy, 1987), multiple sclerosis (Blaivas *et al.*, 1979), spinal injury and spina bifida (Stott and Abrams, 1987) may all damage higher centre control of continence, on the local sacral reflex arc. Furthermore, the associated loss of mobility, dexterity or mental alertness may make reaching the toilet more difficult (A more detailed aetiology of urinary incontinence has already been given in Chapter 2.)

How long has incontinence been present? Is this the first episode of incontinence or the return of a previous problem? Does anything make it worse such as turning on taps, stressful social situations or taking certain foods and drinks? Specific enquiries should be made whether coughing, sneezing, laughing, standing up or lifting, cause urine to leak, which suggests stress incontinence (Green, 1975; Hendrickson, 1981). Although uncommon, 'giggle incontinence' can affect up to 25 per cent of adolescent girls (Mundy et al., 1984). Symptoms occur on laughing and may be those of urgency, or actual voiding. There is no effective treatment for this self-limiting condition. Urodynamic investigations usually show the bladder and urethra to be functioning normally.

Is there any warning of the need to pass urine/of incontinence? Urge incontinence means there is little or no time to reach the toilet, once a bladder contraction has provoked an urgent desire to pass urine (detrusor instability). If the contractions are stronger than urethral closure pressure, incontinence occurs (Brocklehurst, 1990). Body movement (standing, coughing, etc.) can provoke unstable bladder contractions, giving a false impression of stress incontinence (Norton, 1986; Resnick, 1990). It is not uncommon to find a problem of mixed stress and urge incontinence (Jolleys, 1988). Diminished bladder sensation may mean that the first desire to pass urine does not occur until the bladder is full to capacity (Watson and Royle, 1987). This 'neurogenic bladder' may also give rise to symptoms of overflow incontinence, large residual urine volumes and urine infection (Brocklehurst, 1990).

Is there a history of urine infection? A midstream urine specimen (MSU) tested with a dipstick (such as the Microstix 10SG Ames Division, from Miles Laboratory, England) will show the presence of an infection, blood and glucose (Flanagan et al., 1989). Observation of urine colour should also be made for the presence of haematuria, or deposits (Moody, 1990). A history of many urine infections, dysuria and frequency may suggest cystitis and urethritis (Watson and Royle, 1987; McGrother et al., 1986). Other symptoms of urinary infection include pyrexia, increased respiration and pulse rate, headache, nausea, loss of appetite, and general malaise (Watson and Royle, 1987). This urine may appear cloudy and foul smelling. If urine infection is suspected the MSU should be sent to the laboratory for culture and sensitivity to antibiotic treatment.

When dysuria is present, the type of pain should be noted (burning, scalding, prickling, etc.) and whether it occurs before, during or after micturition. The term 'stranguary' is used when dysuria is extreme and accompanied by a diminished urine output (Watson and Royle, 1987).

A patient who complains of perineal or suprapubic pain (often relieved by emptying the bladder) in addition to the irritative symptoms above, may have interstitial cystitis. Biopsy of the bladder wall is essential for confirmation of diagnosis (Raz and Leach, 1983). Urinary incontinence may be non-existent or only occasional.

A poor stream (or flow) of urine on micturition may be due to a weak or absent detrusor contraction. This can result from neurological disease, trauma and certain drugs. Common causes include diabetes mellitis and multiple sclerosis (Mundy *et al.*, 1984), and anticholinergic drugs (Andersson, 1988). Outflow obstruction causing retention of urine may be due to prostatic hypertrophy. Symptoms are those of poor stream, hesitancy, straining to pass urine and post micturition dribble (McGrother *et al.*, 1987b). In some patients detrusor instability is an additional problem secondary to the prostatic obstruction (Mundy *et al.*, 1984).

Frequency of micturition as a symptom is identified by Hilton and Stanton (1981) as 'voiding seven or more times during the waking hours'. Gross frequency is a tiresome and distressing condition and may, or may not be associated with incontinence. An abnormally high frequency rate may be due to detrusor instability (Shah, 1984) or fear of becoming wet (Resnick, 1990). A description by the patient of the number of times the desire is felt to pass urine and of the number of incontinent episodes in 24 hours will complement the frequency/volume chart (Bailey *et al.*, 1990).

Nocturia is the arousal from sleep to pass urine. It may normally be present on occasions following a high fluid intake (Shah, 1984) and is common in the elderly. Nocturnal incontinence is called enuresis (bed wetting) and is common in children and young adults, with no apparent cause (Barry, 1988; Dobson, 1989; Moreton, 1989). A study by Willie (1990) of enuretic children compared with previous sufferers, and children with no symptoms showed no evidence that nocturia was a neurotic disease. In the elderly enuresis may be caused by detrusor instability, or overflow incontinence (Brocklehurst, 1984). Other causes include decreased mobility which prevents the patient from getting out of bed quickly enough, and suppression of the awareness of the desire to rise and pass urine caused by sleeping tablets. Those suffering insomnia for various reasons may pass urine several times during the night simply because they are awake. For most people wetting the bed is the worst aspect or degree of incontinence they could experience.

The number of changes of incontinence pads, or clothing in 24 hours, gives an indication of the severity of the problem. This enquiry also gives an opportunity to assess whether their is any financial burden to the patient by the purchasing of pads (McGrother *et al.*, 1986; 1987a; 1987b). Many people are unaware that incontinence pads are supplied by the National Health Service and buy sanitary towels which are inappropriate for absorbing urine (DHSS, 1986). Even those pads supplied by the National Health Service may be unsuitable or insufficient in quantity (Yarnell and St Leger, 1979; Norton, 1980; Hamilton, 1989).

Considerable extra laundry is generated by wet clothing and bedding, placing a burden on relatives or carers (Vetter *et al.*, 1981). They may not know that laundry services are provided in many areas of the country for those living at home and that there is a collection service for disposal of used pads (Allbeson and Douglas, 1984; Norton, 1986).

Fluid intake can be formally assessed by recording pre-measured amounts on a chart. More often, assessment is made by simply asking the patients how many drinks they would take on an average day, the size of their usual cup or mug, and counting them up. A reasonable intake of between one and two litres in 24 hours is acceptable to most people. However, during hot weather, exercise, on social occasions or after a high salt intake, much more than this may be taken. It is common for incontinence sufferers to cut fluid intake severely in order to try and minimise wetness. This can lead to dehydration and associated problems, particularly in the elderly (Watson and Royle, 1987). Highly concentrated urine may cause local irritation of the bladder mucosa. Conversely, it is never difficult to find the patient who readily admits to drinking up to twenty cups of tea a day! There is nothing wrong with this if there is no problem controlling urine output. If there is, then restricting intake to between six and nine cups in 24 hours would be reasonable (Mundy *et al.*, 1984).

There is a dearth of research on aspects of fluid intake and its effects on incontinence. It is however known that what is consumed can affect continence. Creighton and Stanton (1990) found that drinks containing caffeine (e.g. coffee, tea, chocolate, cola) had an irritant effect upon the unstable bladder in addition to the known diuretic effect. Attention should be given to the timing of drinks taken in relation to incontinence episodes. Insufficient fluid intake or a diet low in fibre may cause constipation or in extreme cases faecal impaction (Bean, 1988), which can prevent effective bladder filling or emptying (Roberts, 1989). A high sodium intake requires the body to produce large volumes of urine in order to excrete the excess salt. Enquiries about diet should include a question about additional salt.

Past medical history may be relevant to the presence of urinary incontinence. Diabetes, cerebrovascular accident and Parkinson's disease (Brocklehurst, 1984), as well as multiple sclerosis (Eardley *et al.*, 1989) are all conditions in which incontinence is a common feature.

A brief history of surgical procedures may provide helpful information relating to the genito-urinary system or neurological system (Mundy *et al.*, 1984). The obstetric and gynaecological history should include (in addition to surgical procedures) the number of pregnancies, any abnormal deliveries and pattern of the menstrual cycle (McFarlane and Castledine, 1984). Postsurgical incontinence is not uncommon. Yarnell and St Leger (1979) found that men that had received prostatectomy, and women who had undergone repair or uterine or vaginal prolapse had urinary incontinence related to their operations.

Social and environmental difficulties can contribute to existing incontinence, especially for the disabled and elderly (Tobin and Riley, 1986). Toilets sited away from general living areas or bedrooms, may discourage the patient from going in good time (Roberts, 1989). The toilet may be cold, unpleasant or difficult to use. Although a study by Vetter *et al.* (1981) found that the degree of urinary incontinence was not significantly related to the siting of toilets, even when outside. In residential homes and hospitals queues for the use of the toilet are sometimes caused by a policy of 'toileting' everyone at set times (Hicklin, 1989). A lack of privacy is a further obstacle to remaining continent. The absence of a toilet seat raiser, grabrail and callbell may deny the opportunity to visit the toilet independently.

Incontinence may prevent social contact because of the constant need to be near a toilet, the sheer size of the amount of bulky pads needed to be kept handy, or the fear of being humiliated by the tell-tale wet patches on clothing or chairs. McGrother *et al.* (1987b) reported that elderly people with urinary incontinence had a level of social contact three times lower than those with no such problem.

A change of environment brought about by admission to hospital, or the necessity for residential care can cause both anxiety and confusion in some elderly patients. The toilets may be difficult to find particularly in older buildings where the Victorian concern for ventilation and hygiene ensured they were well away from the bed areas (Smith and Smith, 1987). Commodes can be very convenient for the staff but may be extremely embarrassing for the user if only a curtain screens the occupant from the rest of the ward. (Possibly a cause of constipation in hospitalised patients?)

In a study of elderly people by Yarnell and St Leger (1979) living accommodation was found to be a factor related to urinary incontinence (80 per cent of elderly hospitalised patients were incontinent compared with 8 per cent living with their families). Those living alone have also been found to have a higher incidence of incontinence than those residing with a spouse or family (McGrother et al., 1987a; 1987b).

Staff attitude may be responsible for promoting incontinence, albeit unwittingly. Individual care calls for large scale reorganisation of working schedules. Fears of increasing demands on carers' time may deter changes being made for such needs as waking patients or residents to pass urine during the night.

Where the patient is living alone and unable to get out there may be little outside support such as a home help, meals on wheels, or family or friends calling during the day. Consideration should be given to how well this person is coping both generally and with the resulting difficulties of being incontinent. Does the house smell of urine? Is there other evidence of inability to cope such as laundry problems and self neglect? Is this person able to get out from the chair to the toilet easily? Is it possible for this person to bath or shower unaided? Would the provision of aids, or alterations, improve the quality of life?

A question about whether or not the patient is a smoker may not appear to be relevant to incontinence. But the presence of a chronic cough may be partly responsible for stress incontinence. It would be pointless to begin intensive treatment for stress incontinence without some effort to stop smoking.

Not everyone who is incontinent finds it intolerable or upsetting. A reason for this attitude may be a lack of awareness due to dementia or acceptance of the condition because of personal values. (Many people think incontinence is an inevitable part of ageing.) Establishing the patient's own attitude to the problem is an indication of potential motivation to participate in securing improvement or cure. A positive attitude towards becoming continent has been shown by Castleden et al. (1984) to be the greatest prognostic factor.

The effects of incontinence on *sexual functioning and relationships* can be devastating. Yet this aspect is frequently ignored by health care workers (Jacobson, 1974). Peplau (1988) argues that if nurses drew from their own experiences of interpersonal problems they would have sufficient skills to help many patients overcome concerns and anxieties and bring about constructive changes. Age is no barrier to the enjoyment of a loving sexual relationship. Many elderly have already made many adjustments to their lifestyle due to decreasing mobility or dexterity. Retirement from work and its associated changes in daily routine may bring a feeling of loss of self-esteem or worth, which can be worsened by problems within a relationship, due to incontinence.

Many women who experience urine loss during sexual intercourse feel so tense and embarrassed that they then avoid sexual contact with their partner (Vierhout and Gianotten, 1990). Despite this being a common problem very few women are prepared to express concern about it or complain (Hilton, 1988). It may therefore only be possible to obtain detailed information about incontinence related to sexual activity at a later stage when the relationship between the patient and nurse has developed sufficiently. Disabled patients may be unaware of the existence of SPOD (Association to Aid Sexual and Personal Relationships of People with Disability), which is an agency established to provide advice and counselling as well as an educational and training resource. The involvement of a partner as carer or 'nurse' may produce conflicts in the relationship resulting in loss of self-esteem and sexual desire for the sufferer (Blannin, 1987). Consideration of this must be included when planning care. Problems could be created through the nurse's failure to include sexual needs in the interview discussion (Jacobson, 1974). Studies by Sutherst (1979) and Hilton (1988) found an association between detrusor instability, stress incontinence and sexual dysfunction. All patients with sexual problems were certain that incontinence was the cause.

An assessment of the patient's mobility and dexterity will indicate whether visiting the toilet is possible without waiting for assistance (Vetter *et al.*, 1981). The reason for impaired function should be established. Painful feet requiring simple chiropody treatment may be all that is making reaching the toilet difficult (Norton, 1986).

Mental impairment is often accompanied by incontinence, and has been found to be a major factor of prognosis (Castleden *et al.*, 1984). An assessment of mental ability should be made. One possible tool for this purpose is the Clifton Assessment Scale (Pattie and Gilleard, 1975; 1976). But it would be wrong to make the assumption that mental illness, or mental disability is always the cause of incontinence without ruling out the presence of a bladder problem or other physical cause. An extensive study by Smith and Smith (1987) into incontinence problems relating to mental illness and mental handicap, focuses on the benefits obtainable through a combined approach of psychological and physical treatments.

There is a large range of drugs prescribed for various bladder conditions associated with incontinence (Brocklehurst, 1984), while those given as part of medical treatment for other reasons may actually cause incontinence, or in certain circumstances worsen a minor problem, particularly if the response to drug therapy is not monitored (Jones-Keister and Creason 1989). Anticholinergic drugs (e.g. imipramine) prescribed to suppress unstable detrusor contractions may cause retention of urine. This type of drug may have been used for the treatment of depression. The nurse needs to be alert to this effect. Night sedation is often prescribed for the elderly person who complains of wakeful nights. Suppression of awareness of a full bladder may result in nocturnal enuresis (Kennedy, 1988). Discovering the reasons for insomnia (anxiety, boredom, sleeping during the day, etc.) may enable the nurse to take appropriate action to secure a good night's sleep for the patient without tablets.

Diuretics given to the patient with cardiac failure can turn a minor problem of 'urgency' into major incontinence (Shepherd *et al.*, 1982). Frequently accompanying complications of decreased mobility may make reaching the toilet in time impossible. Analgesics, particularly those which contain codeine, and are taken over long periods of time for chronic pain, may cause incontinence of urine indirectly by their constipating effect. Excessive laxatives may then be employed as a countereffect. Any antibiotic treatment currently being taken should be noted on any form accompanying a urine specimen to the laboratory. Other treatments not necessarily prescribed (for example creams for skin problems associated with incontinence), should be noted since health problems not previously mentioned by the patient can be highlighted in this way. It is appropriate at this point to ask the patient about any adverse reactions or allergies to any treatments received.

Although many nurses conduct the physical examination of the patient they are assessing, there may be factors which mean this is done instead by the doctor. In addition to assessing general physical condition, the physical examination looks at factors which contribute to incontinence such as chronic cough, genital abnormality, faecal impaction, bladder distention and prostatic enlargement (Eastwood 1989).

Poor vision and impaired hearing are common in the elderly. Allowances need to be made for this by staff in hospital and homes. The elderly person may not hear an invitation to be helped to visit the toilet or be able to see well enough to identify the toilet door signs. Assessment of visual or hearing difficulties enables care staff to anticipate needs, particularly for those patients away from their own homes.

Bowel pattern should always be included in the assessment of urinary incontinence. Constipation is a common complaint of those who are not fully mobile, or who restrict fluid intake in order to reduce wetness. In hospitals and residential homes, lack of privacy and sufficient time to sit on the toilet may encourage constipation, which in turn may cause urinary incontinence (Roberts, 1989). Neurological damage which causes the bladder to fail to contract and empty may cause a similar effect on the bowel. Anticholinergic drugs can also slow bowel contractility.

Skin rashes and soreness around the genital and groin areas can be caused by constant contact with urine soaked clothing or pads. Perspiration caused by wearing plastic pants, or chaffing from badly fitting male urinary appliances can also produce unpleasant skin problems.

Vaginal assessment seeks to exclude atrophic vaginitis (usually accompanied by urethritis) due to oestrogen deficiency, and resulting in sensory urgency in menopausal women (Ritch, 1989). Examination will seek uterine or vaginal wall prolapse, fistula or evidence of stress incontinence (Yarnell *et al.*, 1982). Pelvic floor assessment of muscle strength or ability to contract the pelvic floor muscles, is made digitally. The patient is asked to contract her perivaginal muscles by squeezing the examiner's gloved finger (Brink *et al.*, 1990). A very simple indication of the ability to contract the pelvic floor muscles can be demonstrated by a positive answer to the ability to interrupt midstream flow of urine. Continence requires the pelvic floor and sphincter to be strong enough to resist both the weight of urine in the bladder, and any transient rise in intra-abdominal pressure (such as that caused by sneezing, coughing, laughing) (Stott, 1987). Patients with genuine stress incontinence are usually dry at night and have no symptoms of urgency (Williams *et al.*, 1982). Digital rectal examination will reveal prostatic size, the presence of faecal impaction, and allow assessment of anal sensation and tone (Stott, 1987).

Additional means of assessment

Additional techniques may be required to complement the interview, examination and charting assessment already completed. These may include some of the following outlined below.

The post-micturition residual urine volume can be measured by either inserting a pvc Jaques catheter size 12 charrière (e.g. Bard 'Reliacath') and allowing the urine to drain away (Foley catheters − self-retaining by an inflatable balloon − have been found to be inaccurate for this purpose by Haylen *et al.* (1989)) or by ultrasound scan of the bladder, which is non-invasive and painless, without risk of trauma or infection. Equipment is now available which is specifically for this purpose. It is accurate, portable and simple to use (Bladder-scan, Lewis Medical Limited, London). A study by Bennes *et al.* (1990) suggested that ultrasound should be used more often for assessment of residual urine volumes. Bi-manual palpation of the abdomen is a simple method of estimating residual urine volume. Accuracy though, is dependent on the skill of the person carrying out the assessment (Norton *et al.*, 1989).

Bladder calculi can be detected by straight abdominal x-ray. This same technique will also reveal the presence of faecal impaction. An intravenous pyelogram (IVP) may be required if there are reasons to suspect other implications in the higher renal tract.

A voiding cystourethrogram, is carried out in the X-Ray Department, and gives a visual recording of bladder and bladder-neck function (Mundy *et al.*, 1984).

The pad test has been found to provide a simple, inexpensive and accurate measurement of urine loss during normal daily activity (Walsh and Mills 1981). It was first designed by James *et al.* (1971), and called the 'Urilos-Nappy Test'. This involves the patient wearing a disposable pad containing aluminium strips and dry electrolyte. The pad is worn by the patient for 45 minutes while set activities are performed, and the recorder attached to the pad measures any urine loss that occurs. Further variations on this idea have been developed, although this equipment is still used. Pad weighing tests have been devised. The patient wears a perineal pad for a set period of time, and completes tasks such as walking, coughing, and washing hands, which usually provoke incontinence. In addition large quantities (500–1,000 ml) of fluid are given to patients to drink prior to the test. Studies by Versi and Cardozo (1984) and Frazer *et al.* (1989) consider pad-weighing tests to be valuable in quantifying the patient's urine loss when incontinent.

Urodynamic investigation is the term given to a range of tests which measure bladder and sphincter pressure and capacity, and urine flow rates. Only those tests relevant to the needs of the individual patient need to be selected (Mundy, 1987). There is some argument about the necessity for such tests over the clinical diagnosis obtained in the way that has already been described in this chapter, particularly for elderly patients (Tobin, 1989). The Hilton and Stanton (1981) algorithmic method for assessing urinary incontinence in elderly women showed that very few gained benefit from urodynamic investigations. Eastwood (1989) is in favour of specialist referral centres being reserved for those patients in whom there are management or diagnostic difficulties. It would therefore seem reasonable to pursue invasive or costly investigations only for those patients in whom treatment or management will be influenced in some way by doing so.

Urine flow rate is the most simple urodynamic measurement. The equipment features a special commode chair and collecting funnel. The urine can be directed onto a spinning disc (Urodyn – Dantec Electronics, Bristol) or by an electronic dipstick (Ormed Limited, Welwyn Garden City, Hertfordshire). Both calculate the amount of urine passed in a given time (millilitres per second) and record the flow rate and pattern on a graph. At least 200 ml of urine should be voided to obtain an accurate reading. Flow rates are different between men and women, and vary with age (Shah, 1984). The pattern of flow may be continuous or intermittent and is often characteristic of certain conditions, for example prostatic enlargement causing bladder-neck obstruction.

Ultrasound cystodynamogram (USCD) incorporates ultrasound scanning of the full bladder initially, then as the patient passes urine (in private) a scan is made to assess flow rate and postvoiding residual urine (Chapple and Christmas, 1990). This test is useful for checking postsurgery bladder function.

Simply cystometrogram (cystometry or CMG) measures the pressure generated in the bladder during filling. Standard purpose-built urodynamic equipment (e.g. Ormed Limited and Dantec Electronic Limited) displays the measurement during the test while the pen-recorder charts a permanent record of findings on a graph (Malone-Lee, 1989). The parameters measured by cystometry are intravesical (bladder) pressure, intra-abdominal pressure and detrusor (bladder muscle) pressure. The latter is provided electronically by the urodynamic equipment which subtracts the intra-abdominal pressure from intravesical pressure. This gives a true detrusor pressure reading which is not subject to rises in pressure caused by the patient coughing, talking, moving, etc. Also measured are flow rate and volume voided (Holmes, 1989).

Immediately prior to cystometry the patient is asked to visit the toilet to pass urine. The procedure involves introducing water filled pvc catheters into the bladder and rectum – two into the bladder (one for filling, one for measuring pressure), preferably size 8 charrière nelaton-tip. Alternatively a single double-lumen catheter specially designed for the purpose may be used (Portex Special Products Division of Smiths Industries). The rectal catheter has a terminal balloon containing approximately 3 mls of normal saline. This prevents blockage by faeces. The bladder is filled from the suspended bag of normal saline (at room temperature) via a giving set attached to the bladder catheter. This runs through a peristaltic pump (e.g. a Watson-Marlow pump) which controls the flow. The filling rate is usually around 50 mls per minute, but this can vary in special circumstances (Mundy et al., 1984). A post-micturition residual urine is measured at the time of catheterisation. The investigator is then certain the bladder is empty, and an accurate assessment can be made. During filling the patient is asked to describe bladder sensation: the first desire to void, a strong desire to void, urgency or any pain (Chapple and Christmas, 1990). These descriptions will be compared with the measurements observed. Bladder capacity is determined by either the maximum volume tolerated by the patient, or when leakage occurs due to a rise in detrusor pressure. Cystometry may be performed with a patient lying supine, sitting or standing, depending upon the age, sex and state of health of the patient (Mundy et al., 1984). Ambulatory urodynamics have been found to provide more sensitive results in some patients (James, 1984; McInerney et al., 1990). Detrusor pressure during voiding, and volume voided may be measured after the filling phase of the cystometry.

Measuring urethral pressure and urethral closure pressure provide an assessment of the effectiveness of the urethra in preventing urine leakage. Measurements are made along the length of the urethra as the catheter is withdrawn at the termination of cystometry. The result is termed the urethral pressure profile (UPP), and there are several variations on method (Chapple and Christmas, 1990). Generally it is thought that this test is of little diagnostic value (Brocklehurst, 1984; Malone-Lee, 1989).

Cystometry may be carried out using simultaneous video recording. This is a radiographic test and therefore must be carried out in the X-ray department. The necessity for more staff present may be embarrassing and inhibiting for the patient, resulting in detrimental effects on the test results (Mundy et al., 1984).

Further special medical tests may be required to complete the assessment. They may include blood tests for patients suspected of having diabetes or renal damage. Cystoscopy is indicated where there is no obvious cause for haematuria, severe dysuria or frequency. Biopsy is essential to exclude carcinoma, tuberculous cystitis and interstitial cystitis (Raz and Leach, 1983). A vaginal and urethral swab may confirm infection, or oestrogen deficiency. Cervical smear will reveal cervical carcinoma or abnormal cells (Norton, 1980).

Catheterisation, as with all invasive procedures, carries a certain risk factor of introducing infection into the urinary tract. Sabanathan et al. (1985) found a postcystometry infection rate of 21 per cent among elderly patients. This was in agreement with a previous study by Stamm (1978) who found an infection rate of 20 per cent in patients who had received some form of invasive urinary investigation.

The International Continence Society Committee on Standardisation of Terminology recommends standards which facilitate comparison of results by those providing investigation and treatment for patients with urinary incontinence, and for those carrying out research study (Abrams et al., 1989). Standards and terminology include clinical assessment as discussed in this chapter, evaluation of urine storage by cystometry, urethral pressure measurement and procedures related to micturition (flow, pattern, volume passed, residual urine). Classification of terms used to describe urinary tract dysfunction is set out together with symbols and units of measurement to be used when recording results.

No patient assessment would be comprehensive without a full review of the available history data previously recorded in hospital or GP surgery notes. This information can then be related to the present problems enabling the patient to participate as fully as possible in making informed choices about future care.

Summary

Comprehensive patient assessment provides the basis of good nursing practice. This chapter has explored the methods and approaches of current practice in assessing patients with urinary incontinence; the skills and techniques employed, particular areas of enquiry (by interview, charting and physical examination) which need to be known in order to plan care. Finally more invasive urodynamic investigations, which may be appropriate for some patients, have been discussed.

References

Abrams, P., Blaivas, J., Stanton, S. and Andersen, J. (1989), 'The standardisation of terminology of lower urinary tract function', International Continence Society Committee on Standardisation of Terminology Report.

Allbeson, J. and Douglas, J. (1984), *National Welfare Benefits Handbook* (13th edn), London: Child Poverty Action Group.

Andersson, E. (1988), *Drugs: Disorders of micturition*, London: ADIS Press.

Bailey, R., Shepherd, A. and Tribe, S. (1990), 'How much information can be obtained from frequency/volume charts?' *Neurology and Urodynamics*, International Continence Society, New York: Wiley-Liss.

Barry, J. (1988), 'Night-time despair', *Nursing Times*, 84(14): 82–5.

Bean, N. (1988) 'Simple assessment can save a lot of bother', *Geriatric Medicine*, Community Nursing Supplement (July): 6–7.

Bennes, C., Barnick, C., Curner, A. and Cardozo, L. (1990), 'Normal urodynamic findings in symptomatic women – who to believe, the patient or the test?', *Neurology and Urodynamics*, pp. 118–19.

Blaivas, J., Bhimani, G. and Labib, K. (1979), 'Vesicourethral dysfunction in multiple sclerosis', *Journal of Urology*, 122: 342–7.

Blannin, J. (1987) 'Incontinence: men's problems', *Community Outlook* (Feb): 27–8.

Boedker, A., Lendorf, A., Nielson, A. and Glahn, B. (1989), 'Micturition pattern assessed by the frequency/volume chart in a healthy population of men and women', *Neurology and Urodynamics*, *Proceedings of the International Continence Society*.

Brink, C., Sampselle, C., Wells, T., Diokno, A. and Gillis, G. (1989), 'A digital test for pelvic muscle strength in older women with urinary incontinence', *Nursing Research*, 38(4): 196–9.

Brocklehurst, J. (1984), *Ageing, bladder function and incontinence: Urology in the elderly*, Edinburgh: Churchill Livingstone.

Brocklehurst, J. (1990), 'Urinary incontinence in old age: helping the general practitioner to make a diagnosis', *International Journal of experimental and clinical gerontology*, 36(2): 3–7.

Brown, P. (ed.) (1988), 'Health care and the aged: a nursing perspective', Ch. 6. In *Assessment of the Older Person*, London: Williams & Wilkins.

Campbell, J., Finch, D., Allport, C., Erikson, H. and Swain, M. (1985), 'A theoretical approach to nursing assessment', *Journal of Advanced Nursing*, 10: 111–15.

Caring for People – Community Care in the next decade and beyond (1989) November, London: HMSO.

Castleden, C.M., Duffin, H. and Asher, M. (1984). 'Correlation between the clinical findings and outcome in elderly incontinent patients with unstable bladders'. *Proceedings of the International Continence Society*, 78–9.

Castleden, C.M., Duffin, H., Asher, M. and Yeomanson, C. (1988), 'Factors influencing outcome in elderly patients with detrusor instability', *Age and Ageing*, 14: 303–7.

Castleden, C.M. and Ekelund, P. (1989), 'Alternatives to urodynamics for investigating urinary incontinence', Geriatric Workshop on Incontinence, Kabi Vitrum.

Chalmers, H. (1990), 'Nursing models: enhancing or inhibiting practice?', *Nursing Standard*, 5(11): 34–40.

Chapple, C. and Christmas, T. (1990), *Urodynamics made easy*, Edinburgh: Churchill Livingstone.

Clay, E. (1978), 'Incontinence of urine: a regime for retraining', *Nursing Mirror*, 16 March: 23–4.

Creighton, S. and Stanton, S. (1990), 'Caffeine: does it affect your bladder?', *British Journal of Urology*, 66: 613–14.

DHSS (1986), Report No. 159, *Incontinence Garments: results of a study, health equipment information, health hardware addressed and assessed*, London: HMSO.

Dobson, P. (1989), 'Easing childhood shame', *Nursing Times*, 85: 33, 79–80.

Eardley, I., Kirby, R., Nagendram, C., Lecky, B., Youl, B., Chapple, C., Fowler, C. and MacDonald, W. (1989), 'Where are the lesions that cause the neurogenic bladder in multiple sclerosis?; *Neurology and Urodynamics*, 4(8): 310–11.

Eastwood, H. (1989), 'Incontinence clinics for the elderly: a changing role', Geriatric Workshop on Incontinence, *Geriatric Medicine*, p. 18. Kabi Vitrum.

Faulkner, A. (1987), 'Talking to patients', *Nursing Times*, 82(33): 33–4.

Faulkner, A. (1988), 'Too bad to mention?' *Nursing Times* 84(14): 70–2.

Flanagan, P., Rooney, P., Davis, E. and Stout, R. (1989) 'Evaluation of four screening tests for bacteriuria in elderly people', *The Lancet* (May), 1117–19.

Foster, P. (1989), 'An unrecognised symptom', *Nursing Times*, 84(14): 87–8.

Frazer, M., Haylen, B. and Sutherest, J. (1989), 'The severity of urinary incontinence in women: comparison of subjective and objective tests', *British Journal of Urology*, **63**; 14–15.

Freeman, R. and Baxby, K. (1982), 'Hypnotherapy for incontinence caused by the unstable bladder', *British Medical Journal*, 284: 1831–4.

Frewen, W. (1978), 'An objective assessment of the unstable bladder of psychosomatic origin', *British Journal of Urology*, 50: 246–9.

Gordon, M. (1982), *Manual of Nursing Diagnosis*, Maidenhead: McGraw-Hill.

Green, T. (1975), 'Urinary stress incontinence: differential diagnosis, pathophysiology and management', *American Journal of Obstetrics and Gynaecology*, 122: 368–9.

Hafner, R., Stanton, S. and Guy, J. (1977), 'A psychiatric study of women with urgency and urgency incontinence', *British Journal of Urology*, 49: 211–14.

Hamilton, B. (1989), 'Recognising the problem', *Practice Nurse*, Feb: 369–70.

Haylen, B., Frazer, M. and MacDonald, J. (1989), 'Are urinary catheters we use effective in emptying the bladder? An application of transvaginal ultrasound', *Neurology and Urodynamics*, 8(4): 331–2.

Henderson, V. (1969), *Basic Principles of Nursing Care*, International Council of Nurses.

Hendrickson, L. (1981), 'The frequency of stress incontinence in women before and after the implementation of an exercise programme', *Issues in Health Care of Women*, 3: 81–92.

Hicklin, J. (1989) 'Promoting continence for the elderly', *Nursing the Elderly*, October: 22.

Hilton, P. (1988), 'Urinary incontinence during sexual intercourse: a common, but rarely volunteered symptom', *British Journal of Obstetrics and Gynaecology*, 95: 377–81.

Hilton, P. and Stanton, S. (1981), 'Algorithmic method for assessing urinary incontinence in elderly women', *British Medical Journal*, 282: 940–2.

Holmes, D. (1989), 'Investigative techniques', in Freeman R. and Malvern J. (eds) *The Unstable Bladder*, London: Butterworth.

Jacobson, L. (1974). 'Illness and human sexuality', *Nursing Outlook*, 22(1).

James, E. (1984), 'Ambulatory monitoring in urodynamics', in Mundy, A., Stephensen, T. and Wein, A, *Urodynamics: Principles, Practice and Application*, Edinburgh: Churchill Livingstone.

James, E., Flack, F., Caldwell, K. and Martin, M. (1971), 'Continuous measurement of urine loss and frequency in incontinence patients', *British Journal of Urology*, 43: 233–7.

Jolleys, J. (1988), 'Reported prevalence of urinary incontinence in a general practice', *British Medical Journal*, 296: 1300–2.

Jones-Keister, K. and Creason, N. (1989), 'Medication of elderly institutionalized incontinent females', *Journal of Advanced Nursing* 14: 980–5.

Kennedy, A. (1988), 'Eliminating', in Wright, S. (ed.) *Nursing the Older Patient*, Lippincott Nursing Series, London: Harper & Row.

Lofting, D. (1990), *A Guide to Continence Assessment and Bladder Re-training*, Bath Health Authority.

McCain, R. (1965), 'Nursing by assessment – not intuition', *American Journal of Nursing*, 65: 82–4.

Macaulay, A., Stern, R., Holmes, D. and Stanton, S. (1987), 'Micturition and the mind: psychological factors in the aetiology and treatment of urinary symptoms in women', *British Medical Journal*, 294: 540–3.

McFarlane of Llandaff, Baroness and Castledine, G. (1984), *A Guide to the Practice of Nursing, Using the Nursing Process*, St Louis: C. V. Mosby.

McGrother, C., Castleden, C.M., Duffin, H. and Clarke, M. (1986), 'Provision of services for incontinent elderly people at home', *Journal of Epidemiology and Community Health*, 40: 134–8.

McGrother, C., Castleden, C.M., Duffin, H. and Clarke, M. (1987a), 'Do the elderly need better incontinence services?', *Community Medicine* 9(1): 62–7.

McGrother, C., Castleden, C.M., Duffin, H. and Clarke, M. (1987b), 'A profile of disordered micturition in the elderly at home', *Age and Ageing*, 16: 105–10.

McInerney, P., Vanner, T., Powell, C. and Stephenson, T. (1990), 'Ambulatory urodynamics', *Neurology and Urodynamics*, 9(4): 381–2.

Malone-Lee, J. (1989), 'Urodynamic measurement and urinary incontinence in the elderly', Geriatric Workshop on Incontinence, *Geriatric Medicine*, pp. 4–9. Kabi Vitrum.

Moody, M. (1990), *Incontinence: patient problems and nursing care*, Oxford; Heinemann.

Moreton, J. (1989) 'Nocturnal enuresis', *Practice Nurse*, Nov: 260–2.

Mundy, A., Stephenson, T. and Wein, A. (1984), *Urodynamics: Principles, Practice and Application*, Edinburgh: Churchill Livingstone.

Mundy, A. (1987), 'Urodynamics – an overview', *Hospital update*, 641–4.

Norton, C. (1980), 'Assessing incontinence', *Nursing*, 1(18): 789–91.

Norton, C. (1986), *Nursing for Continence*, Beaconsfield: Beaconsfield Publishing.

Norton, K., Bhat, A. and Stanton, S. (1990), 'Psychosomatic aspects of urinary incontinence in women attending an outpatients urodynamic clinic', *British Medical Journal*, 301: 271–2.

Norton, P., Peattie, A. and Stanton, S. (1989), 'Estimation of residual urine by palpation', *Neurology and Urodynamics*, 8(4): 330–1.

Pattie, A. and Gilleard, C. (1975), 'A brief psychogeriatric assessment schedule: validation against psychiatric diagnosis and discharge from hospital', *British Journal of Psychiatry*, 127: 489–93.

Pattie, A. and Gilleard, C. (1976), 'The Clifton Assessment Schedule – further validation of a psychogeriatric assessment schedule', *British Journal of Psychiatry*, 129: 68–72.

Peplau, H. (1988), *Interpersonal relations in nursing*, London: Macmillan Education (2nd edn).

Raz, S. and Leach, G. (1983), 'Interstitial cystitis', Ch. 26, in Raz, S. (ed.) *Female Urology*, Philadelphia: W.B. Saunders.

Resnick, N. (1990), 'Non-invasive diagnosis of the patient with complex incontinence', *International Journal of Experimental and Clinical Gerontology*, 8(18).

Ritch, A. (1989), 'The use of oestrogen in incontinence in the elderly', Geriatric Workshop on Incontinence, *Geriatric Medicine*, pp. 23–5. Kabi Vitrum.

Roberts, A. (1989), 'Urinary incontinence – systems of life', Senior Systems 35, *Nursing Times*, 85(15): 55–8.

Roper, N., Logan, W. and Tierney, A. (1990), *The Elements of Nursing*, Edinburgh: Churchill Livingstone (4th edn).

Sabanathan, K., Duffin, H. and Castleden, M. (1985), 'Urinary tract infection after cystometry', *Age and Ageing*, 14: 291–5.

Shah, J. (1984), 'The assessment of patients with a view to urodynamics', in Mundy, A., Stephenson, T. and Wein, A. (eds), *Urodynamic Principles, Practice and Application*, Edinburgh: Churchill Livingstone, pp. 53–61.

Shepherd, A., Blannin, J. and Feneley, R. (1982), 'Changing attitudes in the management of urinary incontinence: the need for specialist nursing', *British Medical Journal*, 284: 645–6.

Shuttleworth, K. (1970), 'Urinary tract diseases: incontinence', *British Medical Journal*, 4: 727.

Smith, S. and Smith, L. (1987), 'Continence and incontinence: psychological approach to development and treatment', London: Croom Helm.

Smith, P. and Smith, L. (1989). 'Dark incontinence – the last taboo', The British Psychological Society briefing paper.

Stamm, W. (1978), 'Infections related to medical devices', *Annals of Internal Medicine*, 89: 764–9.

Stott M. (1987), 'Urinary incontinence: what are the considerations?', Medical Dialogue No. 132, London: Barrie Raven Associates.

Stott, M. and Abrams, P. (1987), 'Bladder compliance in patients with spina bifida', *Neurology and Urodynamics*, 6(3): 232–3.

Sutherst, J. (1979), 'Sexual dysfunction and urinary incontinence', *British Journal of Obstetrics and Gynaecology*, 86: 387–8.

Swash, M. (1988), 'Childbirth and incontinence', *Midwifery*, 4: 13–18.

Tattersall, A. (1985), 'Getting the whole picture', *Nursing Times*, 3 April: 55–8.

Tobin, G. (1989), 'Which elderly patients require urodynamic assessment?', Geriatric Workshop on Incontinence, *Geriatric Medicine*, 14–15. Kabi Vitrum.

Tobin, G. and Riley, M. (1986), 'The ten-minute hurdle', *Community Care*, Sept: 18–19.

Totman, R. (1987), *Social Causes of Illness*, London: Souvenir Press (2nd edn).

Versi, E. and Cardozo, L. (1984), 'One hour single pad-test as a simple screening procedure', *International Continence Society Proceedings*, 92–3.

Vetter, N., Jones, D. and Vitor, C. (1981), 'Urinary incontinence in the elderly at home', *Lancet*, 2: 1275–7.

Vierhout, M. and Gianotten, W. (1990), 'Urine loss during sexual activity' *Neurology and Urodynamics*, 9(4), New York: Wiley-Liss.

Walsh, J. and Mills, G. (1981), 'Measurement of the urinary loss in elderly incontinent patients', *Lancet*, 2: 1130–1.

Watson, J. and Royle, J. (1987), *Watson's Medical-Surgical Nursing and related physiology*, London: Bailliere Tindall (3rd edn).

Williams, M., Fitzhugh, C. and Pannil, I. (1982), 'Urinary incontinence in the elderly: physiology pathophysiology diagnosis and treatment', *Annals of Internal Medicine*, 97; 895–907.

Willie, S. (1990), 'Psychological problems in enuretics, former enuretics, and controls', *Neurology and Urodynamics*, Proceedings of the International Continence Society, 446–7, New York: Wiley-Liss.

Yarnell, J. and St Leger, A. (1979), 'The prevalence, severity and factors associated with urinary incontinence in a random sample of the elderly', *Age and Ageing*, 8: 81–5.

Yarnell, J., Voyle, G., Sweetnam, P., Milbank, J., Richards, C. and Stephenson, T. (1982), 'Factors associated with urinary incontinence in women', *Journal of Epidemiology and Community Health*, 36(1): 58–63.

Part 1
Promotion of continence

4 Bladder re-education for the promotion of continence

ANNE P. KENNEDY

Introduction

Introducing a toddler to the joys of the potty can be a trying time for the parent and the child. It is no good starting the process too early, before the child is able to recognise he or she has a full bladder, because the result will be a reflex emptying of the bladder or rectum when the child is placed on the pot. The aim is to get the child to recognise the symptoms of a full bladder and to teach him or her to voluntarily 'hold on' until the appropriate receptacle is correctly positioned and then 'let go'. This is a learning process for the parent as well as the child, the parent has to learn with the child just how much his or her bladder can hold and recognise the signs of an impending bladder contraction. During the process of toilet training the child is rewarded by the genuine pleasure shown by his or her parents when the potty is used correctly. The child also learns it is 'good' to have dry pants and 'bad' to wet them. The child then gradually learns how to increase the capacity of his or her bladder. This then, is toilet training.

In adult life a number of things can contribute to malfunctioning of the bladder and a loss of control over continence. The focus of this chapter is adults who suffer from urinary incontinence and the forms of bladder re-education which can be used to promote their continence. The schemes for bladder re-education presented in this chapter are: bladder training, habit retraining, timed voiding and prompted voiding. It is possible for many people with urinary incontinence to relearn how to gain control over their bladder and they can benefit from bladder training. As in the young, this requires a certain amount of learning and motivation both on the part of the sufferer and the nurse or carer. As well as the bladder, the individual and the nurse need to be re-educated. Those caring for patients unable to motivate themselves or for whom bladder training has failed can achieve external control of the bladder by gaining information on the bladder's capacity and micturition pattern. The incontinence can then be controlled and contained by timed voiding.

This chapter will concentrate on various behavioural approaches to the regaining of continence. The research evidence will be examined to try and clarify which types of patients benefit most from the various types of bladder re-education programmes available.

A standard nomenclature has not yet been developed for the varying types of bladder re-education schemes. At an international workshop on bladder therapies described by Hadley (1986) the various types of bladder regimes for the elderly were categorised (Table 4.1). Basically the types of programmes have one of the two aims as follows:

1. To restore continence by re-educating the bladder to a 'normal' or improved pattern of voiding.
2. To avoid episodes of incontinence by planned voiding regimes.

The first type of programme requires the active participation of the patient, while the second requires the active participation of the nurse or carer.

As well as bladder re-education techniques, other factors in achieving a cure have been included in many studies reported in the literature: drug therapy, psychological therapy and biofeedback techniques which have often made it difficult or impossible to isolate any beneficial effects that can be solely attributed to bladder re-education programmes.

Table 4.1 Bladder re-education programmes

Regimen	Other terms	Change in intervoiding interval during regime	Possible patient types	Approach
Bladder training	Bladder drill Bladder discipline Bladder re-education	Increased	Motivated patients, able physically and mentally to toilet themselves	*Mandatory schedule*: must only void at set times or be wet. Increase interval when dry. *Self-schedule*: gradually increase interval at own discretion – may use toilet if desperate.
Habit retraining	Habit training	Increased or decreased	Motivated staff, helpful for patients with mental and physical disabilities	Assigned toileting schedule (usually 2 hourly). May use toilet if voiding cannot be delayed. Schedule adjusted to fit patient's pattern.
Timed voiding	Scheduled voiding Rigid regime	Unchanged	Motivated staff Spinal cord lesions Patients with mental and physical disabilities	Fixed voiding scheme unchanged. May include techniques to trigger voiding and allow complete emptying of bladder.
Prompted voiding		Prompting schedule unchanged Voiding interval variable	Motivated staff Institutionalised patients with severe mental and physical disabilities	Patient asked to void at regular intervals – only taken to toilet if response positive

Review of the literature

The literature clearly shows that bladder re-education can cure or improve continence for those subjects participating in trials. However, there are several problems in comparing studies because of lack of controls in many, varying criteria for incontinence and cure, and the inclusion of drugs in some studies and not in others. The studies reported are carried out in the main by medical staff with little reported nursing intervention. Hadley (1986) made a detailed review of the literature and found the protocols involved mainly middle-aged women with urge incontinence. Patients with proved stress incontinence were often excluded from studies (Jarvis and Millar, 1980; Jarvis, 1981; 1982) because the studies were designed to deal with the problem of detrusor instability and patients with stress incontinence may benefit from pelvic floor re-education.

Table 4.2 shows results from studies of bladder training where no drugs were used. The results show cure rates (as measured by cessation of incontinence) which range from 44 per cent to 90 per cent. Although drug use has frequently been cited in the literature as comprising part of the cure for bladder instability and incontinence, it may be that in a well-managed regime they are not necessary. Drugs have been used in conjunction with bladder training in several studies but the reasons for use vary. Frewen (1978) and Elder and Stephenson (1980) state anticholinergic drugs and sedatives were used as supportive therapy. Mahady and Begg (1981) used emepronium bromide and chlorodiazepoxide at the start of therapy to give rapid relief of symptoms, drugs were discontinued as soon as symptoms improved. The drugs of choice are generally anticholinergic in action, they are designed to block reflex contractions of the detrusor (bladder) and increase urethral resistance. Anticholinergic drugs include: Imipramine, Propantheline and Emepronium bromide. Smooth muscle relaxants such as Flavoxate hydrochloride are also used. All these drugs have known side effects (Andersson, 1988).

Table 4.2 Bladder training studies without drugs

Source	Number of Patients	Age	Controls	Results[1]
Pengelly and Booth, 1980	25 trial 25 control	10–70	8% cure 20% improved 72% no change	44% cure 28% improved 28% no change
Jarvis and Millar, 1980	30 trial 30 control	27–79	23% cure	90% cure
Frewen, 1982	90	15–75	None	86.6% cure 11.1% improved 2.3% no change
Jarvis, 1982	33	31–63	None	61% cure 39% no change

1. Results show cure in terms of removal of symptoms of incontinence.

Frewen (1978) used detrusor inhibitory drugs in conjunction with bladder training and simple psychological counselling for 40 female patients with a history of urge incontinence and detrusor instability. The drugs are stated to give supportive therapy – the main treatment was considered to be the bladder training. He had a cure rate of 82.5 per cent, however, this was not a controlled study but an objective assessment with no statistical analysis and the cure rate cannot be attributed solely to bladder training due to the other contributing factors. Elder and Stephenson (1980) used Frewen's method in their uncontrolled study of 21 female patients. They found 52 per cent of the patients were cured of the symptoms of urge incontinence and another 33 per cent were much improved. This assessment of treatment was not analysed statistically and bladder training alone cannot be said to have led to the cure. They did report side effects from the use of anticholinergic drugs: dry mouth and oesophagitis. Mahady and Begg (1981) in an uncontrolled long-term study of 48 females used drug therapy only in the early weeks of treatment to give rapid relief from symptoms. The drugs were discontinued as soon as symptoms improved. The most important part of the treatment was the patient's own training of her bladder, 90 per cent of patients were cured, again this cannot be attributed only to bladder training.

Few trials have been reported which directly compare drug therapy with bladder training. In a controlled study, Jarvis (1981) compared inpatient bladder training (25 females) with outpatient drug therapy (25 females) – Flavoxate hydrochloride and Imipramine taken for four weeks. Following bladder training 84 per cent of patients were continent compared with 54 per cent of patients continent after drug treatment, a significant difference. A great many patients had side-effects following drug treatment. The conclusion of the study was that bladder training is the treatment of choice for those with detrusor instability.

A few studies have been made looking at long-term follow-ups of bladder training schemes. Mahady and Begg (1981) annually reviewed 48 females for four years following their bladder training scheme (90 per cent cure). Urge incontinence was cured after an average time of four to five months. The 10 per cent of patients who were still incontinent after up to two years' treatment had a common factor of severe emotional problems and a reluctance to keep charts and attend clinics. Castleden et al. (1985) in an uncontrolled study, looked at a group of 95 elderly patients (33 males and 62 females) with incontinence and detrusor instability who were treated at a continence clinic with bladder training and drug therapy; two-thirds of these patients were significantly improved. This group of patients was contacted two to three years later (Snape et al., 1989) and only 42 per cent of those who had improved were still symptomatically better. They concluded that incontinent elderly patients require continuous supervision preferably by GPs and/or community nurses.

The psychological treatment of the patient is considered to be an important aspect of bladder training by many (Willington, 1975; Frewen, 1978; Elder and Stephenson, 1980; Macaulay et al., 1987). It has always been difficult to find an organic or structural cause (outflow obstruction or neurological disease for example) for most patients with demonstrable bladder instability. Many suppose the condition to be psychosomatic (Frewen, 1978). The effect of the mind on the bladder can easily be seen in those anxiously awaiting the start of an exam or a plane flight. In a group of 40 female patients with unstable bladders studied by Frewen (1978), no structural or organic cause could be found but all of them were found to have an emotive or psychogenic origin for their urinary symptoms. Men only rarely seem to suffer urge incontinence as a psychosomatic symptom. Frewen maintains patients have to understand the psychological components of their urinary symptoms before they can be cured. The results of treatment are said to be directly related to the conditions or influences under which a patient lives (for example, undergoing divorce, coping with a chronically disabled husband). The patient has to change her way or view of life before bladder training can be effective.

Macaulay *et al.* (1987) devised a trial comparing psychotherapy, bladder training and propantheline in a group of 47 females attending a urodynamic clinic in order to clarify the most important therapeutic aspects. All the patients were psychologically assessed before and after treatment. The 47 patients were diagnosed as having detrusor instability or sensory urgency and were randomly allocated to the three groups, 18 to psychotherapy, 15 to bladder training and 14 to receive propantheline. The psychotherapy group were seen weekly by a psychiatrist and given support and counselling. The bladder training was given by a nurse fortnightly. The drug group were given propantheline for three months. Patients kept a bladder diary and had cystometry before and after treatment. The patients were all found to be abnormally anxious and were depressed. The psychotherapy group had significantly improved symptoms of nocturia, urgency and incontinence whereas bladder training and drug therapy only improved frequency and anxiety. Bladder training was thought to be ineffective because it lacked 'warmth, genuineness and empathy'. Psychotherapy was thus shown to be effective in treating urinary symptoms.

Freeman and Baxby (1982) studied the effect of hypnotherapy on removing the symptoms of incontinence and frequency from a group of 50 females with detrusor instability. This study was uncontrolled as the researchers considered it unethical to ask incontinent patients to serve as untreated controls. They cured 58 per cent and improved 28 per cent of the patients, judged by the results from cystometrograms. Seven patients (14 per cent) relapsed during follow-up (three following bereavement). This study shows psychological factors are an important cause of unstable bladders.

Biofeedback is another psychotherapeutic method which has been used to treat detrusor instability. Cardozo *et al.* (1978) cured 40 per cent of 30 patients and improved symptoms in a further 40 per cent. A five year follow-up (Cardozo and Stanton, 1984) on 20 patients, showed mixed results with a high level of relapse. Biofeedback works best with highly motivated women, the disadvantages being that the patient has to be catheterised and the process is time-consuming.

Oldenburg and Millard (1986) compared the psychological status of 53 female patients prior to treatment with bladder training and at an eighteen month follow-up. These patients formed part of a study reported elsewhere (Millard and Oldenburg, 1983). All the patients were found to have a substantial improvement in psychological functioning at eighteen months' follow-up. They conclude that much of the psychological distress was symptomatic of, or exacerbated by, the bladder disorder – the psychological disturbance is causally linked to the urological problem. This is in contrast to Frewen (1978) who believes the psychological problems come first.

The literature concerning other types of bladder re-education, particularly timed voiding, is a bit patchy. Timed voiding regimes are generally used for the elderly. Clay (1978) introduced habit retraining and charting into a rehabilitation ward. She found 12 out of 20 males and 8 out of 11 females were cured of incontinence after thirteen weeks. There were no controls in this study and the patients' type of incontinence was not determined beforehand, so the study is only a demonstration of the method of habit retraining. This form of treatment requires a high degree of motivation from the staff who have to give frequent positive reinforcement to the patients when they use the toilet appropriately.

Tobin and Brocklehurst (1986) made a controlled study of the management of incontinence in local authority homes for the elderly. A study group and a control group were randomly selected from incontinent patients in 30 local authority homes. There were 174 in the study group (29 males) and 104 (19 males) in the control group. The disparity in numbers was because where less than six patients were incontinent in a home, all were included in the study group and no controls were used. The study group were given medical intervention in the form of a medical diagnosis. Those found to have unstable bladders, 93 per cent of females and 97 per cent of males, were all placed on a two-hourly timed voiding toileting regime and given propantheline and flavoxate. No baseline charts were used. Only 3.4 per cent of the females were diagnosed as having genuine stress incontinence and they were shown how to perform pelvic floor exercises, no separate analysis was done for this group. The staff were given no advice on management of the 104 residents in the control group. Patients were reviewed after two months and daytime and nocturnal incontinence were analysed separately. There was no significant difference between the 39 per cent of the study group and the 29 per cent of the control group in reduction of daytime incontinence. There was a significant reduction in nocturnal incontinence, 41 per cent in the study group compared with 23 per cent in the control group. There was no significant difference in reduction of daytime incontinence between the groups possibly because the control group were also toileted more frequently.

A large scale controlled study (Hu et al., 1989) looked at 133 incontinent elderly women in nursing homes whose incontinence was diagnosed by a urologist. They were randomly assigned to a treatment group receiving behaviour therapy for three months: hourly checking and prompting of individuals to go to the toilet or a control group receiving no prompting. The success of the study was measured in reduction of incidence of incontinence, a 26 per cent reduction over baseline was achieved in the study group after six weeks' implementation which was statistically significant. The residents who responded best to the behaviour therapy were those with a high frequency of incontinence during the baseline period, the more cognitively intact and those with normal bladder capacity. This controlled study shows it is possible to reduce incontinence by prompted voiding but only by increasing the workload of the nurses concerned.

Igou (1986) comments on the problems of motivating staff when trying to introduce bladder training schemes. Staff can believe it is faster to do everything for the patient rather than try to motivate the patient to be independent and continent. This type of 'overcare' practised by some nurses and carers encourages total dependence and staff need knowledge in how self-care can be beneficial. To achieve a degree of independence and continence a patient would be expected either to request a visit to the toilet or have toileting times rescheduled to suit his or her bladder. Before patients are initiated into bladder training schemes, nursing staff need to be convinced that their hard work and dedication is vital to the scheme. If they can be made to see the future advantages they will be more motivated to help the bladder training succeed. Igou (1986) says as patients become drier, workloads and morale change and there are economic and psychological benefits. Staff have to be part of the decision making process and be trained and given support in order to get maximum cooperation and good implementation in bladder training schemes. Copperwheat (1985) comments on the importance of communicating with all staff involved and also suggests only retraining one or two patients at a time.

Why does bladder re-education work?

The literature shows that intervention in the form of bladder re-education can have dramatic effects in curing or considerably improving incontinence. The reports show that patients were cured of symptoms of urgency, frequency and incontinence and that these cures were also apparent on objective cystometry recordings, patients were shown to have stable detrusors and a marked increase in bladder capacity. The reasons for these cures are not so apparent.

It may be that bladder re-education improves central nervous system control of micturition reflexes. Lengthening the period between voidings should lead to increased stimulation of bladder stretch receptors. Central nervous system control may be re-established because there is a greater awareness of bladder filling and/or because patients are better able to suppress the urge to void. Functional bladder capacity will therefore increase (Hadley, 1986).

Timed voiding regimes, as practised on the elderly, should be designed to promote normal conditioned reflexes. Willington (1975) describes the systems of reflexes which result in normal micturition. Excitory stimuli are:

1. Full bladder.
2. Sitting on a lavatory seat.
3. The correct position or circumstances.
4. Absence of clothing.

Inhibitory stimuli include:

1. Lack of privacy.
2. Painful stimuli from sitting on a bedpan.
3. Cold.
4. Performing in the wrong place or position.
5. Clean clothes.

In patients with mental and physical disabilities nurses may introduce incorrect inhibitory reactions by, for example, sitting a patient on the toilet after the bladder has been emptied and then making the patient sit there for long periods becoming ever more uncomfortable. If this happens often enough, sitting on the toilet will actually inhibit normal micturition. Positive and negative responses may then get reversed and inhibitory stimuli such as lying in bed or being clothed may encourage voiding. Patients may also be incontinent because they find they get attention then, their incontinence is being rewarded.

To restore normal reflexes and promote continence, nurse and patient have to start with the basic stimulus of a full bladder and then continue with timed voidings which are based on the patient's bladder capacity and previous patterns of incontinence. Micturition should take place in a comfortable and warm toilet. If a patient is incontinent he or she should not receive a great deal of attention but be changed and cleaned with the minimum of contact and conversation.

The nurse or carer often has to be the person to motivate the patient as the elderly sometimes lack self-motivation. Thus it is important to have an enthusiastic and knowledgeable staff when attempting habit training schemes in the elderly.

Client groups

There are certain groups of patients who will probably benefit from a programme of bladder re-education. Before considering a patient for bladder re-education it is necessary to look at both the likely cause for their incontinence and the patient's motivation and ability to cooperate.

Patients suffering from urgency, urge incontinence and detrusor instability are suitable candidates for bladder re-education, but there are no hard and fast rules. As Hadley (1986) notes, bladder re-education regimes may be applicable to patients with stress incontinence as the training may strengthen pelvic floor muscles because the patients learn consciously or unconsciously to tighten their periurethral muscles when trying to increase periods between voidings. This may increase bladder outlet resistance and diminish stress incontinence. No work has been reported on this though and knowledge of the actual physiological effects of bladder re-education is limited. In the majority of papers written on bladder re-education the subjects are middle-aged women with urge incontinence. The best results have been obtained from patients who are well-motivated and have (or are given) an insight into the possible psychological causes of their problems.

In the elderly there is often an underlying disease which leads to an unstable bladder and incontinence, for example, stroke, Parkinson's disease, diabetes, Alzheimer's disease, multiinfarct dementia and spinal cord lesions secondary to degenerative joint disease (Brocklehurst, 1984). Other factors which lead to incontinence in the elderly include mental impairment and physical disability (ibid.) There are a number of reversible causes of incontinence in the elderly which should be dealt with before considering bladder re-education such as: acute urinary tract infection, faecal impaction and use of fast acting diuretics. As yet, no definitive methods of managing the elderly on bladder re-education schemes have been devised but even very debilitated patients have been shown to benefit from training schemes. Bladder re-education programmes can also be helpful for patients following periods of catheterisation (Greengold and Ouslander, 1986).

Timed voiding requires no expensive equipment and does not impose a health risk, it can be carried out in hospital, nursing homes or in the patient's own home. Castleden and Duffin (1981) suggest that timed voiding will not be successful in patients who have unstable bladder contractions occurring at volumes of less than 150 ml. They state all elderly patients should have a cystometric examination to determine bladder capacity before being started on any sort of bladder re-education scheme.

Assessment of patients and use of charts

An initial assessment of the patient should be made which may include a medical examination leading to urodynamic investigations. The aim of the assessment and investigations is to discover what is causing the urinary symptoms and/or the type of incontinence. Other factors documented by Rooney (1989) which need to be considered include the following:

1. The patient's ability to cooperate.
2. The degree of mobility.
3. The degree of disability.
4. Motivation.
5. Home circumstances.

Once it has been decided that a patient is suitable for bladder re-education a baseline record of the patient's continence and incontinence needs to be made. The chart often reveals a pattern of micturition and incontinence. Patients can be trained successfully in hospital although training at home can be just as successful (Frewen, 1982). Rooney (1989) states that patients sent home after a successful inpatient training need to be reassessed in the home surroundings as incontinence problems can recur once old routines and circumstances are taken up again.

It usually takes four to seven days to obtain a useful baseline record from charts. The patient is asked to visit the toilet as normal and mark on the chart whether she was wet or dry and whether she passed urine in the toilet. Some patients have problems with using charts. They can be given a tailor-made chart or be asked to write down on a blank piece of paper the times when they are wet and when they use the toilet. There are many types of chart available and commercial companies selling incontinence aids will often provide them free of charge on request. It is possible to obtain information on fluid intake and output on the same chart if so desired, but this can unnecessarily confuse the patient. A simple chart such as Fig. 4.1 will suffice, particularly for patients in the community.

Ouslander *et al.* (1986) describe the development of an incontinence monitoring

TIME	MONDAY		TUESDAY		WEDNESDAY		THURSDAY		FRIDAY		SATURDAY		SUNDAY	
6 am														
7 am														
8 am														
9 am														
10 am														
11 am														
12 am														
1 pm														
2 pm														
3 pm														
4 pm														
5 pm														
6 pm														
7 pm														
8 pm														
9 pm														
10 pm														
11 pm														
12 pm														
1 am														
2 am														
3 am														
4 am														
5 am														
TOTAL														

Please tick in [ ] column each time you use the toilet.

Please tick in [ ] column every time you are wet.

Fig. 4.1 Continence chart.

record. They state records can serve a number of purposes including the following:

1. The determination and documentation of continence status.
2. The identification of factors associated with incontinent episodes.
3. The planning and monitoring of a bladder re-education programme.
4. The objective assessment of the outcome of treatments such as drug therapy.

They say use of simple charts such as that shown in Fig. 4.1 do not allow recording of other information which might be helpful in diagnosis and treatment, particularly in the elderly. This includes the following:

1. Clear differentiation between incontinent episodes, successful toileting and a dry check without toileting.
2. An assessment of the amount of incontinence.
3. A measurement of voided volume.
4. Whether or not faecal incontinence occurred.
5. The circumstances surrounding the incontinent episode: where it occurred (on way to toilet or in bed) and whether the patient was unaware of or denied the incontinence.

Date	BLADDER				BOWEL		Comments
TIME	Incontinent of urine	Dry	Voided correctly		Incontinent	Normal	
6 am	◊	◊	O	◊ ml			
7 am	◊	◊	O	◊ ml			
8 am	◊	◊	O	◊ ml			
9 am	◊	◊	O	◊ ml			
10 am	◊	◊	O	◊ ml			
11 am	◊	◊	O	◊ ml			
12 am	◊	◊	O	◊ ml			
1 pm	◊	◊	O	◊ ml			
2 pm	◊	◊	O	◊ ml			
3 pm	◊	◊	O	◊ ml			
4 pm	◊	◊	O	◊ ml			
5 pm	◊	◊	O	◊ ml			
6 pm	◊	◊	O	◊ ml			
7 pm	◊	◊	O	◊ ml			
8 pm	◊	◊	O	◊ ml			
9 pm	◊	◊	O	◊ ml			
10 pm	◊	◊	O	◊ ml			
11 pm	◊	◊	O	◊ ml			
12 pm	◊	◊	O	◊ ml			
1 am	◊	◊	O	◊ ml			
2 am	◊	◊	O	◊ ml			
3 am	◊	◊	O	◊ ml			
4 am	◊	◊	O	◊ ml			
5 am	◊	◊	O	◊ ml			
TOTAL							

KEY   Cross correct symbol at the hour closest to the time patient is checked

    = Incontinent, small amount

    = Incontinent, large amount

    = Dry

    = Voided correctly

Fig. 4.2 An incontinence monitoring chart.

Figure 4.2 shows a version of the chart designed, devised to be practical and understandable and to give useful information. The use of symbols is thought to be easier to understand, some versions of the chart use coloured symbols which Ouslander *et al.* (1986) say made for more reliable recording of incidents. They were concerned that a record chart should be easy for untrained staff to understand and use.

Reviewing the baseline chart can give a great deal of information. The patient's problem is shown up and it is easier to make a choice of which form of bladder re-education to select from: bladder training, habit retraining, timed voiding or prompted voiding. For example, small, frequent and regular episodes of incontinence may be due to drugs or anatomic obstruction. Large amounts of incontinence in the morning may be due to a diuretic. Urinary frequency and incontinence at night may be because of mild congestive heart failure or because coffee or tea was taken too close to bedtime. Keeping a chart often in itself proves therapeutic (Norton, 1987).

Running the re-education programme

Once the baseline pattern of continence has been recorded, the chart can be reviewed and a programme for bladder re-education can be established. Such programmes have to be designed for an individual patient. Initially, a decision has to be made on whether to start the patient on a bladder training programme or on a timed voiding schedule. On the whole, this depends on the patient's motivation and ability – a strict bladder training programme requires active and intelligent participation by the patient.

Bladder training

The patient first needs to have a clear understanding of the cause of his or her incontinence and realise that bladder contractions are under the control of the brain. In order to increase motivation, it has been suggested (Jarvis and Millar, 1980) that the patient is introduced to someone who has successfully undergone bladder training. Figure 4.3 shows the typical baseline chart of a woman with urgency and urge incontinence who would benefit from bladder training.

In general the aims of bladder training are the following:

1. To prevent episodes of incontinence.
2. To reduce symptoms of frequency and urgency and progressively increase the interval between voiding to about three to four hours until the patient can void normally without times being set.

There are a number of approaches to achieving these aims (Table 4.1).

TIME	MONDAY		TUESDAY		WEDNESDAY		THURSDAY		FRIDAY		SATURDAY		SUNDAY	
6 am	✓		✓			✓	✓		✓		✓		✓	
7 am	✓	✓		✓	✓		✓	✓	✓	✓	✓			
8 am			✓		✓		✓✓		✓		✓	✓	✓	✓
9 am	✓✓	✓	✓	✓	✓				✓		✓✓		✓✓	
10 am	✓		✓✓			✓	✓				✓		✓	
11 am	✓		✓		✓				✓	✓				
12 am	✓	✓					✓	✓	✓		✓	✓	✓	✓
1 pm			✓	✓	✓✓		✓			✓	✓		✓	
2 pm	✓		✓				✓		✓✓		✓		✓	
3 pm	✓		✓		✓	✓	✓	✓			✓	✓	✓	✓
4 pm	✓✓	✓	✓				✓✓		✓				✓✓	
5 pm			✓✓		✓		✓		✓		✓✓			
6 pm	✓	✓	✓		✓								✓	
7 pm	✓						✓		✓	✓	✓		✓	
8 pm			✓		✓	✓	✓	✓			✓		✓	✓
9 pm	✓		✓	✓	✓✓				✓		✓	✓	✓✓	
10 pm		✓	✓✓		✓		✓		✓					
11 pm	✓		✓	✓	✓		✓		✓		✓		✓	
12 pm														
1 am			✓										✓	
2 am	✓				✓	✓		✓	✓	✓	✓	✓		
3 am							✓							✓
4 am			✓	✓										
5 am					✓									
TOTAL	16	7	20	6	15	5	17	5	15	5	17	5	18	5

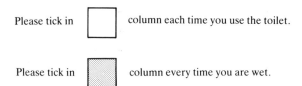

Please tick in ☐ column each time you use the toilet.

Please tick in ▨ column every time you are wet.

Fig. 4.3 Typical chart of patient with urge incontinence.

Mandatory schedule

The patient is given a voiding schedule; the timings based on the baseline assessment, generally one to two hourly. The patient will be told not to use the toilet until the next appointed time even if he or she has to be incontinent. The results will be recorded on a chart by the patient. The patient will be reviewed (daily if in hospital, probably weekly or fortnightly if at home) and when he or she is successful at remaining dry, the periods between voidings will be increased by 15 to 30 minutes. The amount of increase must be easy for the patient to attain so that motivation is not reduced. The process continues until the patient is dry with satisfactorily long periods between voidings. Figure 4.4 shows the type of progression aimed for.

Week 1	Week 2	Week 4	Week 6	Week 8
TIME	TIME	TIME	TIME	TIME
6am	6am	6am	6am	6am
7am 30	7am 45	7am	7am	7am
8am	8am	8am	8am 30	8am
9am	9am 30	9am	9am	9am
10am 30	10am	10am	10am	10am
11am	11am 15	11am	11am	11am
12am	12am	12am	12am	12am
1pm 30	1pm	1pm	1pm 30	1pm
2pm	2pm 45	2pm	2pm	2pm
3pm	3pm	3pm	3pm	3pm
4pm 30	4pm 30	4pm	4pm	4pm
5pm	5pm	5pm	5pm	5pm
6pm	6pm 15	6pm	6pm 30	6pm
7pm 30	7pm	7pm	7pm	7pm
8pm	8pm	8pm	8pm	8pm
9pm	9pm 45	9pm	9pm	9pm
10pm 30	10pm	10pm	10pm	10pm
11pm	11pm 30	11pm	11pm 30	11pm
12pm	12pm	12pm	12pm	12pm
1am	1am	1am	1am	1am
2am	2am	2am	2am	2am
3am	3am	3am	3am	3am
4am	4am	4am	4am	4am
5am	5am	5am	5am	5am
TOTAL	TOTAL	TOTAL	TOTAL	TOTAL

Fig. 4.4 Chart showing progression of patient on bladder training.

Self-scheduling

Again an initial voiding schedule is given to the patient, who will be told to increase gradually the interval between voidings at his or her own rate, but if it is not possible to hold on, the patient will be allowed to use the toilet. The patient will be asked to chart his or her own progress and experiencing and charting a steady improvement should motivate the patient to continue.

In some schedules (Pengelly and Booth, 1980), the patient is given a jug and asked to measure and record the amount of urine passed. The eventual aim being never to void less than 400 ml. To a certain extent, measuring the amount of urine passed should give the patient added motivation providing there is a steady improvement.

The results of previous studies have shown no clear difference between mandatory and self-scheduling schemes (Hadley, 1986). Decisions on which approach to take will depend on knowledge of the patient; more work would be useful to clarify the issue. Possibly the mandatory approach would work better in hospital where a strict watch can be kept on patients and faster results are expected.

Habit retraining

The patient is given a toileting schedule, usually two hourly to start with. The patient is instructed to void at the set times but allowed to use the toilet if necessary. The results are charted and the chart is used to adjust the intervals to suit the individual's voiding pattern. It may be that the patient needs to go two hourly in the morning but only three to four hourly in the afternoon.

Timed voiding

This involves giving the patient a fixed voiding schedule which remains unaltered, generally two hourly. It is used most commonly with the elderly debilitated. Timed voiding can also be used for patients with neurogenic bladders associated with spinal cord lesions. Some patients may also have difficulty in voiding and retention of urine possibly following catheterisation (Greengold and Ouslander, 1986). For these types of patients and those with spinal cord lesions it may be necessary to perform intermittent catheterisation every six to eight hours until the residual urine is less than 100 ml. Techniques to trigger voiding can be taught to the patient. These include running water from a tap, stroking the inner thigh and suprapubic tapping. The patient must be encouraged to empty the bladder completely by, for example, bending forward, applying suprapubic pressure and double voiding.

Prompted voiding

Prompted voiding is a method used with institutionalised patients to try and give them an insight into their bladder's control. The patients are asked at regular intervals if they need to empty their bladders and are only taken to the toilet if they say they do (Hu *et al.*, 1989). Praise is given when toileting is successful and social reinforcement is given to the patients by giving them special attention such as conversation or making them more comfortable if they are found to be dry on checking. It is important always to respect the individual, positive reinforcement of correct behaviour is acceptable ('Well done Mrs Brown, you've managed to use the toilet') whereas negative reactions are definitely not ('You are naughty Mrs Brown, you've wet yourself'). When incontinent, a patient should be dealt with quietly and efficiently.

Patients undergoing most forms of bladder re-education need to be taught methods to overcome the urge to void. Methods include using techniques of perineal pressure, pelvic floor contractions, controlled breathing exercises and various mental distractions such as mathematical problem solving (Millard and Oldenburg, 1983). A simple method is to instruct the patient to count to five when he or she first feels the urge to pass urine before voiding and then to increase this to ten next time and so on until it is possible to postpone micturition comfortably for as long as possible. Millard and Oldenburg (1983) also asked their patients to increase their fluid intake to 2.5 litres a day and to break the habit of voiding 'just in case'. They were encouraged to take longer walks and shopping trips and were discouraged from wearing incontinence pads to stimulate them to try harder.

Bladder re-education schemes have been found to take about three months before the patients have full control over their bladders. Researchers (for example Pengally and Booth, 1980; and Jarvis, 1981) have noted that if there is improvement it is often rapid in the first week or so of treatment and patients need to be encouraged to keep on with their regimes.

During the night, patients are not usually instructed on frequency of micturition. For patients in hospital, the nurse should check the bed at regular intervals and chart the results. It may be necessary to wake the patient once during the night to keep her dry. Jarvis (1982) treated 26 enuretic adult females with bladder training and cured 65 per cent, there was, however, no control group. He postulates that bladder training is a psychomedical technique and so is a good therapy for adult enuresis which is a psychosomatic condition.

Summary

There is evidence that bladder training and habit retraining can be very successful forms of management in the promotion of continence. They work best in achieving continence in patients who are well motivated and who have or are given an insight into their incontinence. They also need to be implemented by a knowledgeable and enthusiastic nurse who will encourage the patient to continue the therapy.

For the elderly institutionalised who seem to have no awareness of their bladder, timed voiding schemes and prompted voiding can be used. It would appear that incorporating some form of behavioural therapy allows the patient to gain awareness of bladder filling and may lead to fewer incidents of incontinence as the patient learns to request a visit to the toilet. Any nurse wishing to institute a form of bladder re-education in the elderly must be aware of the importance of educating all staff and/or carers who will participate in care of the patients. Just one nurse who does not understand what all the fuss is about may undermine the whole therapy.

More nurse-centred work is needed on the best ways of introducing bladder training and timed voiding schemes into areas of long-term care for the elderly. Should a patient-by-patient approach be initiated or should the aim be to have a sweeping reform? What type of behavioural therapy works best for the incontinent elderly and why? Just what level of support do elderly patients need in the community – how often should they be reassessed and by whom? More long-term follow-ups are needed on patients who have undergone bladder re-education in order to pinpoint the types of patient likely to relapse and how they can be helped.

Medical research is needed to achieve the following:

1. Find out just how bladder re-education effects a cure.
2. Elucidate the importance or otherwise of using drugs during bladder re-education.
3. Get greater insight into the psychological factors in detrusor instability and the importance of psychological factors in bladder training.

There is also a need to determine whether patients are best managed in hospital or at home when undergoing strict bladder training. If in hospital, is this a possible justification for having nurse managed beds?

There is obviously a need for further research that investigates the effects of bladder re-education programmes in large well designed randomly controlled trials, which are necessary to determine accurately the benefit which may be attributed to this form of management. As bladder re-education is something which clearly comes under the domain of the nurse, it is surprising there is so little nursing research in this field. It is hoped this will be rectified in the future.

References

Andersson, K.E. (1988), 'Current concepts in the treatment of disorders of micturition', *Practical Therapeutics*, 35: 477–94.

Brocklehurst, J.C. (1984), 'Ageing, bladder function and incontinence', in *Urology in the Elderly*, Edinburgh: Churchill Livingstone.

Cardozo, L.D., Abrams, P.H., Stanton, S.L. and Feneley, R.C.L. (1978), 'Idiopathic detrusor instability treated by biofeedback', *British Journal of Urology*, 50: 521–3.

Cardozo, L.D. and Stanton, S.L. (1984), 'Biofeedback: a 5-year review', *British Journal of Urology*, 56: 220.

Castleden, C.M. and Duffin, H.M. (1981), 'Guidelines for controlling urinary incontinence without drugs or catheters', *Age and Ageing*, 10: 186–90.

Castleden, C.M., Duffin, H.M., Asher, M.J. and Yeomanson, C.W. (1985), 'Factors influencing outcome in elderly patients with urinary incontinence and detrusor instability', *Age and Ageing*, 14: 303–7.

Clay, E.C. (1978), 'Incontinence of urine: a regimen for retraining', *Nursing Mirror*, 146: 23–4.

Clay, E.C. (1986), 'Rehabilitative nursing', in Mandelstam, D. (ed.), *Incontinence and its Management* (2nd edn), London: Croom Helm.

Copperwheat, M. (1985), 'Putting continence into practice', *Geriatric Nursing*, 5(3): 4–8.

Elder, D.D. and Stephenson, T.P. (1980), 'An assessment of the Frewen regime in the treatment of detrusor dysfunction in females', *British Journal of Urology*, 52: 467–71.

Freeman, R.M. and Baxby, K. (1982), 'Hypnotherapy for incontinence caused by the unstable detrusor', *British Medical Journal*, 284: 1831–4.

Frewen, W.K. (1978), 'An objective assessment of the unstable bladder of psychosomatic origin', *British Journal of Urology*, 50: 246–9.

Frewen, W.K. (1982), 'A reassessment of bladder training in detrusor dysfunction in the female', *British Journal of Urology*, 54: 372–3.

Greengold, G.A. and Ouslander, J.G. (1986), 'Bladder retraining program for elderly patients with post-indwelling catheterization', *Journal of Gerontological Nursing*, 12(6): 31–5.

Hadley, E.C. (1986), 'Bladder training and related therapies for urinary incontinence in older people', *Journal of the American Medical Association*, 256(3): 372–9.

Hu, T.W., Igou, J.F., Kaltreider, D.C., Yu, L.C., Rohner, T.J., Dennis, P.J., Craighead, W.E., Hadley, E.C. and Ory, M.G. (1989), 'A clinical trial of behavioral therapy to reduce urinary incontinence in nursing homes', *Journal of the American Medical Association*, 261(18): 2656–62.

Igou, J.F. (1986), 'Incontinence in nursing homes: research and treatment issues from the nursing perspective', *Clinics in Geriatric Medicine*, 2(4): 873–85.

Jarvis, G.J. (1981), 'A controlled trial of bladder drill and drug therapy in the management of detrusor instability', *British Journal of Urology*, 53: 565–6.

Jarvis, G.J. (1982), 'Bladder drill for the treatment of enuresis in adults', *British Journal of Urology*, 54: 118–19.

Jarvis, G.J. and Millar, D.R. (1980), 'Controlled trial of bladder drill for detrusor instability', *British Medical Journal*, 281: 1322–3.

Macaulay, A.J., Stern, R.S., Holmes, D.M. and Stanton, S.L. (1987), 'Micturition and the mind: psychological factors in the aetiology and treatment of urinary symptoms in women', *British Medical Journal*, 294: 540–3.

Mahady, I.W. and Begg, B.M. (1981), 'Long-term symptomatic and cystometric cure of the urge incontinence syndrome using a technique of bladder re-education', *British Journal of Obstetrics and Gynaecology*, 88: 1038–43.

Millard, R.J. and Oldenburg, B.F. (1983), 'The symptomatic, urodynamic and psychodynamic results of bladder re-education programs', *The Journal of Urology*, 130: 715–19.

Norton, C. (1987), 'Improving bladder function', *Geriatric Nursing and Home Care*, 7(6): 22–6.

Oldenburg, B.F. and Millard, R.J. (1986), 'Predictions of long-term outcome following a bladder retraining programme', *Journal of Psychosomatic Research*, 30(6): 691–8.

Ouslander, J.G., Urman, H.N. and Uman, G.C. (1986), 'Development and testing of an incontinence monitoring record', *Journal of the American Geriatrics Society*, 34(2): 83–90.

Pengally, A.W. and Booth, C.M. (1980), 'A prospective trial of bladder training as treatment for detrusor instability', *British Journal of Urology*, 52: 463–6.

Rooney, V. (1989), 'Bladder re-education and timed voiding programmes', *Geriatric Medicine: Geriatric Workshop on Incontinence, Measuring and Managing Incontinence* (a special supplement), February: 26–7.

Snape, J., Castleden, C.M., Duffin, H.M. and Ekelund, P. (1989), 'Long-term follow-up of habit retraining for bladder instability in elderly patients', *Age and Ageing*, 18: 192–4.

Tobin, G.W. and Brocklehurst, J.C. (1986), 'The management of urinary incontinence in local authority residential homes for the elderly', *Age and Ageing*, 15: 292–8.

Willington, F.L. (1975), 'Training and retraining for continence', *Nursing Times*, 71: 500–3.

5   Pelvic floor re-education for the promotion of continence

JOSEPHINE LAYCOCK

Introduction

This chapter describes the contribution of physiotherapy to the management of incontinence. Early reference to the anatomical factors responsible for sustaining continence enables a greater understanding of the sections dealing with pelvic floor exercises, neuromuscular electrical stimulation and biofeedback.

Physiotherapy and nursing overlap in the holistic approach to patient care, especially in the management of incontinence. Many nurses are learning the theory and practicalities of pelvic floor re-education, and physiotherapists are learning the skills of incontinence assessment and the value of the various aids and appliances available to contain incontinence.

Anatomy

Although the mechanisms of continence are not fully understood, an intact anatomy and integrity of nervous pathways is required to co-ordinate the action of the neuromuscular structures of the lower urinary tract and pelvic floor. There are several factors believed to be responsible for maintaining continence, some of which may be influenced by pelvic floor re-education.

Bladder factors
These include bladder compliance and detrusor reflex control. Compliance indicates the change in bladder volume for a change in pressure. High compliance indicates the ability of the detrusor to accommodate high volumes of urine without a significant rise in pressure.

Several reflexes controlling urine storage and voiding are described by Mahoney *et al.* (1977; 1980). Of these, two need special mention:

1. *Perineodetrusor inhibitory reflex*: this involves the reflex inhibition (relaxation) of the detrusor due to tonic activity of the pelvic floor muscles. Reduction in

pelvic tone and power may therefore lead to an overactive detrusor, causing urgency and frequency (Mahoney *et al.*, 1977) often seen in the elderly (Cardozo, 1984). This reflex may be activated by repeated pelvic floor exercises and electrical stimulation.

2. *Detrusosphincteric inhibitory reflex*: this involves the reflex inhibition (relaxation) of the pelvic floor and external urethral sphincter on bladder (detrusor) contraction. Impaired activity of this reflex can produce inability to relax the pelvic floor and external sphincter during micturition, which may be remedied by teaching pelvic floor relaxation exercises.

Bladder neck factors

The position of the bladder neck is controlled by ligamentous supports which arise in part from the pelvic bone and part from the pelvic fascia (Hald, 1984). This fascia is intimately related to the levator ani muscles and may be influenced by pelvic floor re-education. Fascia attached to weakened muscles will undergo degenerative changes, therefore pelvic floor exercises should promote normal physiology of the pelvic fascia (Tchou *et al.*, 1988).

Urethral factors

Adequate compression of the urethral mucosal folds provides the necessary watertight closure pressure for maintaining continence. This compression depends on the competence of the external urethral sphincter and pelvic floor muscles and the anatomical position of the bladder neck and proximal urethra to respond to transmitted abdominal pressure. In addition, vascularity, elasticity and tone of the smooth muscle component will all influence urethral competence in sustaining continence (Stanton, 1984).

The external urethral sphincter is made up from circularly disposed striated muscle fibres of the slow twitch variety, forming a sleeve around the urethra but separate from the levator ani (Gosling *et al.*, 1981). By virtue of the slow twitch population of muscle fibres, this sphincter is capable of maintaining an occlusive action on the urethral lumen for long periods, as slow twitch fibres are not easily fatigued (Gosling, 1979; Pette, 1984). As this sphincter is supplied by motor branches of S 2.3.4 (Juenemann *et al.*, 1988) it is under normal cortical control, and should respond to both pelvic floor exercises and electrical stimulation.

Vascular tissue is said to contribute one-third of the urethral closure pressure (Rud *et al.*, 1980), and would explain the reduction in continence with ageing, when vascularity is reduced (Carlile *et al.*, 1988). This process may be reversed by the application of electrical stimulation, which has been shown to increase vascularity (Currier *et al.*, 1986). This is the result of increased muscle metabolism, due to the electrically elicited muscle contraction (Cummings, 1980). In addition, the pumping effect of pelvic floor muscle contractions (produced voluntarily or by electrical stimulation) will stimulate the circulation in adjoining tissues and so help to maintain or improve a high vascular component of the urethral and periurethral tissues.

The pelvic floor

The muscles, ligaments and fascia comprising the pelvic floor form a sling support at the base of the pelvis. This sheet of muscle is pierced by the rectum posteriorly and the vagina and urethra anteriorly. It serves to support the pelvic and abdominal viscera and provide an additional sphincteric action to maintain urinary and faecal continence. In young active subjects the pelvic floor can be better described as a trampoline-like structure, with elasticity and strength, and the ability to recover after repeated stretching i.e. with lifting, coughing or straining. However, with ageing, obstetric trauma, reduced activity, obesity and repeated stretching, the strength and elasticity are reduced, causing prolapse of pelvic organs and reduced sphincteric action, and a general sagging of this previously taut elastic structure.

The medial periurethral and perivaginal fibres of the levator ani, the pubococcygeus (PC), play an important role in the maintenance of continence by not only providing support to the pelvic viscera, but also by supplying additional occlusive force to the urethral wall particularly during events which are associated with an increase in intra-abdominal pressure, such as coughing and sneezing. Kegel's S.S.S theory (1956) describes the function of the pubococcygeus as: Supportive, Sphincteric and Sexual.

The fibres of the PC have no attachment to the urethra, but insert into the lateral walls of the vagina (Gosling et al., 1981). Consequently, digital palpation per vaginam will ascertain muscle action. Muscle capability may also be evaluated using a perineometer, described by Kegel (1951) and Shepherd et al. (1983).

The pubococcygeus consists of a mixture of fast and slow twitch muscle fibres. Although previously thought to consist of 5 per cent fast twitch (Gosling et al., 1981) recent studies by Gilpin et al. (1989) have shown that on average fast twitch muscle fibres constitute 33 per cent (21–62) of the population. These two fibre types have differing roles to play in maintaining continence and respond to different exercises and different electrical parameters during stimulation.

The action of the PC is one that approximates the coccyx and pubis as the muscle fibres shorten, and in addition causes the vagina to press on the posterior wall of the urethra, and elevate it to the pubic bone. Also, a vaginal sphincteric action is noted on contraction of this muscle. Consequently when teaching pelvic floor exercises, women are instructed to 'squeeze, lift and hold, then relax' ensuring that the muscle fibres are fulfilling their complete role.

The fast twitch fibres, which tire easily, are responsible for the fast reflex response associated with coughing and also for providing a maximum voluntary contraction (mvc). This is important not only during exercises to increase muscle strength, but to enable a subject to quickly and strongly elevate and occlude the urethra prior to a stress provoking act such as coughing, lifting or sneezing. The fast twitch fibres also play an important role in providing a strong maximum contraction to suppress urgency and control detrusor instability, activating the perineodetrusor inhibitory reflex (see section on bladder factors above).

Slow twitch fibres, on the other hand, do not readily tire; they serve a postural function, and can generally be relied on to provide support and sphincteric action for long periods of time. Pelvic floor weakness will reduce the ability of both these components in their important role of sustaining continence.

Many factors may predispose the pelvic floor to weakness, including obstetric trauma (Smith *et al.*, 1989a,b), hormonal influence (Bhatia *et al.*, 1989) and the ageing process (Swash and Swartz, 1988). Obstetric trauma is thought not only to stretch and tear the pelvic floor muscles, but also damage may be incurred by the pudendal nerves, causing partial denervation (Snooks *et al.*, 1984; 1985). Some reinnervation of the denervated muscle fibres is then said to take place, producing polyphasicity on electromyogram (EMG) investigations, showing that more than one muscle fibre is now supplied by a single nerve (Neill and Swash, 1980).

A further cause of pelvic floor muscle weakness is loss of cortical control, and the inability to contract the muscles to command, producing a general lack of awareness and muscle capability. This may be caused initially by postpartum cortical inhibition due to pain, with some women failing to regain the ability to contract the pelvic floor at will. A weakened pelvic floor may result in urinary and faecal incontinence and both these conditions should respond to re-education techniques.

Due to its taboo nature, little is known by the general public of the function of the lower urinary tract and the role of the pelvic floor muscles in controlling micturition and defaecation. Even less is known concerning the sexual function of these muscles. Perry and Whipple (1982) have shown that anorgasmic women with a weak pelvic floor have attained increased sexual enjoyment and orgasm following a course of pelvic floor re-education, and recommend pelvic floor exercises to remedy this problem. Postpuberty girls in some eastern countries are taught pelvic floor exercises by their mothers to ensure the provision of sexual satisfaction to their future husbands, by coordinated muscle contractions during intercourse. These women rarely present with incontinence and one can speculate that their pelvic floor retains its function despite childbirth (Shepherd, 1983).

Client group

Pelvic floor re-education (pelvic floor exercises and electrical stimulation) is prescribed for patients with pelvic floor weakness leading to lower urinary tract dysfunction. Traditionally, women with mild to moderate genuine stress incontinence were identified as the client group most likely to benefit from this form of management, with severe symptomology and prolapse requiring surgery (Kegel, 1951). However, the ability to perform a strong pelvic floor contraction is a useful adjunct to bladder training in the control of urgency and frequency, and can therefore benefit men and women suffering from these symptoms.

The ageing process is characterised by a reduction in all muscle fibres (Swash and Swartz, 1988) causing decreased muscle bulk and concomitant reduction in strength and endurance, which may lead to incontinence. A decrease in vascularity (Carlile *et al.*, 1988) and reduced general activity (Gordon and Logue, 1985), will further dispose an elderly patient to incontinence. These factors may in some cases be reversed by pelvic floor rehabilitation, which should therefore be available to the elderly. Gordon and Logue (1985), in a study on pelvic floor muscle function one year after childbirth, found pelvic power to be significantly related to regular, general exercise and the performance of pelvic floor exercises, when compared with a pelvic floor exercises only group and a control group. This emphasises the need for regular exercise for all age groups.

As long ago as 1951, Kegel recommended the prophylactic treatment of women with poor levator function, especially in the ante- and post-partum periods. This is now generally carried out by physiotherapists specialising in obstetrics and gynaecology, midwives, district nurses, health visitors and nurses working in obstetrics. However, this fails to prevent incontinence in many cases, and perhaps one should examine the French system where pelvic floor rehabilitation is not introduced until six weeks postpartum, when pain, trauma and hormonal levels have normalised (Pigne, personal communication). This is further evidenced by Sleep and Grant (1987) in their study of 1,800 postpartum women recruited 24 hours after vaginal delivery. These women were randomly allocated to one of two groups. Nine hundred received routine postnatal instruction in pelvic floor rehabilitation and 900 were encouraged to follow a more intensive routine and to complete a four-week exercise diary. Assessment at ten days and three months demonstrated no difference between the two groups in terms of prevalence and severity of urinary or faecal incontinence, and the authors recommended that postnatal pelvic floor re-education should be further evaluated. This was again the outcome of five randomised controlled trials in perineal care (Sleep, 1991) and pelvic floor exercises in the postpartum remains a controversial practice.

In many centres in the United Kingdom, due to early hospital discharge, instruction in pelvic floor exercises may be given without assessing the patient's voluntary control, or may be described in a leaflet of exercises and advice handed to the new mother. Improved pelvic floor re-education in the antenatal period, to all women, would help to overcome this short fall in postnatal care.

Kegel (1951) also recommended pelvic floor training before and after surgery involving the pelvic outlet. This was emphasised by Fischer (1983), who recommended a combination of pelvic floor re-education and surgery in the management of incontinence. Both these reports appear to be on the basis of empirical research, but emphasise the need for good muscular control of the pelvic outlet. This is an area often neglected, where nursing input could play an important role.

Further clients to be targeted include all female hospital inpatients on prolonged bed rest (Gomer-Jones, 1963). The resulting muscle atrophy in this group is probably due to the loss of repeated reflex pelvic floor muscle responses to everyday activities and reduced postural action. Especially at risk are the postmenopausal, multiparous subjects on prolonged bed-rest, e.g. orthopaedic patients with fractures of the femur.

The decision to embark on pelvic floor rehabilitation will depend on the patient's motivation and expected compliance to an exercise regime, and the resources available. Selection of all patients will be governed by their ability to understand and remember instructions. It is generally accepted that a combination of exercises, exercise aids (see section on pelvic floor exercises) and electrical stimulation will ensure greater compliance and produce a more favourable outcome than exercises alone (Pigne *et al.*, 1985; Wilson *et al.*, 1987; Laycock, unpublished data). Although at present electrical stimulation is primarily the domain of the physiotherapist, the next decade may well see functional electric stimulation (FES) encompassed in the armament of nurses dealing with the incontinent patient (see section below on electrical stimulation).

Future prevention of incontinence by the teaching of pelvic floor exercises (PFE) to teenage school girls, and later in life at well women clinics, may go a long way to reducing the prevalence of urinary incontinence caused by pelvic floor weakness. Further advice at sport centres, keepfit, aerobics and yoga classes will increase public awareness of the conservative management and prevention of this embarrassing and humiliating problem.

Pelvic floor assessment

Muscle assessment is an integral component of the planning of any exercise programme, to evaluate strength/weakness, fatigue and coordination of the muscle under examination. Weakness is defined as failure to generate the expected force; fatigue is defined as failure to maintain the expected force with continued or repeated contractions (Edwards, 1978). Coordination infers the ability to synchronise muscle action to various commands. When these factors are fully assessed, an individual exercise programme, applying the principles of specificity and overload (see section below on pelvic floor exercises) can be devised for each patient.

Muscle assessment *per se* involves observing and feeling a muscle in the relaxed and contracting state, and evaluating its capability to perform a given task. In limb muscle assessment, this often involves joint movement, which is easily understood by the patient. For example, an instruction to 'straighten the knee' is more easily understood than being told to 'tighten the thigh muscles'. During contraction of the female pelvic floor muscles, the coccyx approximates to the pubis and the vagina and urethra are compressed, retracted and elevated. These movements are very insignificant compared with bending and straightening the knee, and some subjects are unable to understand exactly what is expected when instructed to tighten the pelvic floor. Many patients produce no pelvic floor contraction at all, and others may bear down, instead of squeezing and lifting. Reduced sensation and loss of cortical awareness contribute to this lack of control.

However, many subjects in this category are not incontinent, and so one must presume that postural and reflex responses are intact, and only the ability to contract the pelvic floor to command is lacking. This skill may need to be taught before full assessment is carried out, and hints on increasing muscle awareness are included in the next section. When assessing pelvic floor capability, attention should be drawn to the importance of performing a pelvic floor contraction in isolation, without the involvement of extraneous muscle groups. Commonly, subjects hold their breath, and tighten the abdominals, glutei and thigh adductors, which may mask the pelvic floor action, and increase fatigue. Before assessment an explanation of the procedure should be given to the patient, and agreement obtained to carry out the examination.

Female subjects

To observe and examine the pelvic floor, the subject lays supine, with hips flexed and abducted. The operator first introduces a gloved and lubricated index finger into the distal 5 cm of the vagina, to palpate the rim of the pubococcygeus (Fig. 5.1). This

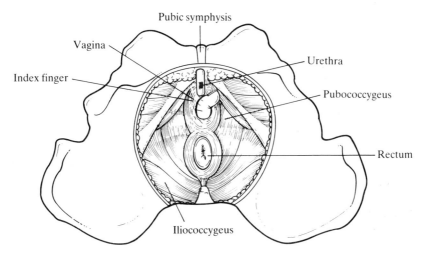

Fig. 5.1 Anatomical drawing showing the position of the examining index finger palpating the pubococcygeus. *Source*: E. Gomer-Jones (1963), 'Non-operative treatment of stress incontinence', *Clinical Obstetrics and Gynaecology*, 6: 222–35.

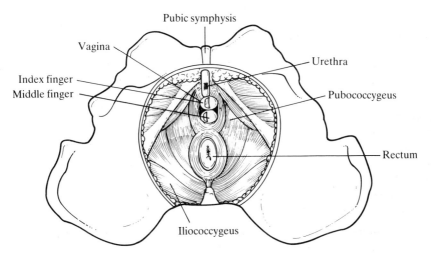

Fig. 5.2 Anatomical drawing showing the index and middle fingers assessing pelvic squeeze. *Source*: E. Gomer-Jones (1963), 'Non-operative treatment of stress incontinence', *Clinical Obstetrics and Gynaecology*, 6: 222–35.

Table 5.1 Oxford grading system for assessing pelvic floor strength

0	Nil
1	Flicker
2	Weak
3	Moderate
4	Good
5	Strong

will determine muscle bulk and any asymmetry, and will detect a change in tone as the subject contracts and relaxes the muscle. Next, the index finger and middle finger are introduced (index only if the introitus is narrow) into the vagina; the patient is asked to 'squeeze and lift' on the examining fingers, and hold for up to ten seconds (Fig. 5.2). Assessment takes place with the fingers in the antero-posterior (A-P) position, and also spread laterally. The A-P position will detect lift and movement of the coccyx towards the pubis: the lateral position enables palpation of the PC, and evaluation of its lift and squeeze potential (Brink *et al.*, 1989). To record muscle strength, a modified Oxford grading system is recommended, as shown in Table 5.1.

To assess fatigue, the hold time in seconds is recorded.

Example 1:

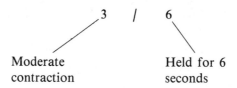

3 / 6

Moderate contraction   Held for 6 seconds

It is then necessary to determine the number of repetitions the subject can produce to further evaluate endurance and to set a target for daily home exercises.

Example 2:

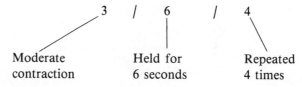

3 / 6 / 4

Moderate contraction   Held for 6 seconds   Repeated 4 times

– it is recommended that four seconds' rest is given between each contraction (Laycock *et al.*, 1991)

A full assessment will include evaluation of the function of both the fast and slow twitch components of the levator ani. The slow fibres are responsible for the endurance qualities, i.e. 'hold' time and number of repetitions, the fast twitch fibres are recruited whenever a maximum voluntary contraction, or speed, is required. This can be assessed by recording the number of fast one second contractions (flicks) the patient can perform. A complete assessment may be represented as follows:

Example 3:

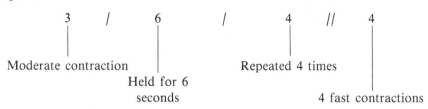

This assessment scoring method has established validity, interrater and test–retest reliability (ibid.). Coordination is an important factor in muscle function, and this is assessed by evaluating the response to commands to contract and relax, both quickly and slowly.

An alternative method has been described by Brink *et al.* (1989) and has established reliability and validity. However, this method lacks flexibility and it is not always possible to classify some subjects. Furthermore, this scoring system does not examine the two main components of the levator ani (fast and slow twitch) and moreover, the authors fail to develop their technique into a simple exercise programme.

Self-digital assessment should be encouraged for patients on an exercise programme, to enable self-monitoring of progress. However, there is often reluctance to perform this self examination, and in these cases, the patient's feelings should be respected. It may also help to concentrate the mind on pelvic floor contraction if the patient closes his or her eyes.

Pelvic floor muscles are under hormonal influence (Bhatia *et al.* 1989) and many patients report more severe incontinence the week before, and during, menstruation. In view of this, it is more meaningful to reassess a patient at the same stage in the menstrual cycle as the original assessment.

The assessment detailed above enables the planning of a home exercise programme. Table 5.2 proposes guidelines for treatment selection (Laycock, 1989).

Table 5.2 Treatment selection for pelvic floor re-education

PELVIC FLOOR GRADING		
Biofeedback	0 1 2	Electrical stimulation
	3 4 5	Pelvic floor exercises

The perineometer

This equipment is used to assess pelvic floor function, as an exercise aid to give resistance and also as a biofeedback device. Generally, a perineometer consists of a vaginal probe sensitive to pressure changes. This is connected to a manometer, which indicates the squeeze exerted by the perivaginal muscles.

The Bourne Perineometer (Fig. 5.3) is available in two sizes with replacement condoms preventing transference of infection between users. This is a very useful aid to pelvic floor muscle assessment, as both the strength, hold time and number of repetitions can be evaluated. As it is more sensitive than the digital method, a more accurate result will be obtained.

The biofeedback effect is used to encourage the subject to produce a stronger squeeze (higher meter reading) and hold for longer; a perineometer can also be used to manage patients with difficulty in coordinating relaxation. It is very important when using a perineometer to first ascertain digitally that the correct pelvic floor action is being performed. This is because extraneous muscle action such as tightening the abdominals and/or glutei, or inappropriate action, such as bearing down, will compress the pelvic viscera against the vaginal probe and produce a positive meter reading.

As a home exercise aid, a perineometer has been shown to enhance motivation and compliance (Shepherd *et al.*, 1983, Stoddart, 1983) and although Castleden *et al.* (1984) in their study did not improve the success of physiotherapy, they concluded that it did have an important role in instructing patients in the correct use of the pelvic floor muscles.

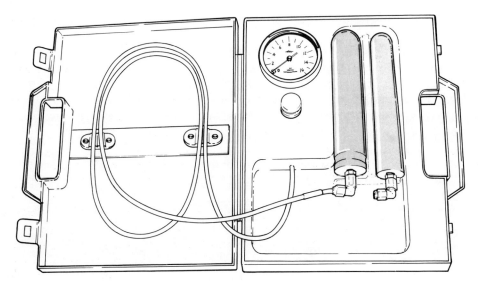

Fig. 5.3 The Bourne Perineometer.

Male subjects

The male pelvic floor is best assessed in the left lateral position, with hips and knees flexed. The action of the pelvic floor to compress and elevate the urethra and anal canal is explained to the patient, and examination using the index finger (gloved and lubricated) introduced into the anal canal will identify and evaluate this, by palpation of the puborectalis and external anal sphincter. In addition, two fingers placed posterior to the scrotum and pressed into the perineum will detect a pelvic floor contraction. The patient in both cases is instructed to squeeze, lift, hold and then relax.

Pelvic floor exercises

History

One of the earliest accounts of pelvic floor re-education was reported by Kegel (1948a,b, 1951) of an uncontrolled study of 500 women, in which he concluded that 'all patients suffering from simple urinary incontinence demonstrated loss of function or atrophy of the pelvic floor muscles, especially the pubococcygeus, in some cases simulating paralysis'. He described the condition as a 'syndrome of lack of awareness of function and co-ordination of the pubococcygeus muscle', and noted that 30 per cent of women could not elicit a contraction on command. The remaining women when requested to draw up and draw in, could produce only a weak squeeze. The contractions were measured on a perineometer, with continent women exerting a pressure equal to 30–60 mm Hg and incontinent subjects exerting as little as 0–5 mm Hg.

To remedy this problem, over a six to eight week period, Kegel advocated 20 minutes' exercises with a perineometer, three times per day, and five contractions every half hour. Weekly checks were essential to ensure correct muscle action and maintain motivation. Of the 500 patients in his study, 84 per cent became continent, including obese and elderly subjects. These results have not generally been matched by other workers in the field. Klarskov *et al.* (1986) report 42 per cent satisfied and not requiring surgery (number in study = 50); Kujansuu (1983) describes a trial in which 54 per cent reported subjective improvement (number in study = 24).

Further study of Kegel's results showed that some patients required nine to twelve months to attain continence, and perhaps this accounts for the superior outcome of his study as the other workers assessed all subjects within two to three months. Furthermore, Kegel instructed his patients personally and this could have increased motivation and compliance; also perhaps surgical intervention in the 1950s was not an attractive alternative, further enhancing motivation. In addition, Kegel's patients used a perineometer for resistive home exercises three times each day, and this was not included in the other studies reported above. The use of a perineometer would ensure activation of the fast and slow twitch muscle fibres and the biofeedback effect would encourage the patient to practise regularly, and work the muscles maximally. Kegel's study reported on 500 patients, but a control group would have added more credence to his results, as pelvic floor power could have been improved and incontinence reduced, with weekly muscle assessment and increased general awareness of perineal function.

Kegel's methods were adopted by Gomer-Jones (1963) who emphasised the need to teach awareness of the pubococcygeus, and its role to draw in, draw up and retract the perineum. Importance was laid on the ability to hold this position, and relax the muscles completely, during half-hourly exercise sessions. Gomer-Jones maintained that more than ten contractions at each session would produce fatigue and was therefore contraindicated. Recent studies (Laycock *et al.*, 1991) suggest that individual exercise programmes are needed to ensure maximum effort without fatigue, depending on pelvic floor muscle assessment.

Kegel's methodology provides the basis of pelvic floor rehabilitation as practised today in many parts of the world, both in community and hospital settings. An enthusiastic instructor and motivated patient have been shown to be necessary ingredients for success.

Muscle awareness

Kegel (1948a,b) and Millard (1987) report that 30 per cent of incontinent women are unable to contract their pelvic floor to command, and these subjects need careful tuition to comprehend the required exercise. The following hints may help to re-educate the correct muscle action, which involves the ability to squeeze, lift, hold, and relax the pelvic floor.

1. First teach contraction of the posterior pelvic floor muscle fibres, as if preventing the passage of wind from the bowel: most patients can perform this action easily.
2. Next teach contraction of the anterior fibres as if preventing the passage of urine from the bladder. The subject should imagine passing urine and attempt to stop the flow.
3. Stop test. The patient should practise stopping the flow of urine, once per day (ibid.). It may only be possible to slow the stream at first but this helps to identify the correct muscles. This exercise is best practised at the second void of the day and then performed progressively later in the day as the muscle strengthens and fatigue is reduced.
4. Teach the patient to retract the perineum away from an imaginary pin about to be stuck into the area anterior to the anus.
5. Instruct the subject to close his or her eyes, then to suck their thumb at the same time as they contract the pelvic floor. The squeezing and retraction of the lips in thumb sucking is a similar action to the squeezing and retraction of the contracting pelvic floor muscles.
6. The use of digital palpation by the operator or self-palpation by the patient is valuable, by spreading the fingers in a scissor-like action, the PC is stretched and increased sensation produced.
7. When teaching and assessing the correct muscle action, first request a short,

gentle squeeze. This may avoid the use of extraneous muscle groups often coopted when a maximum contraction is required. Once the correct muscle action is produced, and the subject is aware of this, a stronger and longer contraction is introduced.

8. To further encourage lift, and improve coordination, subjects may control the pelvic floor rise and fall by imagining it as an elevator, first lifting a little way (to the first floor), and gradually lifting in stages to an imaginary fifth floor, and then slowly relaxing the muscle and allowing the 'elevator' to descend, one floor at a time, back to the ground floor; further relaxation may be attained by imagining the elevator descending to the basement. (Patients are more likely to learn awareness of squeeze and lift, than actually feeling the muscles contracting, and so this should be emphasised.)

Physiology of muscle action

To produce a physiological change in any muscle, it is necessary to exercise regularly, and to satisfy the principles of overload and specificity. Overload describes the technique of gradually increasing the output produced by the muscle, i.e. power, hold time and the number of repetitions, always working the muscle to its limit, and then extending the limit. It is therefore necessary to determine each patient's capability and then plan an individual exercise programme. It is not satisfactory to instruct every patient to contract the muscles maximally for five seconds, five times every hour. Some patients are unable to hold a pelvic floor contraction for five seconds, and would therefore become demotivated; other patients, able to hold a strong contraction for seven to ten seconds, would not be 'overloading' their capability, and would not produce a physiological effect. The proven method of muscle rehabilitation involves assessing the muscles' capability and gradually, through regular exercise, overloading this by increasing the strength, hold time and the number of repetitions. Continuous overload will involve continuous reassessment and alteration of the exercise programme. Specificity involves using the different muscle components in a specific way, and the muscle as a whole to perform specific action (Table 5.3).

Table 5.3 Pelvic floor re-education

Fibre type	Specific function	Exercise type	Aims
Slow twitch	Postural	Endurance: High repetition Low resistance	1. To increase length of squeeze. 2. To increase number of repetitions.
Fast twitch	1. Reflex contraction during stress. 2. Active reinforcement during stress.	Strengthening: Low repetition High speed and resistance	1. To increase strength of squeeze. 2. To increase speed of contraction.

The aims of regular exercise are to achieve the following:

1. Increase cortical awareness.
2. Increase circulation.
3. Stimulate reflex activity.
4. Hypertrophy existing muscle fibres to:
   (a) increase resting tone,
   (b) increase active strength,
   (c) increase endurance,
   (d) improve coordination.

In the case of the pelvic floor complex, this will:

(a) increase urethral compressive forces,
(b) possibly better support the proximal urethra to respond to transmitted abdominal pressure,
(c) reduce the downward movement of the perineum during increased abdominal pressure, such as when coughing.

Exercise programme

The levator ani is a sheet of muscle spanning the base of the pelvis. In many subjects with weak musculature, this sheet becomes very thin and easily tires. It is therefore necessary to exercise the muscle 'a little and often', as despite its predominance of slow twitch fibres, the reduced muscle bulk renders it easily fatigued. The fast and slow twitch muscle fibres respond to different exercises, as shown in Table 5.3. Slow twitch fibres are activated by endurance exercises, i.e. high repetition rate and low speed and resistance. Fast twitch fibres are activated by fast phasic contractions, i.e. low repetition and high speed and resistance. Resistance can be given by the use of vaginal cones, or a perineometer, or the withdrawal of a vaginally located Foley catheter (see section below on vaginal cones).

To satisfy the principle of specificity, all these factors should be considered when planning an exercise programme. To avoid confusion, it may be necessary to introduce one new exercise only at each session; however, it probably helps compliance and motivation to add variety to the exercise regime, and to stress the importance and rationale behind the need to include different types of exercises.

Home exercise programme

Example 1

Assessment:

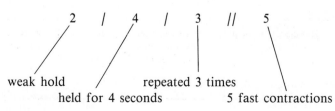

Exercise programme:

1. Assessment values provide targets for each exercise session, to be repeated a minimum of eight times each day.
2. Four second contractions repeated three times (with a four second rest between contractions).
3. This group of three contractions is repeated five times at each session (with a one minute rest between each group) (Laycock *et al.*, 1991).
4. Also once per day: five fast contractions and the stop test.

Total number of contractions per day = **125**

Example 2

Assessment:

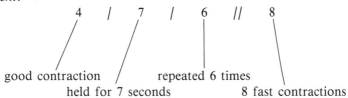

Exercise programme:

1. Assessment values provide initial target for each exercise session, to be repeated a minimum of eight times per day.
2. Seven second contractions repeated six times (with a four second rest between contractions).
3. This group of six contractions is repeated five times at each session (with a one minute rest between each group) (ibid.).
4. Also, once per day: eight fast contractions and the stop test.

Total number of contractions per day = **247**

These two examples clearly show the different exercise regimes of subjects with differing muscle capability; continuous reassessment will necessitate an alteration in the programme to satisfy the principle of overload. An exercise diary (Fig. 5.4) (Laycock *et al.*, 1991), with the exercise programme clearly stated, helps as a reminder to exercise and the correct exercises to do at each session.

Do's and don'ts

Do

1. Exercise regularly, at least eight times per day.
2. Exercise intelligently, using the muscles to squeeze and retract the perineum, holding for the specified time, and relaxing completely.
3. Stop test once per day. Initially, the second void of the day is recommended, but as muscle power increases, this should be practised progressively later in the day.
4. Avoid overtiring the muscles by allowing at least one hour between each session.

Name..

Date ....   Next Appointment ....

Use the diary to record each time the exercises are performed. Times may vary, but allow at least one hour between sessions. See example.

1. Write the actual times when the maximal slow contractions are performed. For you this will be:

.... slow contractions, lasting

.... seconds, with a 4 second rest between each contraction.
        This routine is repeated

... 5 ......times, with a

... 1....... minute rest in between each routine.

Do this 8 times each day.

2. Tick when session of .... fast contractions is performed, each day.

3. Mark with an asterisk * when you do the stop test, once each day.

When you can interrupt your urinary flow midstream at the second void of the day, start to perform the stop test later and later in the day.

Example	Mon	Tues	Wed	Thur	Fri	Sat	Sun
8.15							
9.30 *							
11.0							
12.0 √							
2.30							
4.30							
6.0							
8.30							

Fig. 5.4 Exercise diary.

5. Always tighten the pelvic floor muscles before and during a stress provoking act, such as coughing.

Don't
1. Don't hold the breath during a contraction.
2. Don't use extraneous muscles, such as the abdominals, glutei or thigh adductors.
3. Don't lose heart. Results may take two to six months. Remember, everyone has bad days, especially around period time. Once continence has been established, one session of exercises per day should be encouraged as a lifelong habit.

Vaginal cones

Introduced by Plevnik (1985), weighted vaginal cones are available in sets of five (Fig. 5.5, and see Appendix). The feeling of losing the cone causes the user to contract the pelvic floor in an effort to retain it in the vagina. Cones are used for assessing muscle capability and as an exercise aid. Plevnik (1985) reported that 80 per cent of a trial group (number in study = 10) increased the resting strength of the pelvic floor muscles and 100 per cent increased the active strength, using cones. Stanton *et al.* (1986) reported 67 per cent clinical success (number in study = 15) in a study using cones in the management of stress incontinence and Peattie *et al.* (1988) reported 80 per cent subjective and 60 per cent objective improvement in the cone group, in a clinical trial comparing pelvic floor exercises with cone therapy (number in study = 37). Bridges *et al.* (1988) have also shown this method to be effective in reducing the symptoms of GSI (genuine stress incontinence). This study compared the effect of cone therapy versus interferential therapy (number in study = 69). Improvement of 78.2 per cent (cones) and 90 per cent (interferential therapy) was reported, with cones shown to be more cost effective.

After an explanation of their function, the user is instructed to introduce the lightest cone into the vagina, in the position of a tampon. She then walks around for up to two minutes; if the cone is retained during this time, it is withdrawn by applying tension on the 'tail' and bearing down. The next heaviest cone is then introduced and the procedure repeated until a cone of a certain weight slips out. This cone is then used for ten minutes, twice per day, to exercise the pelvic floor, with the subject performing household tasks while retaining the cone. It is advisable to wear pants for this procedure and the cone should be repeatedly repositioned each time it slips out. When the cone can be retained for ten minutes, it is replaced by the next heaviest cone.

To increase the exercise value of vaginal cones, patients can practise retaining the appropriate cone during coughing and jumping, or any stress provoking act which causes incontinence. This will reinforce the reflex pelvic floor contraction associated with increases in intra-abdominal pressure and the muscle power necessary to retain the cone may eventually be sufficient to prevent urine leakage.

Vaginal cones are designed for one-patient use and careful washing and drying between use will ensure the necessary cleanliness for this purpose. If the cones are to be reused by other women, cleaning with soap and water, followed by disinfection in

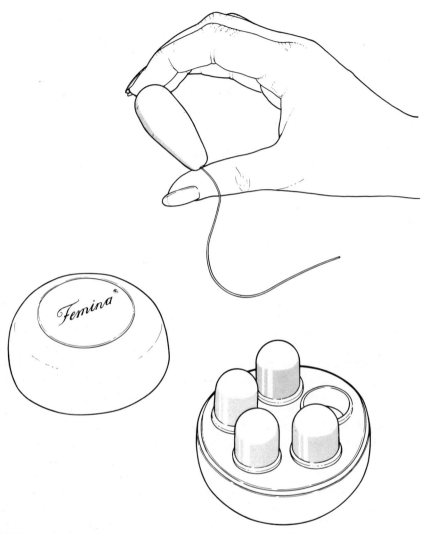

Fig. 5.5 Vaginal cones.

1000 ppm av Cl_2 NaDCC or sodium hypochlorite (community), or 2% glutaraldehyde (hospital) followed by thorough rinsing will be an effective bactericidal and virucidal disinfection process. If these products are not available 70% alcohol may be used instead. (Report by Hospital Infection Research Laboratory, 1989.)

Cones are generally accepted by women of all ages and their use is said to improve compliance to an exercise programme (Peattie *et al.*, 1988). Their use is contraindicated during menstruation or vaginal infection. Clients should be seen at least once every two weeks to reinforce the regime and monitor progress. General pelvic floor exercises should be practised in addition to the use of cones.

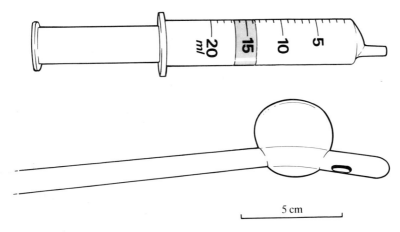

5 cm

Fig. 5.6 Inflated Foley catheter for pelvic floor resistive exercises.

If cones are not available, resisted exercises, working the fast twitch component of the pelvic floor musculature, can be given using a vaginally located Foley catheter (Fig. 5.6), (Laycock, 1987). This is inflated (with air or water) and placed in the vagina in the position of a tampon; the patient is then instructed to tighten the pelvic floor in an attempt to prevent the operator withdrawing the catheter. The feeling of the cuff stretching the pubococcygeus stimulates a muscle contraction and also produces a biofeedback effect. Increased withdrawal force and speed will necessitate a stronger and faster response from the patient, thus enhancing muscle power and coordination. Self-resistance is then introduced and the patient encouraged to practise for ten minutes, twice per day, in the privacy of her own home. As with vaginal cones, the catheter is used in conjunction with general daily pelvic floor exercises. Its use has the advantage over cones of being cheaper (the cheapest catheter will suffice) and the cuff can be inflated to accommodate various vaginal widths; also, graded pressure can be applied, according to the patient's capability. However, a pilot study (Laycock, unpublished data) showed that patients preferred the use of cones to the catheter method.

Electrical stimulation

History

The effect of an electric current applied to the body is no new phenomenon. Greek fishermen in 500 BC felt the electric discharge from black torpedo fish in their nets and Hippocrates in 420 BC proposed a boiled portion of this fish for his asthmatic patients. In AD 16, the Greek physician Pedanius Dioscorides recommended the use of a live torpedo fish in the treatment of prolapsus ani (Kellaway, 1947), which must surely be the forerunner of electrical stimulation for the weakened musculature of the pelvic floor. In more modern times, often confusing reports of different types of electrical stimulation used in the management of incontinence can leave health professionals in a quandary as to 'what is what' and which is the best.

Background

An active muscle contraction is elicited by impulses travelling in the peripheral efferent nerves from the anterior horn cell to the neuromuscular junction where a chemical reaction causes the muscle fibres to shorten. The frequency of these impulses varies depending on the type of muscle fibre to be supplied: i.e. slow twitch fibres receive 10 to 20 pps (pulses per second) and fast twitch fibres receive 30 to 60 pps (Eccles *et al.*, 1958). This process can be mimicked by passing an electric current along the efferent nerves at these low frequencies i.e. 10 to 60 pps (electrically referred to as Hertz (Hz.)). The ensuing muscle contraction is a useful adjunct to pelvic floor exercises in the rehabilitation of weakened pelvic floor muscles and is extremely beneficial for patients who are unable to contract these muscles to command, as it may teach the correct action.

Another variable to be considered is the intensity (amplitude) of the current, as this must be sufficient to excite the nerves. However, the sensory nerves as well as the motor nerves are activated at these low frequencies, causing discomfort, and the intensity will therefore be limited by the subject's tolerance. Electric currents are applied to the body via electrodes (generally two) and their position is very important to ensure that the route of least resistance is selected and the appropriate muscle or muscle group stimulated. Stimulation of the pelvic floor and external urethral sphincter, via branches of the pudendal nerve (S. 2.3.4.), also activates the perineodetrusor inhibitory reflex (see section above on anatomy) and reduces bladder instability (Lindstrom *et al.*, 1983; Fall, 1984; Eriksen *et al.*, 1989).

There are no side-effects to electrical stimulation of the pelvic floor and contraindications include pregnancy, the wearing of a pacemaker, and pelvic malignancy. Electrical stimulation should only be applied to patients who are able to understand the procedure and who can report any discomfort. Electrotherapy can be applied in several different ways, including Faradism, Interferential Therapy and Functional Electric Stimulation.

Faradism

Traditionally, Faradism has been used by physiotherapists to stimulate weakened skeletal muscles and Scott *et al.* (1969) describe its use in the treatment of weakened pelvic floor muscles. In essence, two electrodes are placed over the muscle or nerve to be stimulated and the current passes from one electrode to the other, exciting all the nerve and muscle cells in its path. If the muscle is small or inaccessible, one 'active' electrode is placed over the muscle and the second 'indifferent' electrode sited in the near vicinity. When applying Faradism to the pelvic floor, the active component is either a cylindrically shaped vaginal or anal electrode, or a small pad placed over the perineal body (between the anus and the vagina). A large indifferent electrode is placed over the lower abdomen or over the sacral region. A current (in milliamps, mA) of sufficient intensity is applied at 50 Hz, which will produce a tetanic contraction, i.e. the muscle fibres remain contracted while the current lasts. The current is surged, which means that the intensity is gradually increased, held for the requisite time (say five seconds) and then reduced to zero, allowing a rest period. This procedure is repeated several times, giving the subject the feeling of the perineum tightening and lifting. The subject then 'joins in' with this exercise and thus learns the correct muscle action. Faradism causes discomfort, especially under the indifferent electrode and has been superseded in many centres by interferential therapy and functional electric stimulation, which produce less sensory stimulation for the same motor effect. It is interesting to note that the vagina and perineum are less sensitive than most other areas of the body, and consequently high currents can be tolerated in these areas (personal observations).

Interferential therapy

This form of electrotherapy stems from the concept of two currents 'interfering' with each other in the tissues and hence the name 'interference current', now known as interferential therapy (IFT). IFT was developed to overcome the discomfort associated with other low frequency currents such as Faradism. Low frequency currents encounter a high resistance at the skin/electrode interface and a high voltage is required to drive the current through the skin to the tissues beneath. High frequency currents (2,000 Hz to 10,000 Hz) on the other hand, can pass through the skin more easily, but need modifying to be effective in stimulating neuromuscular structures. There are various ways of modifying this high frequency current and IFT produces its modification by incorporating two currents of different frequencies − say 4,000 Hz and 4,020 Hz. These currents pass easily through the skin into the underlying tissue and if so arranged, will interfere with each other, producing a beat frequency equal to the difference of the two currents, i.e. 20 Hz in this example (Fig. 5.7), which will activate skeletal muscle. It simply remains to crossfire the currents in such a way that the interferential effect takes place in the appropriate tissues. This is achieved by attaching four electrodes to the relevant area of the body. In the case of the pelvic floor, the traditional method, often using suction electrodes, has been adopted in many centres (McQuire, 1975; Savage, 1984) (Fig. 5.8).

In modern equipment, the 'interference' effect can be produced electronically inside the machine, enabling the same effect using two electrodes (Fig. 5.9), (Laycock and Green, 1988; Switzer and Hendricks, 1988) or a vaginal probe housing two electrodes in one unit (Fig. 5.10). A vaginal electrode is more effective than external transcutaneous electrodes in stimulating the pelvic floor, irrespective of the type of current used. This is because the stimulating electrodes are closer to the nerves supplying the muscle fibres; in addition, the sensory nerve supply of the vagina is less

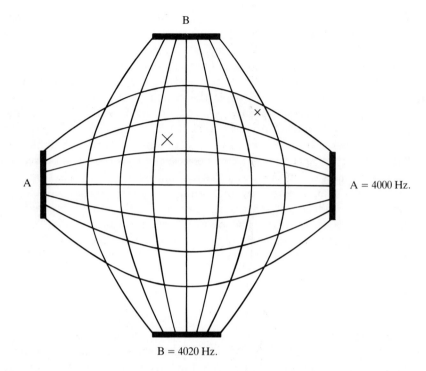

Fig. 5.7 Interferential effect in a homogeneous medium. X (frequency) = 20 Hz.

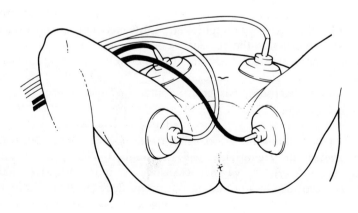

Fig. 5.8 'Traditional' interferential electrode position.

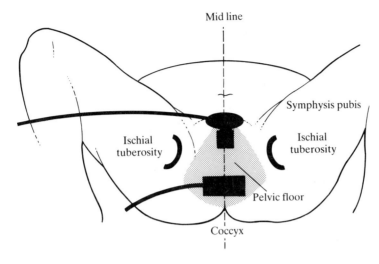

Fig. 5.9 Bi-polar interferential application to the pelvic floor.

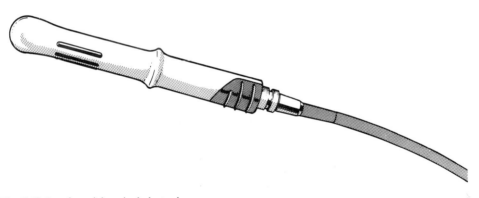

Fig. 5.10 Interferential vaginal electrode.

than to the perineum, and consequently greater current intensity can be tolerated, producing an enhanced motor effect.

A recent clinical study (Laycock, unpublished data) comparing PFE with IFT, showed that approximately 50 per cent of women in each group were cured or very much improved by treatment; a further 20 per cent showed some improvement (number in study = 40). This study utilised IFT in isolation, whereas in practice, IFT would always be an adjunct to PFE.

Wilson *et al.* (1987) described a study of physiotherapy for GSI in which 60 women were assigned to one of four groups, for six weeks' treatment: group 1 – hospital based PFE; group 2 – hospital based PFE and Faradism; group 3 – hospital based

PFE and IFT; group 4 – PFE at home. Approximately two-thirds of the hospital treated patients (groups 1 to 3) experienced marked or moderate improvement at six months, 27 per cent were dry or almost dry. There was no marked difference between the three hospital treated groups, but those patients receiving electrotherapy had a better attendance record. Approximately a quarter of the home-treatment patients noted some improvement. This study confirms that of Scott and Hsueh (1979) who attributed their results using electrotherapy to better patient motivation with the more impressive equipment.

One may therefore question of validity of electrotherapy in the light of Wilson's (1987) and Laycock's (1987) reports and perhaps the emphasis of pelvic floor re-education should be on repeated patient/nurse (physiotherapist) contact to reinforce motivation and compliance, using pelvic floor exercises as the initial modality of management.

Functional electrical stimulation

Originally, this form of stimulation was developed for the management of paraplegic patients, with repeated (three to four hours daily) stimulation, resulting in functional movement. The term FES is now applied to both long-term sub-maximal stimulation (several months) (Farragher *et al.*, 1987; Kidd and Oldham, 1988) and short-term, maximal stimulation (several weeks). Its use in the management of incontinence, using vaginal or anal electrodes (Fig. 5.11) and a small battery operated home unit, (Fig. 5.12) has been developed by many workers, including Plevnik *et al.* (1986); Fall (1984); Fall *et al.* (1986); Eriksen *et al.* (1987 and 1989).

Plevnik *et al.* (1986) reported on a study using maximum current intensity (up to 100 mA) applied for 30 minutes per day for one month on 310 patients suffering from urinary incontinence. The results showed cure or improvement in 56 per cent. Fall *et al.* (1986) report on a study of 40 women with mixed urinary incontinence; 25 patients were improved and another 8 had excellent results, following long-term (several months') vaginal stimulation for several hours per day. The results were more favourable in patients with bladder hyperactivity.

Different effects are produced by altering the frequency of any electrical stimulation unit. A frequency of 35–50 Hz is selected if muscle awareness and ability to contract the pelvic floor is the main problem; 10–20 Hz is generally used for daily long- or short-term FES, in the treatment of GSI. A frequency of 5–10 Hz has been found to be more effective for the management of detrusor instability (Ohlsson, 1986).

With the increase in the cost of 'hands-on' therapy time, it may prove more economical to provide an FES unit for home use (see Figs 5.11 and 5.12 and Appendix). In Europe and Scandinavia, this service is provided by doctors, nurses and physiotherapists and a similar service may well develop in the United Kingdom. In addition, a battery operated neuromuscular stimulator operating at 40 Hz with a vaginal or anal electrode, may help nurses and physiotherapists to teach pelvic floor contractions to clients unable to produce an active contraction.

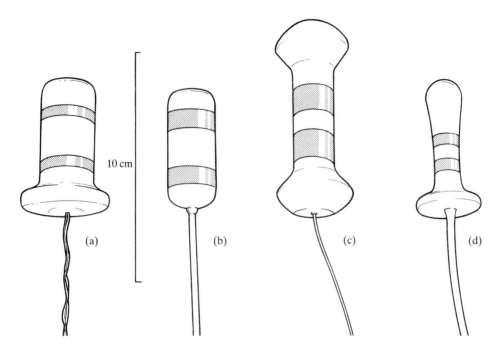

Fig. 5.11 Various electrodes for use with Functional Electrical Stimulation: (a) vaginal; (b) vaginal; (c) vaginal; (d) rectal.

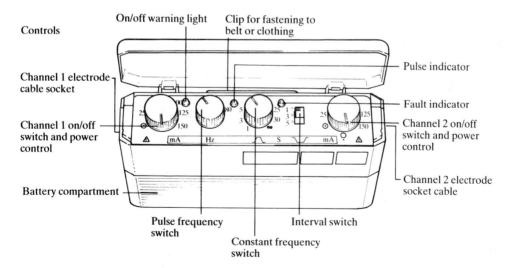

Fig. 5.12 Electrical stimulation unit (Enraf Nonius, ENS 931, Delft, The Netherlands).

Biofeedback

This is a technique whereby the subject is able to receive visual, audio or other sensory information relating to a body function, otherwise difficult to appreciate. In the management of incontinence, biofeedback has been used during cystometry to control detrusor instability (Cardozo, 1984) and in pelvic floor rehabilitation to reinforce muscle contractility and coordination (Kegel, 1951; Burgio *et al.*, 1986).

Biofeedback can be a useful technique for patients who are unable to understand the concept of pelvic floor contraction and relaxation; also, once the action has been performed correctly, biofeedback is an effective stimulus to encourage the patient to greater muscular effort. Any device which enables appreciation of the pelvic floor squeeze and lift, will provide a biofeedback effect.

In simple terms, self-digital vaginal palpation will provide information on the squeeze and lift capability of a contraction and this should be encouraged in all patients. A further simple biofeedback technique involves the 'stop test', which relates the effect of a pelvic floor contraction during voiding on urine flow rate. This helps many patients to appreciate the correct action and avoid the use of extraneous muscles, for example the accessory use of the abdominals may increase urine flow rate. The biofeedback effect of the stop test will also enhance a subject's ability to relax the pelvic floor muscles, which is important for patients who encounter difficulty in this direction, and pelvic floor relaxation exercises can be used as a useful adjunct in the management of dyspareunia and non-neurogenic detrusor/sphincter dyssynergia.

An enhanced biofeedback effect is enabled using a perineometer, with the subject observing the meter. In this way, strength of squeeze and hold time can be modified in response to a visual stimulus. An audio/visual stimulus is often used with an EMG monitoring perineometer, with the sound output increasing as the contraction increases in power and more motor units are recruited. Some sophisticated units allow additional EMG electrodes to be placed over the abdominal muscles, giving information regarding unwanted abdominal muscle activity.

This dual biofeedback effect, i.e. the appreciation of both pelvic floor and abdominal muscle activity, is also enabled using Femina Cones. The correct pelvic floor contraction will improve cone retention and inappropriate action of the abdominals or 'bearing down' will cause the cone to be ejected. This effect is also produced using the vaginally placed Foley catheter method as part of pelvic floor exercises. Biofeedback can therefore increase cortical awareness of pelvic floor contraction and possible extraneous muscle activity.

Future role of the nurse

The future role of the nurse and in fact all health professionals, should be directed to prevention of incontinence and the promotion of continence.

Prevention of incontinence

Hospital and community based nurses have an important role to play in the prevention of incontinence, in two main areas, namely mobility and teaching pelvic floor exercises.

Mobility

The tone of the pelvic floor is maintained by repeated reflex contractions and postural changes. This may be sufficient to maintain muscle tone above the threshold of incontinence and sustain continence for a whole lifetime. Hence exercises of all kinds, e.g. walking, running and cycling etc., will help to ensure healthy pelvic floor musculature (Gordon and Logue, 1985). Many people, unknowingly, may be close to the continence threshold and it takes only a small reduction in muscle tone to tip the balance, resulting in incontinence.

It is therefore important to ensure maximum mobility and activity for all age groups, especially the elderly. By repeatedly standing, walking around and sitting down the pelvic floor will be activated. It is important that the patient and carers are aware of this.

Pelvic floor exercises

There are many instances where PFE can be included in the nurse's role. These include cervical cytology and family planning clinics and well women centres. Hospital based nurses could be involved in teaching PFE to pre- and postoperative patients undergoing gynaecological surgery and all women on prolonged bed rest.

District and practice nurses, midwives and health visitors will find many appropriate opportunities to teach PFE, not only to postnatal and elderly patients, but to those who are on treatment for various conditions. It is perhaps relevant to add here that a vaginal assessment is necessary to ascertain the correct muscle action; patients cannot generally be relied upon to identify this themselves.

Many women believe that urinary incontinence is an inevitable outcome of childbirth and ageing and do not think that it necessitates professional intervention. Others believe nothing can be done to cure their incontinence and some are too embarrassed to bring it to the attention of their nurse or GP, and careful and sympathetic questioning by a district or practice nurse may highlight many hidden cases. Mild cases of incontinence may be cured or may be prevented from becoming severe by early intervention and these patients are often highly motivated to practise daily pelvic floor exercises.

Promotion of continence

Detailed assessment of urinary incontinence is necessary before a meaningful treatment is commenced. However, a strong pelvic floor is a prerequisite for continence and the nurse can safely teach pelvic floor exercises to all incontinent patients. It is also important to explain to relatives and carers the value of pelvic floor re-education to ensure continued care.

Continence advisers are familiar with the importance of the pelvic floor musculature, and this chapter addresses the importance of muscle assessment and re-education, by providing a clearer understanding of the physiological processes involved. With the present economic climate, fewer patients will be eligible for free pads and pants, and this may well promote a move towards the introduction of more self-help methods of dealing with incontinence, where appropriate.

Summary

Pelvic floor re-education is provided by many different health professionals, some of whom are unfamiliar with general muscle re-education methods. This chapter deals with the relevant anatomy and physiology and describes muscle assessment in detail. This enables the planning of individual exercise programmes with specific exercises detailed. The use of vaginal cones and perineometers is discussed and basic electrotherapy principles are presented. It is recommended that all nurses become familiar with the theory and application of pelvic floor rehabilitation in the prevention of incontinence and for the promotion of continence.

Appendix

1. Bourne perineometer.
   Available from: Doncast
   56 Chaldon Common Road
   Chaldon
   Caterham
   Surrey   CR3 5DD

2. Femina Cones.
   Available from: Colgate Medical Ltd
   1 Fairacres Estate
   Dedworth Road
   Windsor
   Berkshire   SL4 4LE

3. Interferential Vaginal Electrode.
   Available from: Nomeq
   23/24 Thornhill Road
   North Moons Moat
   Redditch
   Worcs   B98 9ND

4. FES. Incontinence Stimulation Unit.
   Available from: Nomeq
         23/24 Thornhill Road
         North Moons Moat,
         Redditch
         Worcs B98 9ND

References

Bhatia, N.N., Bergman, A. and Karram, M.M. (1989), 'Effects of estrogen on urethral function in women with urinary incontinence', *American Journal of Obstetrics and Gynecology*, 160: 176–81.

Bridges, N., Denning, J. and Olah, K.S. (1988), 'A prospective trial comparing interferential therapy and treatment using cones in patients with symptoms of stress incontinence', *Neurourology and Urodynamics*. 7(3): 267–8.

Brink, C.A., Sampselle, C.M., Wells, T.J., Diokno, A.C. and Gillis, G.L. (1989), 'A digital test for pelvic muscle strength in older women with urinary incontinence', *Nursing Research*. 38(4): 196–9.

Burgio, K.L., Robinson, J.C. and Engel, B.T. (1986), 'The role of biofeedback in Kegel exercise training for stress urinary incontinence', *American Journal of Obstetrics and Gynecology*, 154: 58–63.

Cardozo, L. (1984), 'Detrusor Instability', in Stanton, S.L. (ed.), *Clinical Gynecologic Urology*, St Louis: C.V. Mosby.

Cardozo, L.D. and Stanton, S.L. (1984), 'Biofeedback: a five year review', *British Journal of Urology*, 56: 220

Carlile, A., Davies, I., Ribgy, A., and Brocklehurst J.C. (1988), 'Age changes in the human female urethra: a morphometric study', *Journal of Urology*. 139: 532–5.

Castleden, C.M., Duffin, H.M. and Mitchell, E.P. (1984), 'The effect of physiotherapy on stress incontinence', *Age and Ageing*, 13: 235–7.

Cummings, G. (1980), 'Physiological basis of electrical stimulation in skeletal muscle', *Certified Athletic Trainers Association Journal*, 3: 7–12.

Currier, D.P., Petrelli, C.R. and Threlkeld, A.J. (1986), 'Effect of graded electrical stimulation on blood flow to healthy muscle', *Physical Therapy*, 66: 937–43.

Eccles, J.C., Eccles, R.M. and Lundberg, A. (1958), 'The action potentials of the alpha motoneurones supplying fast and slow muscles', *Journal of Physiology*, 142: 275–91.

Edwards, R.H.T. (1978), 'Physiological analysis of skeletal muscle weakness and fatigue', *Clinical Science and Molecular Medicine*, 54: 463–70.

Eriksen, B.C., Bergmann, S. and Eik-Nes, S.H. (1989), 'Maximal electrostimulation of the pelvic floor in female idiopathic detrusor instability and urge incontinence', *Neurourology and Urodynamics*, 8: 219–30.

Eriksen, B.C., Bergmann, S. and Mjolnerod, O.K. (1987), 'Effect of anal electrostimulation with the "Incontan" device in women with urinary incontinence', *British Journal of Obstetrics and Gynaecology*, 94: 147–56.

Eriksen, B.C. and Eik-Nes, S.H. (1989), 'Long-term electrostimulation of the pelvic floor: primary therapy in female stress incontinence', *Urology International*, 44: 90–5.

Fall, M. (1984), 'Does electrostimulation cure urinary incontinence?', *Journal of Urology*, 131: 664–7.

Fall, M., Ahlstrom, K., Carlsson, C.A., Erlandson, B.-E., Frankenberg, S. and Mattiasson, A. (1986), 'Contelle: pelvic floor stimulation for female stress-urge incontinence', *Urology*, 3: 282–7.

Farragher, D., Kidd, G.L. and Tallis, R. (1987) 'Eutrophic electrical stimulation for Bell's palsy', *Clinical Rehabilitation*, 1: 265–71.

Fischer, W. (1983), 'Physiotherapeutic aspects of urine incontinence', *Acta Obstetrics and Gynaecology Scandinavia*, 62: 579–83.

Gilpin, S.A., Gosling, J.A., Smith, A.R.B. and Warrell, D. (1989), 'The pathogenesis of genito-urinary prolapse and stress incontinence of urine: a histological and histochemical study', *British Journal of Obstetrics and Gynaecology*, 96: 15–23.

Gordon, H. and Logue, M. (1985), 'Perineal muscle function after childbirth', *The Lancet*, July: 123–5.

Gosling, J. (1979), 'The structure of the bladder and urethra in relation to function', *Urologic clinics of North America* 6(1): 31–8.

Gosling, J., Critchley, H.O.D. and Thompson, S.A. (1981), 'A comparative study of the human external sphincter and periurethral levator ani muscles', *British Journal of Urology*, 53: 35–41.

Hald, T. (1984), 'Mechanism of continence', in Stanton, S.L. (ed.), *Clinical Gynecologic Urology*, St Louis: C.V. Mosby.

Hospital Infection Research Laboratory, Dudley Road Hospital, Birmingham. Personal correspondence with T. Churchward. October, 1989.

Gomer-Jones, E. (1963), 'Non-operative treatment for stress incontinence', *Clinics in Obstetrics and Gynecology*, 6: 220–35.

Juenemann, K.P., Lue, T.F., Schmidt, R.A., and Tanagho, E.A. (1988), 'Clinical significance of sacral and pudendal nerve anatomy', *Journal of Urology*, 139: 74–80.

Kegel, A.H. (1948a), 'Progressive resistance exercise in the functional restoration of the perineal muscles', *American Journal of Obstetrics and Gynecology*, 56: 238–48.

Kegel, A.H. (1948b), 'The Nonsurgical treatment of genital relaxation', *Annals of the Western Journal of Medicine and Surgery*, 2: 213–16.

Kegel, A.H. (1951), 'Physiologic therapy for urinary stress incontinence', *Journal of the American Medical Association*, 146(10): 915–17.

Kegel, A.H. (1956), 'Stress incontinence of urine in women: physiologic treatment', *Journal of the International College of Surgery*, 4: 487–99.

Kellaway, P. (1947), 'The part played by electric fish in the early history of bioelectricity and electrotherapy', *Bull History of Medicine*, 20: 112–37.

Kidd, G.L. and Oldham, J.A. (1988), 'An electrotherapy based on the natural sequence of motor unit action potentials: a laboratory trial', *Clinical Rehabilitation*, 2: 125–38.

Klarskov, P., Belving, D., Bischoff, N., Dorph, S., Gerstenberg, T., Okholm, B., Pedersen, P.H., Tikjob, G., Wormsler, M. and Hald, T. (1986), 'Pelvic floor exercises versus surgery for female urinary stress incontinence', *Urology International*, 41: 129–32.

Kujansuu, E. (1983), 'The effect of pelvic floor exercises on urethral function in female stress urinary incontinence: a urodynamic study', *Annals of Surgery and Gynaecology*, 72: 28–32.

Laycock, J. (1987), 'Graded exercises for the pelvic floor muscles in the treatment of urinary incontinence', *Physiotherapy*, 73: 371–3.

Laycock, J. (1989), 'Algorithm for physiotherapy management of incontinence', *Neurourology and Urodynamics*, 8(4): 353–4.

Laycock, J., Farragher, D., Gardner, J., Herbert, J., Morris, J. and Woodward, A. (1991).

'Standardisation of physiotherapy clinical practice in the management of female urinary incontinence', *Physiotherapy* (in press).

Laycock, J. and Green, R.J. (1988), 'Interferential therapy in the treatment of incontinence', *Physiotherapy*, 74: 161–8.

Lindstrom, S., Fall, M., Carlsson, C.A. and Erlandson, B.-E. (1983), 'The neurophysiological basis of bladder inhibition in response to intravaginal electrical stimulation', *Journal of Urology*, 129: 405–10.

Mahoney, D.T., Laferte, R.O. and Blais, D.J. (1977), 'Integral storage and voiding reflexes', *Urology*, 1: 95–105.

Mahoney, D.T., Laferte, R.O. and Blais, D.J. (1980), 'Incontinence of urine due to instability of micturition reflexes' (Part 1 and Part 2), *Urology*, 3: 229–388.

McQuire, W.A. (1975), 'Electrotherapy and exercises for stress incontinence and urinary frequency', *Physiotherapy*, 61(10): 305–7.

Millard, R.J. (1985), 'Interferential therapy in the treatment of urinary stress incontinence', *Proceedings ICS* (London): 444.

Millard, R.J. (1987), *Overcoming Urinary Incontinence*, Wellingborough: Thorsons, p. 21.

Montgomery, E. and Shepherd, A.M. (1983), 'Electrical stimulation and graded pelvic exercises for genuine stress incontinence', *Physiotherapy*, 69(4): 112.

Neill, M.E. and Swash, M. (1980), 'Increased motor unit fibre density in the external anal sphincter muscle in ano-rectal incontinence: a single fibre EMG study', *Journal of Neurology, Neurosurgery and Psychiatry*, 43: 343–7.

Ohlsson, B.L. (1986), 'Effects of some different pulse parameters on bladder inhibition and urethral closure during intravaginal electrical stimulation: an experimental study on the cat', *Medical and Biological Engineering and Computing*, 24: 27–33.

Peattie, A.B., Plevnik, S. and Stanton, S.L. (1988), 'Vaginal cones: a conservative method of treating genuine stress incontinence', *British Journal of Obstetrics and Gynaecology*, 95: 1049–53.

Perry, J.D. and Whipple, B. (1982), 'Vaginal myography', in Graber, B. (ed.), *Circumvaginal Musculature and Sexual Function*, New York: S. Karger.

Pette, D. (1984), 'Activity-induced fast to slow transitions in mammalian muscle', *Medicine and Science in Sports and Exercise*, 16(6): 517–28.

Pigne, A., Cotelle, D., Kunst, D. and Barrat, J. (1985), 'Physiotherapy and functional electro-stimulation in the post partum', *Proceedings ICS* (London): 265–6.

Plevnik, S. (1985), 'New method for testing and strengthening of pelvic floor muscles', *Proceedings ICS* (London): 267–8.

Plevnik, S., Janez, J., Vrtacnik, P., Trsinar, B. and Vodusek, D.B. (1986), 'Short-term electrical stimulation: home treatment for urinary incontinence', *World Journal of Urology*, 4: 24–6.

Rud, T. (1981), 'The striated pelvic floor muscles and their importance in maintaining urinary continence', in *Female Incontinence*, New York: Alan Liss, pp. 105–12.

Rud, T., Andersson, K.E. and Asmussen, M. (1980), 'Factors maintaining the intraurethral pressure in women', *Investigative Urology*, 17: 343–7.

Savage, B., (1984), *Electrotherapeutics*, London: Faber and Faber, pp. 94–7.

Scott, B.O., Green, V.M. and Couldrey, B.M. (1969), 'Pelvic Faradism: investigation of methods', *Physiotherapy*, 55(8): 302–5.

Scott, O.M., Vrbova, G., Hyde, S.A. and Dubowitz (1986), 'Effects of electrical stimulation on normal and diseased human muscle', in Nix, W.A. and Vrbova, G. (eds), *Electrical Stimulation and Neuromuscular Disorders*, Berlin and Heidelberg: Springer-Verlag.

Scott, R.S. and Hsueh, G.S.C. (1979), 'A clinical study of the effects of galvanic vaginal muscle stimulation in urinary stress incontinence and sexual dysfunction', *American Journal of Obstetrics and Gynecology*', 135: 663–5.

Shepherd, A.M. (1983), 'Management of urinary incontinence; prevention or cure', *Physiotherapy*, 69(4): 109–10.

Shepherd, A.M., Montgomery, E. and Anderson, R.S. (1983), 'Treatment of genuine stress incontinence with a new perineometer', *Physiotherapy*, 69(4): 113.

Sleep, J. (1991), 'Perineal care; a series of five, randomised controlled trials', In Robinson, S. and Thomson, A.M. (eds) *Midwives, Research and Childbirth* (vol 2), London: Chapman and Hall.

Sleep, J. and Grant, A. (1987), 'Pelvic floor exercises in postnatal care', *Midwifery*, 3: 158–64.

Smith A.R.B., Hosker, G.L. and Warrell, D.W. (1989a), 'The role of pudendal nerve damage in the aetiology of genuine stress incontinence in women', *British Journal of Obstetrics and Gynaecology*, 96; 29–32.

Smith, A.R.B., Hosker, G.L. and Warrell, D.W. (1989b), 'The role of partial denervation of the pelvic floor in the aetiology of genito-urinary prolapse and stress incontinence of urine: a neurophysiological study', *British Journal of Obstetrics and Gynaecology*, 96: 24–8.

Snooks, S.J., Barnes, P.R.J. and Swash, M. (1984), 'Damage to the innervation of the voluntary anal and periurethral sphincter musculature in incontinence: an electro-physiological study', *Journal of Neurology, Neurosurgery and Psychiatry*, 47: 1269–73.

Snooks, S.J., Badenoch, D.F., Tiptaft, R.C. and Swash, M. (1985), 'Perineal nerve damage in genuine stress urinary incontinence: an electrophysiological study', *British Journal of Urology*, 57: 422–6.

Stanton, S.L. (1984), 'Urethral sphincter incompetence', in Stanton, S.L. (ed), *Clinical Gynecologic Urology*, St Louis: C.V. Mosby.

Stanton, S., Plevnik, S. and Peattie, A. (1986), 'Cones: a conservative method of treating genuine stress incontinence', *Proceedings ICS* (Boston): 227.

Stoddart, G.D. (1983), 'Research project into the effect of pelvic floor exercises on genuine stress incontinence', *Physiotherapy*, 69(5): 148–9.

Swash, M. and Schwartz, M.S. (1988), *Neuromuscular Diseases* (2nd edn), London: Springer-Verlag.

Switzer, D. and Hendriks, O. (1988), 'Interferential therapy for the treatment of stress and urge incontinence', *Irish Medical Journal*, 81: 30–1.

Tchou, D.C.H., Adams, C., Varner, R.E. and Denton, B. (1988), 'Pelvic-floor musculature exercises in treatment of anatomical urinary incontinence', *Physical Therapy*, 68(5): 652–5.

Wilson, D.P., Al Samarrai, T., Deakin, M., Kolbe, E. and Brown, A.D.G. (1987), 'An objective assessment of physiotherapy for female genuine stress incontinence', *British Journal of Obstetrics and Gynaecology*, 94: 575–82.

Part 2
Management of incontinence

6 Aids and appliances for incontinence

ALAN M. COTTENDEN

Introduction

Over the last ten years the number of companies marketing pads and appliances has grown phenomenally as the hidden problem of incontinence has gradually emerged into the open. Never before has the choice of wares and, therefore, the potential for meeting the needs of a particular sufferer been so great. But it is now quite impossible for a nurse − even one specialising in incontinence − to be familiar with more than a small proportion of the plethora of products on offer. What, then, can the nurse do faced with the common tasks of identifying the best aid for an individual or recommending which equipment should be bought in bulk for use in a hospital or health district?

A search of the literature for information on a particular pad or appliance will usually be disappointing. Few are subjected to proper clinical trials and still fewer trials are ever published. Furthermore, products are changing all the time and so results are often out of date soon after − or even before − they are in print.

Accordingly, the pages that follow devote little space to detailed description of products that can no longer be bought. Rather the emphasis is on identifying the key characteristics and requirements of different groups of products and patients respectively. The needs of incontinent people are unchanging and with a little effort their documented experiences with old products can be fashioned into valuable guidelines for getting the best out of the new designs that have superseded them.

This chapter will concentrate on absorbent products and male and female urine collection appliances. Literature on catheters and legbags is reviewed in the following chapters.

Absorbent products

Absorbent products may be conveniently classified into four groups: disposable bodyworns, disposable underpads, reusable bodyworns, and reusable underpads.

Disposable bodyworns

The most comprehensive trials of bodyworn pads and pants have been those published by Journet (1981), Malone-Lee *et al.* (1982) and Fader *et al.* (1986; 1987). However, the literature also contains accounts of a number of smaller but still very useful projects.

Journet (1981) trialed the fifteen different pad and pant systems described in Table 6.1 with the help of 45 handicapped children, mostly under 15 years old. Sixty per cent were doubly incontinent while the remainder were incontinent of urine only. Each child tested each of a selection of six of the products for a month. Each product was tested by at least 10 children. Questionnaires were used to gather performance data from parents on: ease of application and removal, fit and comfort, absorbency, overall acceptability, and whether or not the products were leakproof.

Nine of the products consisted of a pad held in place by some form of separate plastic pant. As a group they performed badly on every parameter and so it is not surprising that few products of this type are in use today.

The two products which used more normal, textile pants instead of plastic ones were more successful – especially the Kanga system (developed by Willington *et al.*, 1972) in which a disposable pad is held in a waterproof pouch in the pants. The absorbency and leakage properties were deemed disappointing but acceptability, fit, comfort, and ease of putting on and taking off were rated highly. Marsupial systems like this are still widely used by incontinent people – handicapped and able bodied.

As a group the all-in-one diapers were most successful. All were judged easy to put on and take off and all scored highly on acceptability. Interestingly, the diaper without

Table 6.1 Test products in Journet's study (1981)

Pads with separate plastic pants:
IPS pads and pants (IPS Hospital Supplies Ltd)
Inco roll and drop-front pants (Robinson and Sons Ltd)
Inco roll and pull-on pants (Robinson and Sons Ltd)
Sandra pull-on pants and pads (Henley's Group)
Sandra drop-flap pants and pads (Henley's Group)
Maxi snibb and pads (Molnlycke Ltd)
Feel free pull-on pants and pads (Contenta)
Extra large Readinaps (Robinson and Sons Ltd)
Golden Babe overnight nappies and pants (Smith & Nephew Medical Ltd)

Pads with separate textile pants:
Kanga doublet pads and pants (Kanga Hospital Products Ltd)
Kanga pads and pants (Kanga Hospital Products Ltd)

All-in-one diapers:
Cosifits (Robinson and Sons Ltd)
Peaudouce (Peaudouce (UK) Ltd)
Snugglers (Curity)

Plastic-backed pad and stretch net pants:
Maxi plus pads and stretch pants (Molnlycke Ltd)

elastication at the legs (Snugglers) was deemed superior in both fit and comfort to the two with elastics. The best results for leakage and absorbency were found among these three products. Disposable diapers have improved enormously in the decade since this study – particularly with respect to increased absorbency and lower bulk (helped by the advent of superabsorbent polymers), better fit, and improved ergonomics due to features like resealable tapes and better elastication at the legs.

The remaining test product was a rectangular plastic-backed pad to be held in place by stretch net pants. This was one of the forerunners for what is now a common design approach and it performed quite well on comfort and ease of application and removal but fit, absorbency and leakage performance were disappointing. Most products of this kind in use today are shaped rather than rectangular and, like diapers, many now contain some superabsorbent polymer.

Journet (1981) concluded that no single product was suitable for all handicapped children and that it was vital that a choice be offered for experimentation. The extent to which a child was able to help with his or her own management was a key factor in product selection. If the child was able to manage a simple product independently this was often better than a more complex one requiring assistance. Where possible the child should be fully involved with the choice of pad. The needs and constraints of parents, guardians and schools should also be taken into account.

Shepherd and Blannin (1980) compared the performance of three different pad and pant systems with 20 incontinent people of whom the majority lived in their own homes. They were aged 4 to 84 and 18 were female. Each used each pad and pant system for a month. Given the variety of their pathologies (spina bifida, mental subnormality, cerebrovascular accident and dementia) the number of testers was too small to produce very significant results but some valuable insights on user requirements and preferences were obtained. Kanga Standard marsupial pants and pads (Kanga Hospital Products) proved the most popular. They were comfortable and durable but some found the pads bulky and difficult to position and remove. The Molnlycke rectangular plastic-backed pads held in place with stretch net pants proved to be difficult to handle for those who had had strokes and for some parents of disabled children. Those with sufficient mobility and manual dexterity to manage putting them on and taking them off found them comfortable. The Sandra pants and A&D pads (Henley) were the most unsatisfactory. The pants were made largely of plastic and the incidence of skin irritation, sweating and general discomfort was high. However, they provided the best protection for the four disabled children who were totally incontinent. Again, the key conclusion from the study was that no single garment will suit everyone.

Bainton et al. (1982) conducted a crossover trial of Kanga Standard pads and pants (Kanga Hospital Products) against Sandra Pants (Henley) with Bambi pads (Smith & Nephew) with 51 incontinent women in the community. Their ages ranged from 25 to 95 but most were over 65. Each used each system for a month, one half testing in reverse order to the other. The two systems were found to be equally effective at preventing leakage through to wearers' clothes. However, 49 of the women judged the Kanga pants to be more comfortable than the Sandra pants (p < 0.01). By contrast, the Bambi pad was found to be significantly more comfortable than the Kanga pad (p < 0.05). Twenty-seven of the women preferred the Bambi, 11 preferred the Kanga, and 13 rated them equally. In interviews with the testers the reasons for their preferences became clear. The Sandra pants were made largely from plastic and 46 women specifically mentioned that they were hot and clammy to wear. By contrast the textile Kanga pants were praised for their comfort and softness. The reason for the lower popularity of the Kanga pad was its bulk, some women fearing that it would show through their clothes, especially trousers.

Malone-Lee *et al.* (1982) tested eight different pad and pant systems (Table 6.2) with 113 subjects. Sixty lived in the community, while 53 came from a total of five Part III homes. Ages ranged from 30 to 100 but most testers were in their 70s and 80s. Of the 113 subjects, 22 had slight incontinence (enough to significantly wet their underwear); 51 had moderate incontinence (enough to significantly wet their underwear and clothing); and 40 had heavy incontinence (enough to spread beyond their clothing). Prior to the study only 9 had been receiving incontinence pads from community supplies. Of the remainder, 47 had been using privately bought baby pads; five, sanitary pads; and 51, pieces of cloth or tissues.

Subjects were asked to try each product for a month in turn and their views on product performance (and/or their carers' views if appropriate) were gathered by structured interview. Attention was focused on acceptability, leakage, odour, skin problems and difficulties with washing, drying or changing the garment. Refusal to wear any test product and premature withdrawals before the end of the prescribed test period were also noted. Most of the testers tried all eight systems.

One of the products consisted of a rectangular pad held in place by plastic pants while a second involved a similar pad secured by a plastic snib (shaped plastic sheet tied at the waist). As in Journet's study (1981) with handicapped children, these were judged to perform badly, about three-quarters of testers electing to discontinue use before the end of the test period. The snib product failed principally because it was awkward to apply; the plastic pant product principally because of the infantile appearance. Complaints of excessive sweating were common with both.

Four of the products consisted of a plastic-backed pad secured with stretch net pants. Three of the pads were rectangular, the other (the Tenaform pad) hour-glass

Table 6.2 Test products in Malone-Lee *et al.*'s study (1982)

Pads with separate plastic pants:
Sandra plastic pants and insert pads (Henley's Group)
Maxi snibb and pads (Molnlycke Ltd)

Plastic-backed pads and stretch net pants:
Comfort insert pads 2245 and 2260 and stretch pants (Ancilla (UK) Ltd)
Maxi plus pads and stretch pants (Molnlycke Ltd)
Tenaform pad and stretch pants (Molnlycke Ltd)
Dandeliner and stretch pants (Smith & Nephew Medical Ltd)

Marsupial pads and pants:
Kanga Lady pants and Single pads (Kanga Hospital Products Ltd)
Kanga Standard pants and Standard pads (Kanga Hospital Products Ltd)

---

shaped. The Ancilla pad was reported to be uncomfortable due to its considerable width (220 mm) and abrasive surface. This was the only pad of the eight to consistently cause skin problems (for 15 per cent of testers). The main complaint with the Smith & Nephew system concerned the pants. These were reported to slip and roll at the waist and to fray with use. In addition both systems were reported to leak frequently.

The other two products of this type were the most popular with residents in Part III homes. Of the 41 who expressed a preference – often in conjunction with care assistants – 36 chose the shaped, plastic-backed pad (Molnlycke Tenaform) and stretch pants as their favourite of the eight. It was acceptable to practically all testers. Many commented on its good absorbency and comfort and reported that it was easy to change. Although the product is no longer available in this form it has been superseded by many others based on the same design. These are probably the most commonly used products for heavy incontinence in UK hospitals today. The remaining five Part III home residents chose the Molnlycke Maxiplus pad as their favourite. Good comfort and absorbency were reported. Similar pads are still on the market.

The last two test products consisted of rectangular pads to be used with marsupial pants. The Kanga Standard combination proved disappointing, largely because of the considerable bulk of the pad. Many wearers and carers had trouble changing it too. By contrast the Kanga Lady pant and Single pad was easily the most popular product among lightly and moderately incontinent women living in the community. The absorption capacity proved inadequate for heavy incontinence. Excellent reports were received with respect to leakage, ease of changing and acceptability. Both of the Kanga products are still commercially available and in wide use.

Interestingly, no odour problems were reported with any of the test products. Seven of the eight were the favourite of at least one community resident underlining Journet's (1981) plea to treat incontinent people as individuals with different priorities and requirements.

Fader et al. (1986; 1987) have conducted the most comprehensive and wide-ranging trial to date involving a total of twenty-six different pad and pant systems (Table 6.3) and 137 testers. They divided the pads into three categories following the advice of suppliers' sales literature. Group 1 products were for light day time incontinence; group 2 for heavy day time incontinence; and group 3 for heavy night time incontinence. Testers – or their carers, if necessary – selected which group(s) of products they wished to try.

The mean age of the 34 testers in group 1 was about 70 and all but one were women. Of the 101 testers in group 2, 79 were women and the mean age of the group was about 80. Of the 47 testers in group 3, 45 were also in group 2 and 39 were women. Interestingly, the severity of a tester's incontinence correlated highly with his or her mobility and level of independence. Ninety-seven per cent of group 1 testers were able to change their own pads without help and all of them could walk without assistance. The majority lived independently in the community. By contrast only around 5 per cent of testers in groups 2 and 3 could change their own pad and only a quarter could walk unassisted. Almost all of them were resident on long-stay hospital wards or in Part III homes. Accordingly, Fader et al. (1986; 1987) suggested that assessing for

Table 6.3 Test products in Fader *et al.*'s study (1986; 1987)

Group 1

Marsupial pads and pants:
Kanga Lady pants and Single pads (Kanga Hospital Products Ltd)
Sandralux pants (Henley's Group) and Single pads (Kanga Hospital Products)

Inco roll and pants:
Moltexal interliner roll and pants (Brevet Hospital Products)

Plastic-backed pads and stretch pants:
Dandeliner (Smith & Nephew Medical Ltd)
Tenette Plus (Molnlycke Ltd)
Sanitary towel (Johnson & Johnson (UK) Ltd)
Daisy (LIC Ltd)
Molinea, small (Paul Hartmann AG)
Tranquility (Henley's Group)
Cumfie, small (Vernon Carus Ltd)

Group 2

Plastic-backed pads and stretch pants:
Tenaform, normal (Molnlycke Ltd)
Polypad (Undercover Products International Ltd)
Interliner (IPS Hospital Supplies Ltd)
Molinea, large (Paul Hartmann AG)
Incocare (Robinson & Sons Ltd)
Cumfie, large (Vernon Carus Ltd)
Cumfie, medium (Vernon Carus Ltd)

All-in-one diaper:
Slipad (Peaudouce (UK) Ltd)

Wingfold pads and stretch pants:
Doublet (Kanga Hospital Products Ltd)
Incontinette (Ancilla (UK) Ltd)

Marsupial pads and pants:
Kanga Standard (Kanga Hospital Products Ltd)
Urocare (IDC (UK) Ltd)

Group 3

Plastic-backed pads and stretch pants:
Tenaform, super (Molnlycke Ltd)

All-in-one diaper:
Tenders (Ancilla (UK) Ltd)

Wingfold pads and stretch pants:
Diaper (IPS Hospital Supplies Ltd)
Deopad (LIC Ltd)

mobility and independence would give a good first indication of the size of pad likely to be appropriate for an individual.

Each test subject trialed each of the test products in his or her chosen group in random order for about seven days per product. Patients' or carers' assessments of pad and pant performance were gathered using questionnaires covering: overall reaction, leakage, confidence, dry and wet comfort, ease of application and removal, staying in place, coverstock/absorbent break-up, odour, effects on skin, reaction to pad dimensions and absorbency, and pant fit. Incidences of premature withdrawal from testing any product were also noted.

In keeping with Journet's (1981) and Malone-Lee *et al.*'s (1982) results with subjects able to express a preference for themselves, each of the products in group 1 was liked very much by at least 20 per cent of testers. However, some emerged as clear favourites. The most popular was Kanga Lady marsupial pants with Kanga single pads. This scored well on all parameters except for ease of pad positioning and removal. Conversely, it performed exceptionally well for staying in place securely once positioned. The next most popular was the Brevet tissue roll which wearers had to cut to their preferred length before fitting into pants containing a waterproof panel. This system scored at least reasonably well on all test parameters but wearers particularly appreciated the freedom to choose the 'pad length' that suited them best. In consequence no tester reported that this product had any effect at all on which clothes she felt able to wear.

All the remaining group 1 pads were plastic-backed. Four of the seven (one a sanitary towel) were rectangular and contained just fluff pulp as absorbent. Interestingly, these were the four least popular pads of the ten, each for a different reason. Not surprisingly, the sanitary towel was found to have an inadequate absorption capacity − it was only included in the project because many incontinent women make use of them. The Molinea pad was judged too wide (190 mm) and too thin (6 mm) and performed badly for both comfort and leakage. The Dandeliner achieved the greatest freedom from leakage but at the expense of excessive bulk so that it attracted the lowest scores for comfort and restriction on the clothing testers felt able to wear. Cumfie performed badly on comfort, apparently because of its rather incompliant structure, and the tendency for the pulp to break up and the coverstock to split in use.

Tranquility, a very thin (6 mm) rectangular pad containing tissue paper impregnated with superabsorbent powder drew an interesting response: it was second only to the Kanga Lady/Kanga Single pad for the number of testers liking it very much but, paradoxically, more testers strongly disliked it than any other product. This polarity was not mirrored in any other performance parameter − such as comfort or leakage − but a considerable number of subjects withdrew prematurely from testing the product due to dissatisfaction with the accompanying pants within which it was a fiddly task to secure a pad. Accordingly, the polarity may have been between those who liked the pad and those who disliked the pants.

The remaining two products in group 1 were shaped, with a waist at the centre. The Tenette Plus contained only fluff pulp absorbent while the Daisy also contained superabsorber. The Daisy attracted a similar polarity of overall reaction to the other superabsorber-containing product, Tranquility. It performed reasonably well for all performance parameters except for leakage on which it scored badly. Surprisingly, given their contoured shape, both performed badly on comfort. Trials on more recent products (Philp *et al.*, 1989a; 1989b; 1989c) have shown that shaping can make a very positive contribution to comfort and so it is probable that the poor performance recorded in the Fader *et al.* (1986; 1987) study was due to the shortcomings of what amounted to early implementations of a good design idea.

Neither odour nor skin damage emerged as significant problems with any of the ten pad and pant systems. In general, the dry comfort and leakage properties of this group of products were good while wet comfort was universally poor.

Subsequently Cottenden *et al.* (1987) analysed the Fader data in search of correlations that would elucidate the relationships between different clinical and technical performance parameters. Overall pad reaction correlated strongly with confidence (p < 0.01); impact on the clothes testers felt able to wear (p < 0.05) and wet comfort (p < 0.05), and more weakly (p just > 0.1) with dry comfort and leakage incidence. Confidence varied greatly between pads and seemed largely to reflect the freedom from leakage afforded (p < 0.01). The greatest single factor affecting the freedom of testers to wear whatever clothes they wished was pad length (p just > 0.1). Dry comfort was determined largely by pad width (p < 0.001) and pad length (p < 0.01) while the compliance of pads to lateral compression was also important.

The incidence of leakage of pads correlated significantly (p < 0.1) with the absorption capacity of the central portion of pads as measured in the laboratory; the more absorbent material there, the greater the freedom from leakage. Freedom from leakage was also enhanced by a rapid penetration of urine into the pad (p < 0.05). Fader *et al.* (1986; 1987) concluded that group 1 testers tended to select products which were of low bulk, comfortable and effective, and closely resembling normal underwear.

The results from group 2 and group 3 tests were somewhat simpler. None of these products contained any superabsorber. The Tenaform normal − a shaped, plastic-backed pad − emerged as the clear favourite in group 2. It was associated with low leakage and was deemed to be easy to put on and take off. The Slipad all-in-one diaper was the next most popular, largely because of the freedom from leakage which its large bulk conferred. However, many carers reported difficulties with putting it on their patients and some were concerned by the infant connotations of a diaper-style design.

Of the remaining ten pads in group 2, six were rectangular and plastic backed. None was very popular but the Cumfie (large) was best due, apparently, to its good absorption capacity. Its tendency to slip from position was its main weakness. The two wingfold pads were unpopular largely due to difficulties in putting them on and taking them off. The unpopularity of the two marsupial systems was essentially caused by the unpleasantness to nursing staff of removing used pads from their patients' pant pouches.

In their analysis of Fader *et al.*'s (1986; 1987) data, Cottenden *et al.* (1987) identified significant correlations between overall pad reaction and leakage incidence (p < 0.01) and confidence (p < 0.05). Ease of pad removal also made an important contribution (p just > 0.1). Incidence of leakage correlated highly (p < 0.001) with the absorption capacity of the central portion of pads as measured in the laboratory. They also established (Cottenden, 1988b) that wingfolding and shaping reduced the frequency of severe leakage compared with simple rectangular designs while elastication had a still greater beneficial effect. Fader *et al*. (1986; 1987) concluded that group 2 patients appeared to require pad and pant systems that could be easily changed by their carers and which could cope with large amounts of urine without leaking.

The results for group 3 were similar to those for group 2. The Tenaform super – a shaped plastic-backed pad – emerged as the clear favourite scoring very well on incidence of leakage, and ease of putting on and taking off. The wingfold and all-in-one diaper designs tested with this group suffered from the same limitations as the corresponding products in group 2.

In the five years since Fader *et al*. (1986; 1987) chose their test products, shaped pads and all-in-one diapers have become the most popular design choices for group 2 and group 3 categories of users. Not surprisingly, given their poor performance in the Fader study, rectangular and wingfold products have declined in popularity. It is now commonplace to find superabsorbent powders included in both shaped pads and diapers.

In subsequent years the research team at St Pancras Hospital in London used variations on the basic Molnlycke Tenaform shaped pad design in a series of studies on the mechanisms of pad performance. Malone-Lee *et al*. (1988) tested pads which were identical in all respects except for having six different coverstock facings. Two of the materials – based on rayon fibres – were highly hydrophilic, while a third – apertured polyethylene film – was highly hydrophobic. The three remaining materials – one based on polyester and two on polypropylene fibres – had intermediate properties. Twenty-three heavily incontinent patients on geriatric long-stay hospital wards tested pads with the six coverstocks in random order for four weeks each and had fortnightly skin examinations.

No significant differences in skin health were observed between pads with different coverstocks. Thus doubt was cast on the trend at the time away from rayon and towards polypropylene for pad coverstocks. Interestingly, this trend has since slowed and, in some countries, begun to reverse in the face of heightening concern for green issues. Rayon is much more biodegradable than polypropylene. The study had two principal limitations which have not so far been addressed. Firstly, the test pads contained only fluff pulp absorbent: the results might have been different if pads had also contained superabsorbers. Secondly, the testers were not sufficiently alert to be able to express an opinion on pad comfort. It would be valuable to repeat the project with alert testers.

Clancy and Malone-Lee (1991) trialed four variations on the Molnlycke Tenaform pad to discover the impact of different combinations of fluff pulps with a superabsorber on leakage performance. The severity of leakage from some 5,500 used pads of the four designs was noted as they were removed from subjects on geriatric long-stay hospital wards. The results were complex but illustrated that, firstly, including some superabsorber in a pad did not guarantee a good product. Secondly, however, the absorption properties of fluff pulps could be enhanced if the properties of the superabsorber and its distribution in the absorbent core were carefully chosen.

Hanley *et al*. (1988) conducted an elegant comparative crossover trial of two marsupial pad and pant systems which highlighted the potential inaccuracies inherent in uncontrolled trials. For historical reasons incontinent people in North Lothian in Scotland had been receiving IDC Urocare marsupial pads and pants prior to the trial while those in South Lothian had been receiving products of a similar design from Hygicare. Test subjects were recruited into four groups, two from each area. During a first four week period, half of the subjects received the product usually supplied to those resident in the other area, while half continued to use their usual product. During the second four week period the reverse took place.

Seventy-six testers completed the trial, 36 from North Lothian (mean age 72, standard deviation 20) and 40 from South Lothian (mean age 75, standard deviation 17). Only nine were men; four from North Lothian, five from South Lothian. The response in the two areas was quite different. Whereas patients in South Lothian found no significant differences between the two garments, those in North Lothian rated the Hygicare garment better on comfort ($p < 0.01$), leakage ($p < 0.001$), odour ($p < 0.01$) and avoidance of skin problems ($p < 0.01$). Since the two groups of testers were extremely well matched for age and sex, were cared for by the same group of Community Nurses and came from areas of similar social structure the researchers suggested that the explanation for these results was to be found in the Hawthorne effect. In the Hawthorne studies recounted by Roethlisberger and Dickson (1939) it was demonstrated that people tend to respond favourably to all innovations, whether or not the innovations themselves represent improvements, because of the attention given to them when participating in the trial.

Hanley *et al*. (1988) suggested that the Hygicare product was in fact better but that its superiority over the IDC Urocare product was masked in North Lothian by the Hawthorne effect causing them to look favourably upon the latter since it was new to them and the apparent cause for the extra attention they received. Conversely, in South Lothian, the superiority of the Hygicare product was enhanced and exaggerated by the Hawthorne effect. This is a frustrating limitation since asking those already experienced with incontinence products to test something new seems, on the face of it, to be a sensible approach to evaluation. It is a good way to discover major faults and gross improvements but will not provide a sound basis for making major buying decisions. The Hanley study serves as a warning to treat with caution the results of trials in which a new product is compared only with that already in routine use. Trials initiated and/or supported by the supplier of the new product are even more problematic since they are susceptible to a double portion of Hawthorne effect with both test subjects and trial nurses receiving extra attention. This is an annoying, but nevertheless real, barrier for companies seeking objective assessment of their products.

A considerable number of uncontrolled trials of disposable absorbent body worn pads have been published (Tam *et al*., 1978; Beber, 1980; Watson, 1980; Orr and Black, 1982; Orr and Sykes, 1982; Kelly, 1982; Watson, 1983; Boulton and Kazemi, 1984; Turner, 1987; Dawson and Wilkinson, 1988; Mackin and Webb, 1990) but, because they were uncontrolled, their findings need to be treated with caution and are of limited clinical value.

Merret *et al.* (1988) conducted a small but methodologically interesting controlled comparative trial of two disposable pads: Depend from Kimberly Clark and Softeze Moderate from Sancella. The test subjects were six longstay psychogeriatric patients in their 70s (four women and two men) who had previously been using washable pads. They used the Depend for a week followed by the Softeze for a further week. Subjective opinions of nurses were quantified using a visual analogue scale from 0 to 9. No severe skin problems were encountered but the Softeze was judged to be more comfortable and a little kinder to the skin. Both disposable pads reduced nursing time for pad changing and unpleasantness for nurses compared with the product worn previously. Less clothing was sent for laundry but the accompanying cost saving was exceeded by the increase in product costs.

Philp *et al.* (1989a; 1989b; 1989c) compared the performance of the six small, plastic-backed pads for light incontinence described in Table 6.4. Four were rectangular (two with a superabsorber, two without), and two were shaped (one with a superabsorber and one without). Twenty women living independently in the community tested each product for a week in turn in random order. Their ages ranged from 14 to 90 and their opinions on pad performance were gathered by informal interview and questionnaire with attention particularly focused on leakage, comfort, staying in place and whether or not the pad showed beneath clothing. The two shaped pads, Tenette and Serenity, emerged as the clear favourites but, importantly, 40 per cent of testers would not have been willing to continue using each of these two products after the trial. Each of the six pads except Restful was at least one person's favourite but the two traditional, rectangular pulp-filled pads were generally the least popular. The two rectangular pads containing superabsorber usually obtained intermediate ratings.

Major differences were found between the age groups in relation to the pads. Almost all older women (over 65) liked Tenette but disliked Serenity while almost all the younger women (under 65) rated Serenity highly. Freedom from leakage is a fundamental requirement of a pad and yet the two products which were most effective at preventing leakage – Serenity and Tenette – were reported to leak often by a quarter of testers. The least effective pad – Restful – was reported to leak often by

Table 6.4 Test products in Philp *et al.*'s study (1989a; 1989b; 1989c)

Pads containing just fluff pulp absorbent:
Tenette extra (Molnlycke Ltd)
Cumfie, small (Vernon Carus Ltd)
Restful 200 (IDC (UK) Ltd)

Pads containing superabsorbent polymers:
Serenity, regular (Johnson & Johnson USA)
Conveen, regular (Coloplast Ltd)
Super strola, large (IPS Hospital Supplies Ltd)

---

nearly half. Taken as a group, the three products containing superabsorber were no more effective at reducing the frequency of leakage than the three without. However, leakages from Serenity were judged to be generally smaller in quantity than for any of the other five pads.

Wet and dry comfort varied considerably between products but the two shaped pads performed best. The impressive surface dryness of Conveen in laboratory tests (Cottenden *et al.*, 1989), did not translate into good wet comfort in the experience of users. The incompliance of Conveen when it was wet masked the potential benefits of a dry surface. In others of the pads a tendency to break up or twist when wet contributed to poor wet comfort.

Philp *et al.* (1989a; 1989b; 1989c) concluded that the presence of a superabsorber in a pad by no means guaranteed freedom from leakage and good wet comfort. However, the potential of superabsorbers to enhance pad performance in these respects was considerable.

The design, evaluation and informed purchase of pads would be much easier if there were standards; that is, laboratory tests which were known to be good predictors of clinical performance. With the help of an International Standards Organisation working group, Cottenden (1990a; 1990b; 1990c) is currently coordinating an international project to create a standard for freedom from leakage for pads designed to cope with heavy urinary incontinence. Six different pads – each in three sizes and absorbencies – have been selected to represent the range of designs and materials in current use and have been assessed for leakage by some 35 technical and user test centres from a dozen countries. It will be some time before an International Standard emerges from the work but it is already clear that some simple laboratory tests for estimating the functional absorption capacity of pads produce results which correlate very well with user test data. Analysis of the user test data has also shown differences in the leakage properties of pads of different designs at low urine volumes (less than 50 ml of urine, say). About 30 per cent of rectangular pads, 10 per cent of shaped pads and 5 per cent of all-in-one diapers with less than 50 ml of urine in them leaked at least a little bit. For large urine volumes (over 300 ml, say) performance was dominated by the quantity of absorbent in the pad. Performance at intermediate volumes was governed by the two factors in combination.

Disposable underpads

Disposable underpads generally contain either fluff pulp or multiple layers of cellulose wadding as absorbent, are backed with polyethylene, and faced with a water-permeable non-woven coverstock. Some designs include a layer of cotton and/or rayon linters between coverstock and wadding while some manufacturers have begun experimenting with the inclusion of some superabsorber. In the past, coverstocks were usually made from hydrophilic rayon fibres but, supposedly to improve wet comfort, most are now made from polypropylene, which is hydrophobic. Lengths, widths, thicknesses and weights vary considerably and pads may be sealed on two or four sides with the additional option of the polythene being folded over on top of the absorbent along two edges with the objective of impeding lateral leakage.

The literature on disposable underpads is sparse. Motivation to trial specific products is low since most of the design features can be easily altered by the manufacturer who will often be willing to produce pads to the preferred specification of bulk buyers. The lack of literature is sad since large quantities of these products are used at great expense and there is virtually no published data to aid purchasing decisions. Liversy and Krushner (1978) estimated the consumption of the UK health service at 120 million pads for 1972, for example. A further discouraging factor for would-be trialists is that underpads are widely misused (Ramsbottom, 1982); the practice of packing incontinent patients with several underpads at a time is still common.

The UK Department of Health and Social Security has attempted to assist buyers by publishing a specification (DHSS, 1972) which suggests a minimum absorption capacity of 44 ml of water per 100 cm^2 of pad. Thomas and Hubbard (1979) have also designed a laboratory apparatus for measuring the absorption capacity and surface dryness of pads under pressures calculated to simulate those under a supine patient.

It seems that the only published comparative trial of different underpads is that due to Henderson and Rogers (1971). They tested four designs: A and B contained 17-ply cellulose wadding beneath a layer of cotton linters while C and D contained 19-ply cellulose wadding. A and C were 60 cm × 40 cm while B and D were 60 cm × 45 cm. Eighteen hospitalised women, mostly in their 70s and 80s, tested each in turn for a week. A and B were found to be softer and to cause fewer skin reactions. C and D tended to adhere to the skin, to disintegrate and to rustle noisily when moved. The two smaller sized pads were deemed adequate for most patients while the larger ones were appreciated for more restless testers. Projects in which disposable underpads have been compared with reusable products are described in the section on reusables.

Underpads are supplied as non-sterile items and some workers (for example, Bradbury, 1985) have drawn attention to the risk of infection, particularly from pads containing recycled paper. Leigh and Petch (1987) and Sprott et al. (1988) conducted microbiological studies on a range of pads. Both studies identified low levels of bacterial contamination but concluded that the risk to patients was minimal unless they were immunocompromised in some way. Accordingly, disposable underpads should not be used in surgical or obstetrical situations or when patients have broken skin.

Reusable bodyworns

The use of makeshift washable cloth pads for incontinence disappeared from most hospitals and homes many years ago with the advent of specially designed disposable products. But in recent years washable garments – in the form of either pads to be secured by separate pants, or of all-in-one designs – have been emerging as commercial products. Initially, the impetus came from laundries – mostly in North America – which rented the products to hospitals along with their laundry services.

The main attraction to hospitals was the hope of reduced costs but the dioxin scare in 1989 (Sadler, 1989; Haddad, 1990) and the enormous growth in interest in environmental issues since the late 1980s has motivated many health care agencies to look afresh at the reusables alternatives (Seaman, 1988).

The environmental damage which can be caused by wood pulping processes has received considerable media coverage along with concern over the growing shortage of landfill sites for disposal. There has been much ill-informed 'green' journalism and a good deal of panic response from disposables manufacturers anxious to protect their markets. Dubious claims to 'biodegradability' and 'environmental friendliness' have been rife on packaging when neither term has any universally agreed meaning. More recently, government agencies and trades associations on both sides of the Atlantic have been addressing the environmental questions surrounding disposables in a more coordinated fashion (Department of Trade and Industry, 1990; Noonan, 1990; 1991). For example, a solid waste policy based on a hierarchy of waste management approaches has been adopted by the Environmental Protection Agency in the United States (Noonan, 1991). This recommends the following in order of decreasing desirability: source reduction (i.e. use as little material as possible in the first place), composting/recycling/reuse of waste materials, incineration and landfilling.

Various attempts to compare the environmental impact of disposable and reusable products have been made (Noonan, 1990; Franke, 1991), mostly sponsored by manufacturers of disposables. A valid comparison has to take a so-called 'cradle to grave' approach so that the energy and environmental costs of manufacture, reuse (washing and drying) and disposal are all taken into account. Published comparisons have generally indicated that environmental costs of using disposables or reusables are somewhat similar.

Many workers have attempted to compare the relative financial costs of managing incontinence with disposable or reusable products. Some have considered the introduction of reusables where disposables have been used, others the other way round. Most have added a proviso that any cost saving should not be at the expense of quality of care for patients. Grant (1982) compared an undescribed washable incontinence pad – which had been in routine use before the trial – with an undescribed disposable diaper. The thirty test subjects were from a psychogeriatric hospital. No significant difference in skin health were found between the two products but the superior convenience of the disposable product was judged not to justify their extra cost relative to reusables.

Haeker (1985) compared an undescribed washable product in routine use before the trial with an undescribed disposable diaper in trials with 26 residents in an 'intermediate care facility'. The disposable caused more skin problems. Stone (1986) subsequently reported that, although use of disposables in the Haeker study had almost halved the quantity of laundry generated, the centre reverted to reusables because of skin problems and because the reusables left them more time to spend with residents.

For her trial Dolman (1988) recruited from a Part III home 11 residents (10 of them women) who had all been using Kanga marsupial pants and pads. During an initial two month period testers used one of two new disposable products depending on which suited them best: some used an all-in-one diaper (Slipad from Peaudouce), and others a shaped pad secured with stretch net pants (Tenaform from Molnlycke). During the second two month period patients changed to ACS Medical reusable insert liners held in place with either a polyester mesh support pant or drop-front snap-on briefs, depending on individual needs. The study involved too small a sample of testers to produce conclusive results but Dolman (1988) made a number of useful observations. The disposable products were found to be comfortable, easy to handle, kind to the skin and to create less laundry as compared with the reusables. Disadvantages of the disposable were greater expense, the need for storage of a stock and lack of dignity for those wearing the diaper-like all-in-one. Dolman (1988) concluded that the extra expense of the disposables was justified by their superior performance.

Hu *et al.* (1989; 1990) conducted a study to compare the costs and benefits of a disposable product (Promise pads and stretch net pants from Scott Health Care Products) and the reusable cloth diapers and underpads previously in routine use. (Promise pads in the United States are similar to Tenaform pads by Molnlycke in Europe.) Data on the frequency, volume and type of incontinence of residents in a nursing home were used to select 34 matched pairs of testers. One of each pair continued using the cloth products for five weeks while the other member of each pair changed to the disposable pad. Thus the trial was controlled in so far as the two groups of testers were matched pairs, but uncontrolled in the sense that half of them were using a new product and half continuing with their old. It was found that subjects using the reusables soiled two to three times more clothes and bedclothes. The skin of 65 per cent of the disposables users improved over the five weeks compared with only 3 per cent of the cloth product users. During interview carers scored the disposables as superior on freedom from leakage, containment of odour and bedding protection. There was no significant difference between the per day product costs for the two forms of management but the laundry costs associated with the disposable pad were significantly ($p < 0.01$) lower.

Not surprisingly, a full spectrum of conclusions has been reported in the disposables versus reusables debate. However, several useful observations can be made. Firstly, it is surely not possible to draw blanket conclusions from trials comparing one particular disposable with another particular reusable. Secondly, cost comparisons inevitably depend upon the durability of the reusable. This in turn will depend upon how carefully it is used and laundered and on the criteria for determining when to discard it. Thirdly, financial calculations will depend a great deal on how carer time and laundry services are costed. Reusables carry a further 'cost' in terms of risks and inflexibility. For example, equipping an individual or an entire ward with reusables represents a commitment to their use for a considerable period. Expensive mistakes can be made if the choice turns out to have been wrong or frustration can ensue if a better product becomes available soon after the purchase has been made. Nevertheless the potential of reusable bodyworn products remains high and largely unexplored. It is to be hoped that more comprehensive studies will be performed in the future. There appear to be no published trials in which different reusable bodyworn products are compared.

Philp and Cottenden (1988) and Cottenden and Philp (1988) have described the development of Kylie pants – reusable absorbent pants for lightly incontinent men and women. Their aim was to provide an alternative to disposable pads which gave greater discretion and normality and freedom from the regular ordering, storing and disposal associated with single use items.

Reusable underpads

As with reusable bodyworns, the majority of trials involving reusable underpads have compared their performance with disposable underpads or drawsheets. Most trials have been uncontrolled in the sense of comparing a new reusable with an established disposable. Of all reusable underpads the Kylie bedsheet by Nicholas Laboratories Ltd has been subjected to by far the greatest number of tests: either in its original form of a needlepunched rayon absorbent layer with a hydrophobic (yellow) nylon facing; or, latterly, a combined rayon and polyester absorbent layer with a hydrophobic (pink) brushed polyester facing. In both versions it is used with a separate waterproof sheet.

Silberberg (1977) reported the first trial on the Kylie sheet (nylon-faced version). Each of 32 bedbound, elderly, female patients was managed with each of three absorbent products for a seven day period. The first product was the Kylie sheet; the second, the Kylie sheet impregnated with an antimicrobial agent; the third, the cotton drawsheet in routine use before the trial. The frequency of bed changes with Kylie sheets was less than half that for the drawsheet. They were also judged to keep skin drier; to be associated with fewer cases of erythema; and to reduce odour. No distinct advantage could be attributed to the antimicrobial agent except a possible further suppression of odour.

In a similar study Burton (1979) compared Kylie sheets with the linen drawsheets already in routine use in a long-stay hospital ward. Twelve elderly men were divided into two equal groups. The first used the Kylie sheet for twenty-eight days followed by the draw sheet for a similar period; the second tested the products in the reverse order. Draw sheet usage produced almost 50 per cent more items for laundry and for every Kylie sheet used, 2.6 draw sheets were required. The Kylie sheet also performed better on odour, skin dryness, erythema and wrinkling and creasing. Prinsley and Cameron (1979) obtained similar results in a similar trial involving 23 geriatric patients.

Broughton (1979) compared the performance of the Kylie sheet (nylon-faced version) with the drawsheets and disposable bed sheets already in established use with 18 patients from a psychogeriatric ward. They were divided into two groups, the first used the Kylie sheet for two weeks followed by a further two weeks with drawsheets and disposable pads while the second group used them in reverse order. He reported a 45 per cent reduction in items needing laundering when the Kylie sheet was used, and estimated a 40 per cent reduction in costs. Skin health was also better when the Kylie sheet was used.

Scoffin, a laundry manager, described his experiences in introducing Kylie sheets into a health district (Scoffin, 1980). He found that during the six months immediately following its introduction the use of disposable pads fell to approximately 17 per cent of its previous level. During the subsequent six months, however, it climbed back to 57 per cent. Clearly calculations based on the initial figure of 17 per cent would have yielded unduly optimistic predictions concerning costs. He established that the Kylie sheet would withstand at least 100 washes and that, in his situation at least, a minimum of 12 sheets per patient were needed to ensure a steady supply.

Pottle (née Smith) has conducted several studies involving the Kylie sheet (Smith, 1979; 1985; 1986; Pottle, 1986). The first (1979) compared the nylon-faced version with the disposable bodyworn pads in established use. The original protocol ran into some problems of logistics but some data were gathered for both hospital and community use. One hospital used the Kylie sheet for over a year enabling an estimate of comparative cost for the two management approaches to be made. Use of the Kylie sheet was estimated to be be over four times cheaper than management with disposables due largely to reductions in the frequency of bed changes and the quantity of items for laundry.

Smith subsequently published the results (1986) of a small study in which six subjects in the community tried a lightweight version of the Kylie sheet (300 g instead of 600 g) with a polyester facing in place of the nylon. Five of the testers had previously been using the heavier product. Improvements in washing, drying, comfort and staying in position were reported. In a similar comparison involving five hospital patients (Pottle, 1986) she subsequently found the lightweight Kylie sheet was of inadequate absorbency for this group. Although both these studies were too small to produce conclusive results which can be applied with confidence to other populations, they both draw attention to key factors to be borne in mind when the use of reusable bedpads is being considered.

Finally (Smith, 1985) she compared a 600 g Kylie sheet with polyester facing with disposable bedpads (Hygi pad from Undercover Products, and Polyweb pad from Smith & Nephew) used with and without a washable hydrophobic cover sheet (Everdri from Undercover Products). The Hygi pad was a 60 cm square plastic-backed pad containing ten layers of cellulose wadding; the Polyweb pad was of the same size but had a layer of cotton and rayon linters between the coverstock and fourteen layers of cellulose wadding; and the Everdri was made from a brushed polyester fabric. Five subjects from each of three hospitals tested each combination for one or two weeks. The views of ward nurses on product performance were obtained by questionnaire offering multiple choice answers to standard questions. The Kylie sheet was judged superior to all the other methods of management on all parameters; that is, absorbency, effects on skin, wrinkling and odour. Smith estimated that using the Kylie sheet produced a saving of around 30 per cent on costs as compared with any of the other methods tested.

Jones (1982) reported a project in which twelve subjects (7 women, 5 men, eleven aged over 75) in the community or nursing homes used no absorbent bed sheet for a period of a month, and then used Kylie bed sheets for a further month. Carers were asked to record their observations on structured forms. Attention was particularly focused on odour, skin condition, comfort, restlessness, bed wetness, sheet wrinkling, washing and drying problems, and overall assessment of product benefit. The Kylie sheet was associated with a significant reduction in odour (p < 0.01) and in the frequency with which bed and night clothes had to be changed (p < 0.01). No significant differences in skin condition, comfort, restlessness or bed wetness were found (p > 0.05). Some 80 per cent of carers reported no problems with washing and drying. All carers had access to domestic washing machines but those without spin dryers reported problems. Some useful data on the durability of the Kylie sheets was also presented: 90 per cent of the original batch of 43 sheets were still usable after 70 washes (seven months' use based on three sheets per patient used in rotation); 80 per cent after 140 washes (fourteen months); and 50 per cent after 190 washes (nineteen months). Jones (1982) rightly pointed out that the situation for hospital use would be quite different. Revealingly, he reported that it had been difficult to break residential care staff of their habit of changing their patients' sheets routinely during the night even when use of the Kylie sheet removed the need. He also described their reluctance to put patients to bed naked below the waist – an advisable practice if urine was to be confined to the Kylie sheet.

Williams *et al.* (1981) described the first clinical trials of Kylie sheets (nylon-faced version) in the United States. Thirty-six hospitalised patients (25 women, 11 men, 34 aged over 60) were involved, Approximately half continued to use the established disposable underpad for a fourteen day observation period followed by Kylie sheets for a subsequent fourteen days. The remainder used the products in reverse order. The disposable pad consisted of plastic-backed cellulose wadding with a cotton and nylon facing. Carer observations were recorded on daily sheets. Significant (p < 0.001) reductions in skin wetness, product creasing, frequency of linen changes and urine odour were associated with the Kylie sheet. The reduction in bed changes was 43 per cent. In a subsequent two week period the skin wetness of four patients was noted each time their Kylie sheet was changed and the weight of the soiled one measured. The mean weight of urine in sheets when the skin was judged to be dry was 162 g (standard deviation 142, maximum 425); and 270 g (standard deviation 116, maximum 765) when it was wet. An estimated cost saving of 40 per cent was calculated for Kylie sheets usage taking laundry and product costs into account. The calculation appears to have assumed a Kylie sheet lifetime of 200 washes.

Meier (1986) compared the performances of the Kylie bed sheet (polyester-faced version) and the Gericare reusable underpad. The latter had a cotton facing and integral waterproof backing. The test subjects were 12 women and 12 men over the age of 60 from two psychogeriatric units. The products they used prior to the study were not disclosed. Each subject used each of the two test products for seven days. Use of the Gericare product yielded about twice as much bed linen laundry as the Kylie sheet and kept patients' skin dry on about ten times fewer occasions. The Gericare product was only about a third of the price of the Kylie sheet but Meier (1986) judged that the extra cost would be recouped rapidly in reduced laundry costs.

Clancy (1989a; 1989b) evaluated a range of bed protectors focusing particularly on urine leakage, skin condition, odour, and ability of pads to stay in place on the bed. Each of the 70 test subjects was heavily incontinent of urine at least three nights per week. Forty-one were resident on three long-stay wards for the elderly while the other

29 lived in the community. The products on trial were used in a different order on each ward and in random order in the community, and each was used exclusively for either one week (community) or two (hospital). Five systems were tested: the Dundee reusable bedpad (Gimson-Tendercare), consisting of a cotton facing, polyester absorbent and integral butyl waterproof backing; the Kylie sheet (Nicholas Laboratories Ltd) in the polyester-faced version; a cotton drawsheet; a fluff pulp disposable underpad (Ancilla UK Ltd) and shaped, fluff pulp filled bodyworn pads (Tenaform Super, Molnlycke Ltd) held in place with stretch net pants (Tenafix, Molnlycke Ltd). Clancy (1989a; 1989b) found that more items of bed linen were changed when the disposable bedpad was used than for any other system. If a patient was wearing the bodyworn pad a drawsheet was just as effective as any other disposable or reusable underpad at preventing leakage onto the bottom sheet. The Kylie sheet leaked less frequently than the Dundee but the latter was reported to stay in place on the bed better and to be less likely to smell. In the community fewer significant differences were found between the two reusables but in general the Kylie was preferred. The disposable underpad was not popular in either setting. Subjects' skin condition changed continually throughout the project but such changes were not associated with any particular product.

Few people would now dispute that in the case of heavy urinary incontinence reusable bedpads usually provide better protection for both bed and patient than either disposable underpads or drawsheets. A more pertinent question for today's nurses concerns the decision whether or not to change from using disposable bodyworn pads to reusable bedpads. The driving force for posing the question is generally the hope of cost savings but the task of comparing costs is far from trivial.

The cost per patient per day for reusables depends on initial product costs, product lifetime, frequency of pad changes and laundry costs. Depending on laundry turnaround times, between five and twelve bedpads will be needed for each patient. The lifetime of pads will depend, primarily, on the materials they contain, how carefully they are washed and dried, and the criteria used for discarding them. For pads containing an integral plastic backing it is usually the durability of the backing that determines lifetimes. Severe faecal staining may be another reason for discarding and manufacturers generally recommend that their products are not used with those who are regularly incontinent of faeces. In theory, the frequency of changing reusable bedpads should be lower than that for disposable bodyworns since they generally have much higher absorption capacities. However, if ward routines are inflexible potential savings will often not be fulfilled in practice without sustained effort from nurse managers. The cost of washing and drying is often set at a particular cost per item by hospital laundries but real costs can be somewhat higher because pads may take in excess of half an hour to dry in a standard dryer. Obviously, pads without an integral backing dry faster since hot air has access to both sides of the absorbent layer. Laundry costs for bed linen should also be considered. These will depend on the efficiencies with which the products − reusable or disposable − prevent leakage onto the bed.

The cost per patient per day for disposable bodyworns depends on product costs, frequency of pad changes and costs of disposal − generally by incineration for hospitals, and into landfill sites for the community. Environmental considerations were discussed in the section on reusable bodyworns. Given this complexity it is quite impossible to draw firm and universal conclusions with regard to the relative costs of reusables as a group compared with disposables as a group.

Another factor in the choice concerns organisation and convenience. Disposables have to be ordered regularly, stored, delivered and disposed of. Reusables are less problematic in these respects but the effort required to create and maintain effective arrangements for laundering should not be underestimated; indeed, without the active support of laundry staff (or the ready availability of good washing and drying facilities in the community) the introduction of reusables is ill advised. A further concern for some would-be buyers of reusables is the potential for cross-infection between different users: a pad used by one patient on a ward may be used by another when it returns from the laundry.

If the decision to buy reusables is made there are still more problems to face since only three (Meier, 1986; Clancy 1989a; 1989b) of the thirty or forty different products on the market have been subjected to a controlled trial which has been published. Reusable underpads clearly have an important role to play in managing incontinence. However, a great deal more data are required if buyers are to be able to make informed choices both between disposables and reusables, and between different reusable products.

Collection appliances

Male collection appliances

Male collection appliances fall into two broad categories. Firstly, there are those generally termed bodyworn urinals. They usually comprise a semi-rigid rubber cone held in place over the penis with the help of belts and straps and attached to a leg drainage bag. Although these designs have been around for a long time the literature on them is restricted to brief coverage in general articles on incontinence devices. Norton (1985), for example, advises that they should be fitted by an experienced appliance fitter and that wearers must have sufficient manual dexterity to manage them properly. If there is a slight retraction of the penis, a pubic pressure flange may counteract the tendency to retraction. Blannin (1985) counsels that a high standard of personal hygiene is a vital requirement for this category of aid. Cottenden (1988a) records that bulkiness, soreness, sweatiness and fiddliness are frequent complaints of users.

The second category comprises what are generally termed condoms, sheaths or external catheters. They consist of a thin, close-fitting, latex sheath which is usually held in position by means of skin adhesive, an elastic strap, or – in the early versions – surgical tape. They drain into a leg bag. They are a much newer class of products and they have attracted more literature, some describing the advantages and limitations of the class in general, some comparing different products of similar type. Newman and Price (1985) reviewed the experiences of 60 patients with spinal cord injuries who had used external catheters for an average of 48 months each (range 1 to 159 months). The specific products used were not declared. Just over half of the men were found to have positive urine cultures at the time of their last follow-up. Positive cultures were more common among quadriplegics than paraplegics and in those with complete lesions than incomplete. Radiography revealed that 27 of the 34 patients with no urinary tract abnormalities prior to using external catheters had developed them. The most common changes were bladder trabeculation (26), bladder diverticulitis (14) and reflux (4). Patient histories and examinations revealed tendencies towards poor hygiene and inattention to adequate bladder emptying. Equipment obstruction was common because of twisting or improper placement of drainage apparatus. Newman and Price (1985) concluded that, with care, external catheters may accomplish adequate drainage and sterile urine but the hazards of infection and overdistension should be countered by medical monitoring and sustained patient education. However, these results need to be interpreted with caution since some of the bladder problems encountered may have had little to do with the use of external catheters. Comparisons with similar groups using alternative forms of management for their incontinence would need to be made to establish links between products and problems.

Several authors have catalogued informally the experiences of their patients with external catheters and issued warnings on possible complications. Golji (1981), for example, estimated that 15 per cent of his spinal cord injured patients who used external catheters developed some kind of penile or urethral complication and classed them as irritative, allergic or compressive in aetiology. Mild skin rash, erythema and allergic reaction to skin adhesive or condom material were the most common. Tissue damage due to the hard roller ring at the proximal end of the condom or due to tapes or straps to secure the condom in place were potentially the most dangerous. Jayachandran et al. (1985) listed a similar series of warnings from their experiences. They highlighted the need to ensure that devices did not become twisted distal to the penis leading to outflow obstruction and the danger of urinary tract infection. They also stressed the importance of maintaining adequate hygiene of the genitalia; of changing condoms at least daily to relieve pressure and inspect the skin; and varying the site of application of straps and adhesive on the penis if possible.

Bransbury (1979) studied allergy to condoms and adhesives. Some of the products she studied have been changed or discontinued since but she established an interesting protocol of patch testing which produced positive results for at least one material in just over half of the 50 men tested. In addition 40 per cent of external catheter users contacted by letter claimed to have experienced symptoms or signs of contact allergy to either a condom and/or adhesive.

Hirsh et al. (1979) set out to discover whether external catheters caused urinary tract infection (UTI). No UTI (defined as bacteriuria $> 10^3$ colonies per ml) developed in any of 79 men who were established as infection free at the start of the study and who were prospectively categorised as 'cooperative'. By contrast, 8 of 15 who were prospectively categorised as 'uncooperative' – in the sense of tugging at the appliance pulling it off and kinking the tubing, for example – developed a UTI within 9.6 days.

Johnson (1983) conducted a retrospective study of 64 elderly men on an extended care unit. Thirty-five of them (group A) used external catheters; 24 leaving them undisturbed while 11 frequently manipulated, twisted and pulled at their condoms. The remaining 29 men (group B) did not use external catheters and constituted a control group. Groups A and B were well matched for age, disease and length of hospital stay. The rate of UTI (defined as bacteriuria $> 10^5$ colonies per ml) in group A during their period of hospitalisation (mean length 35 months) was 63 per cent; while for group B (mean period of hospitalisation 57 months) it was 14 per cent. No significant difference was found between UTI rates in those who did and did not interfere with their appliances.

Ouslander *et al.* (1987) examined the relative frequency of urinary tract infection and bacteriuria among male nursing home patients managed with and without external catheters. They prospectively followed four cohorts of men; those wearing external catheters continuously (30); those wearing them just at night (19); those whose incontinence was managed without the use of external catheters (13); and those who were continent (30). They were followed for a mean of 5.4 months. Of the men using catheters continuously 87 per cent had at least one episode of bacteriuria ($> 10^5$ colonies per ml) and 40 per cent at least one incident of symptomatic UTI. These rates were significantly higher than those for continent men or incontinent men not using external catheters. Levels were intermediate for those using external catheters only at night. For comparison they calculated the incidence per patient month at risk for 54 patients managed by indwelling catheter and produced a figure of 0.21. The corresponding value for those using external catheters continuously was 0.08.

There is no major published study comparing different designs of external catheters but there have been several comparative trials involving a small number of products and test subjects. Leval and Louis (1978–9) described the introduction of a new condom adhesive strip (Urihesive from E.R. Squibb & Sons) among 18 paraplegic men who had previously been securing their condoms with Elastoplast tape. They reported that condoms secured with Urihesive stayed in place longer, resulted in fewer skin lesions and did not restrict urine flow through the urethra.

Gonzalkorale and Lawless (1987) recounted their experiences in trying the InCare sheath (InCare Medical Products) with 22 hospitalised elderly men the majority of whom had been using the Macrodom sheath (Macarthy's Surgical Ltd) previously. The Macrodom sheath was a simple device secured in place with surgical tape. The InCare sheath was more sophisticated, including an integral adhesive coating, anti-reflux valve and a wider bore outlet than the Macrodom. Nursing staff recorded their observations on an initial two week period with Macrodoms followed by a further two weeks with the InCare sheath. The average wear time for Macrodoms was 12.3 hours compared with 33 hours for InCare sheaths. Only one tester had longer wear times with Macrodoms. Nurses took some time to learn how to use the InCare sheath and their results during the second week of trial were better than in the first, an observation which has important implications for the choice of test period with unfamiliar products.

The InCare sheaths were six times as expensive as Macrodoms but Gonzalkorale and Lawless (1987) estimated that, if the cost of surgical tape, skin care products, pads and linen changes were taken into account along with the longer wear times for InCare sheaths, then they were cheaper per patient day.

With the help of six elderly hospitalised men, Watson (1989) compared the performance of three different sheath drainage systems: system A; the Simpla Bubble-U sheath and adhesive strip with Simpla Trident long tube leg bag or Simpla 2000 ml S2 drainage bag (Simpla Plastics Ltd); system B; the Conveen sheath and Uriliner adhesive strip with the Conveen 600 ml leg bag (Coloplast Ltd) or Simpla 2000 ml S2 drainage bag; and system C; the Conveen Sheath and Uriliner adhesive strip with the Seton 750 ml leg bag (Seton Ltd) or Simpla 2000 ml S2 drainage bag. Each sheath was available in a range of sizes. The Simpla sheath had a reinforced funnel and bubble at the outlet designed to impede twisting and kinking and an outlet lumen of 8 mm. The Conveen sheath had no reinforcement or bubble and a 6.5 mm outlet lumen. Each man used each system for a week in random order and nurses recorded their observations on questionnaires.

The average times for which the sheaths of the three systems stayed in place were: A, 17 hours; B, 12 hours; and C, 13 hours. The differences between the performance of A and B was significant ($p < 0.01$) but the differences between C and either A or B failed to reach significance at the $p = 0.05$ level. None of the subjects had to be withdrawn from the trial because of broken skin. Few problems were encountered with any of the systems distal to the sheath indicating that product selectors should focus their attention primarily on the sheath itself. Watson indicated that his sample size was too small to produce any firm conclusions but pointed out that different systems worked best for different people. Accordingly, it is reasonable to suggest that patients should be free to choose the sheath and drainage system they find the most effective for them.

In a subsequent study Watson and Kuhn (1990) compared system A (Simpla Bubble-U sheath and adhesive strip with Simpla Trident long tube leg bag or Simpla 2000 ml S2 drainage bag (Simpla Plastics Ltd)) from his earlier study (Watson, 1989) with another system; system D, say, comprising the Conveen sheath and uriliner (Coloplast Ltd) with the Simpla Trident long tube leg bag or Simpla 2000 ml S2 drainage bag. Six men used each of the two systems in turn for five non-consecutive days. A crossover design was adopted with half the subjects using each system first. The sheath in system D stayed in place significantly ($p < 0.05$) longer than the sheath in system A – the mean times were 22.5 and 17 hours respectively. System A stayed on for a mean time of 17 hours in both studies and Watson and Kuhn (1990) therefore suggested that the results from system B (Conveen sheath and Uriliner adhesive strip with the Conveen 600 ml leg bag or Simpla 2000 ml S2 drainage bag) in the first study could be compared with the results for system D (Conveen sheath and uriliner with the Simpla Trident long tube leg bag or Simpla 2000 ml S2 drainage bag) in the second. Since the mean wear times for these two systems were 12 and 22.5 hours respectively and the same sheath was used in each he concluded that the choice of drainage bag could have a substantial impact on the length of time for which a given sheath would stay in place. Accordingly, experimenting with combinations of sheaths and bags from different suppliers could be fruitful.

Female collection appliances

The female anatomy presents the inventor of collection appliances with a much greater challenge than the male. The patent literature is replete with designs but none to date has attained commercial success or widespread use. At the heart of the problem is the difficult requirement of providing a psychologically acceptable, comfortable and leakproof seal with the body without skin irritation or undue risk of tissue damage.

Pieper *et al.* (1989) have provided an excellent review of efforts to date to meet this requirement. Some counsel that female collection appliances are an unattainable pipedream while others pin their hopes on new materials with unprecedented levels of biocompatibility. Whoever is right, there is no sign of the answer on the horizon as yet.

Summary

Almost all the trials reviewed in this chapter conclude that 'no one product suits everybody'. Indeed, what is ideal for one person may be disastrous for another. Accordingly, it is both absurd and unacceptable to dispense pads and appliances without a proper assessment of the individual, the individual's incontinence, abilities and disabilities, lifestyle and environment – and those of the individual's carer(s) too, if appropriate. Wherever possible, a range of products should be offered for experimentation.

Some products are more susceptible to misuse than others but all will work best if those using them – wearers and carers – receive proper instruction and ongoing support. Periodic review and reassessment is also important.

Since only a tiny minority of products on the market has been subjected to proper controlled trial, most buying decisions currently have to be made on the basis of pooled experience, anecdotal evidence and small, uncontrolled trials. There will always be a need for good trials but they are time-consuming and the cost of covering the entire range of products and keeping up with all new developments would be astronomical. Accordingly, there is a need for trials to be designed in such a way as to yield information which can be extrapolated to whole classes of products rather than just being limited to the specific products tried. For example, what are the merits and demerits of using shaped pads secured with net pants compared with all-in-one diapers? Secondly, the whole incontinence community – manufacturers, suppliers, buyers, carers and wearers – would benefit from a coordinated network of centres willing to trial products to a common protocol and pool their findings for the benefit of all.

References

Bainton, D., Blannin, J.B. and Shepherd, A.M. (1982), 'Pads and pants for urinary incontinence', *British Medical Journal*, 285: 419–20.
Beber, C.R. (198), 'Incontinent', *American Journal of Nursing*, March: 483–4.
Blannin, B. (1985), 'A guide to selecting incontinence aids', *Geriatric Medicine*, Feb.: 20–4.
Boulton, S.W. and Kazemi, M.J. (1984), 'Evaluating disposable briefs', *American Journal of Nursing*, Nov.: 1413 and 1439.

Bradbury, S.M. (1985), 'Incontinence pads and clostridium infection' (letter), *Journal of Hospital Infection*, 6(1): 115.

Bransbury, A.J. (1979), 'Allergy to rubber condom urinals and medical adhesives in male spinal injury patients', *Contact Dermatitis*, 5: 317–23.

Broughton, N. (1979), 'The Kylie: a ward trial of this absorbent drawsheet', *Nursing Times*, July: 1140–1.

Burton, B. (1979), 'Keeping the incontinent patient dry', *Nursing Mirror*, May: 25–9.

Clancy, B. (1989a), 'No more guesswork! Choosing incontinence products', *The Professional Nurse*, June: 455–6.

Clancy, B. (1989b), 'Bed protectors: no easy choice', *Nursing Times*, 85(33): 70–5.

Clancy, B. and Malone-Lee, J.G. (1991), 'Reducing the leakage of body-worn incontinence pads', *Journal of Advanced Nursing*, 16: 187–93.

Cottenden, A.M. (1988a), 'Incontinence pads and appliances', *International Disability Studies*, 10: 44–7.

Cottenden, A.M. (1988b), 'Incontinence pads: clinical performance, design and technical properties', *Journal of Biomedical Engineering*, 10: 506–14.

Cottenden, A.M. (1990a), 'The ISO pad leakage project: progress report', *Proceedings INDEX 90 Congress, Baby products and adult protection*, Geneva, April.

Cottenden, A.M. (1990b), 'The ISO pad leakage project: findings to date', *INDA Journal of Nonwovens Research*, 2(2): 23–8.

Cottenden, A.M. (1990c), 'The ISO pad leakage project: results and conclusions', *Proceedings INSIGHT '90 Adult Incontinence Products Conference*, Toronto, Nov., I, 1–21.

Cottenden, A.M., Fader, M.J., Barnes, K.E., Jones, T.M. and Malone-Lee, J.G. (1987), 'The clinical performance of incontinence pads in relation to technical testing', *Proceedings INSIGHT '87 Adult Incontinence Products Conference*, Toronto, Sept., II: 1–30.

Cottenden, A.M. and Philp, J. (1988), 'Innovation for incontinence', *Journal of District Nursing*, Oct.: 7–10.

Cottenden, A.M., Philp, E.J., Butchers, D. and Garside, J. (1989), 'Comparative clinical and technical study of six absorbent products for lightly incontinent adults', *Proceedings INDA-TEC '89 International Nonwoven Fabrics Conference*, Philadelphia, June, 219–39.

Dawson, B. and Wilkinson, E. (1988), 'Ward based comparison of two continence care products', *Care-Science and Practice*, 6(4): 105–6.

Department of Trade and Industry (1990), 'The disposal of hygiene products', *Proceedings of a workshop at Warren Spring Laboratory*, Stevenage, November 1990.

DHSS (1972), *Specification for: disposable incontinence underpad*, TSS/D300,000, June.

Dolman, M. (1988), 'The cost of incontinence', *Nursing Times*, 84(31): 67–9.

Fader, M.J., Barnes, K.E., Cottenden, A.M. and Malone-Lee, J.G. (1986), 'Incontinence garments: results of a DHSS study', *Health Equipment Information*, 159.

Fader, M.J., Barnes, K.E., Malone-Lee, J.G. and Cottenden, A.M. (1987), 'Choosing the right garment', *Nursing Times*, 15 April: 78–85.

Franke, M. (1991), 'Approach of a multinational company to assist management of solid waste: a research program for baby diapers', *INDA Journal of Nonwovens Research*, 3(1): 41–3.

Golji, H. (1981), 'Complications of external condom drainage', *Paraplegia*, 19: 189–97.

Gonzalkorale, M. and Lawless, J. (1987), 'Looking for the perfect fit', *Nursing Times*, 83(40): 38–9.

Grant, R. (1982), 'Washable pads or disposable diapers?', *Geriatric Nursing*, July/Aug.: 248–51.

Haddad, C. (1990), 'Marketing disposables in a green consumer climate', *Proceedings INDEX 90 Congress, Baby products and adult protection*, Geneva, April.

Haeker, S. (1985), 'Disposable vs. reusable incontinence products)', *Geriatric Nursing*, Nov./Dec.: 345–7.

Hanley, J., Beveridge, M., Aitken, C., Dick, T., Prescott, R. and Hunter, J. (1988), 'Clinical trial of incontinence garments: recognition of the possible influence of the Hawthorne effect', *Clinical Rehabilitation*, 2: 285–90.

Henderson, D.J. and Rogers, W.F. (1971), 'Hospital trials of incontinence underpads', *Nursing Times*, 4 Feb.: 141–2.

Hirsh, D.D., Fainstein, V. and Musher, D.M. (1979), 'Do condom catheter collecting systems cause urinary tract infection?', *Journal of the American Medical Association*, 242(4): 340–1.

Hu, T., Kaltreider, D.L. and Igou, J. (1989), 'Incontinence products: which is best?', *Geriatric Nursing*, July/Aug.: 184–6.

Hu, T., Kaltreider, D.L. and Igou, J. (1990), 'The cost-effectiveness of disposable versus reusable diapers: a controlled experiment in a nursing home', *Journal of Gerontological Nursing*, 16(2): 19–24.

Jayachandran, S., Mooppan, U.M.M. and Kim, H. (1985), 'Complications from external (condom) urinary drainage devices', *Urology*, XXV(1): 31–4.

Johnson, E.T. (1983), 'The condom catheter: urinary tract infection and other complications', *Southern Medical Journal*, 76(5): 579–82.

Jones, I.G. (1982), 'A community trial of absorbent incontinence sheets', *Health Bulletin*, 40(6): 279–85.

Journet, C. (1981), *DHSS aids assessment programme: incontinence aids for handicapped children*, HMSO.

Kelly, L.S. (1982), 'Incontinence: cost effective management in a psychogeriatric ward', *British Journal of Geriatric Nursing*, Sept./Oct.: 9–10.

Leigh, D.A. and Petch, V.J. (1987), 'Sterility of incontinence pads and sheets' (letter), *Journal of Hospital Infection*, 9 Jan: 91–3.

Leval, J. de and Louis, J.C. (1978–9), 'Urihesive: a new aid in the management of urinary incontinence in male paraplegic patients', *Paraplegia*, 16: 299–302.

Liversy, B. and Krushner, J.A. (1978), 'Incontinence: knowing and caring', *Journal of Community Nursing*, 1(3): 31–2.

Mackin, B. and Webb, T. (1990), 'Evaluating bodyworn continence pads', *Nursing Standard*, 4(19): 36–9.

Malone-Lee, J.G., Butchers, D., Cottenden, A.M., Fader, M.J. and Barnes, K.E. (1988), 'A clinical study of absorbent products', *Proceedings INDA TEC '88*, Fort Lauderdale, Florida.

Malone-Lee, J.G., McCreery, M. and Exton-Smith, A.N. (1982), *A community study of the performance of incontinence garments*, DHSS Aids Assessment Programme, HMSO.

Meier, V. (1986), 'Absorbent draw-sheets', *Australian Nurses Journal*, 15(10): 46–7.

Merrett, S., Adams, L. and Jordan, J. (1988), 'Incontinence research provides some answers', *Australian Nurses Journal*, 18(2): 17–18.

Newman, E. and Price, M. (1985), 'External catheters: hazards and benefits of their use by men with spinal cord lesions', *Archives of Physical Medicine and Rehabilitation*, 66 (May): 310–13.

Noonan, E. (1990), 'Disposing of the disposables', *Nonwovens Industry*, July: 20–6.

Noonan, E. (1991), 'Green report sets guidelines, causes reactions in disposables industry', *Nonwovens Industry*, January, 52–6.

Norton, C. (1985), 'Incontinence in the elderly', *Nursing Times*, 30 Jan.: 17–20.

Orr, J. and Black, E. (1982), 'A boost to morale', *Nursing Mirror*, 14 July.

Orr, J. and Sykes, B. (1982), 'Dry nights', *Nursing Mirror*, 21 July.

Ouslander, J.G., Greengold, B. and Chen, S. (1987), 'External catheter use and urinary tract infections among incontinent male nursing home patients', *Journal of the American Geriatrics Society*, 35(12): 1063–70.

Philp, J. and Cottenden, A.M. (1988), 'Light relief', *Nursing Times*, 84(31): 72.

Philp, J., Butchers, D. and Cottenden, A.M. (1989a), 'Are you sitting comfortably?', *Nursing Times*, 85(7): 68–72.

Philp, J., Butchers, D. and Cottenden, A.M. (1989b), 'Absorbing facts', *Journal of District Nursing*, Aug.: 5–8.

Philp, J., Cottenden, A.M. and Butchers, D. (1989c), 'Pads for people', *Journal of District Nursing*, Sept.: 4–6.

Pieper, B., Cleland, V., Johnson, D.E. and O'Reilly, J.L. (1989), 'Inventing urine incontinence devices for women', *IMAGE: Journal of Nursing Scholarship*, 21(4): 205–9.

Pottle, B. (1986), 'When the sheets were changed', *Nursing Times*, 26 Nov.: 64–6.

Prinsley, D.M. and Cameron, K.P. (1979), 'Management of urinary incontinence', *Medical Journal of Australia*, 1: 578–9.

Ramsbottom, F.J. (1982), 'The use of incontinence underpads in hospital', *Nursing Times*, 3 Nov.: 1868–9.

Roethlisberger, F.J. and Dickson, W.J. (1939), *Management and the worker: an account of a research program conducted by the Western Electric Company, Hawthorne works*, Chicago: Harvard University Press.

Sadler, C. (1989), 'Sullied whiteness', *Nursing Times*, 85(12): 16–17.

Scoffin, G.J. (1980), 'Conditions improved in test bed hospital', *Laundry & Cleaning News*, 22 Feb.

Seaman, C. (1988), 'Do disposables belong in your healthcare product mix?', *Textile Rental*, Oct.

Shepherd, A.M. and Blannin, J.P. (1980), 'A clinical trial of pants and pads used for urinary incontinence', *Nursing Times*, 5 June: 1015–16.

Silberberg, F.G. (1977), 'A hospital study of a new absorbent bed pad for incontinent patients', *Medical Journal of Australia*, 16 April: 582–6.

Smith, B. (1979), 'A dry bed – and save on costs', *Nursing Mirror*, 31 May.

Smith, B. (1985), 'A comparative trial of urinary incontinence aids', *British Journal of Clinical Practice*, 39(8): 311–19.

Smith, B. (1986), 'New Kylie development', *Journal of District Nursing*, May: 9–10.

Sprott, M.S., Kearns, A.M. and Keenlyside, D. (1988), 'A microbiological study of absorbent pads', *Journal of Hospital Infection*, 12: 125–9.

Stone, T. (1986), 'Reusable reigns', *Clean Scene*, 26 July.

Tam, G., Knox, J.G. and Adamson, M. (1978), 'A cost-effectiveness trial of incontinence pants', *Nursing Times*, 20 July: 1198–200.

Thomas, S. and Hubbard, J.K. (1979), 'A laboratory evaluation of incontinence underpads', *Nursing Times*, 5 July: 1136–9.

Turner, G.N. (1987), 'An evaluation of the usefulness of an incontinence aid incorporating a wetness indicator', *British Journal of Clinical Practice*, 41(8): 876–8.

Watson, A.C. (1980), 'A trial of Molnlycke pants and diapers', *Nursing Times*, 5 June: 1017–19.

Watson, A. (1983), 'Kanga pads on trial', *Nursing Mirror*, 10 Aug.: 48–50.

Watson, R. (1989), 'A nursing trial of urinary sheath systems on male hospitalized patients', *Journal of Advanced Nursing*, 14: 467–70.

Watson, R. and Kuhn, M. (1990), 'The influence of component parts on the performance of urinary sheath systems', *Journal of Advanced Nursing*, 15: 417–22.

Williams, T.F., Forester, J.E., Proctor, J.K., Hahn, A., Izzo, A.J. and Elliott, G.A. (1981), 'A new double-layered launderable bed sheet for patients with urinary incontinence', *Journal of the American Geriatrics Society*, XXIX(11): 520–4.

Willington, F.L., Lade, C.M. and Thomas, A.M. (1972), 'Marsupial pants for urinary incontinence', *Nursing Mirror*, 18 Aug.: 40–1.

7 Intermittent self-catheterisation

ANN WINDER

Introduction

'Intermittent Self Catheterisation has reduced infection hazards and greatly improved the lives of many patients with disorders of micturition' (Lapides *et al.*, 1972). Many patients have benefited over the years by using this technique of intermittent self-catheterisation (ISC) and it has enabled them to control their bladders rather than their bladders controlling their lives. It is a simple technique to teach. However, the instructor must have a good understanding of bladder dysfunction and an adequate knowledge of normal voiding patterns for it to be a satisfactory and safe practice. It is unfortunate that there are few research papers specifically related to the clinical aspects of this method of care and its long-term effects on the patient. This chapter provides guidelines on all aspects of patient care related to teaching intermittent self-catheterisation. As this technique becomes more generally accepted and the numbers of patients increase, so our knowledge grows and we develop easier methods to help those who require it.

Historical perspective

Clean intermittent self-catheterisation is attracting increasing attention as a form of treatment for patients with problems of urinary incontinence and bladder dysfunction. It requires great motivation with the patient being well prepared both physically and psychologically. History has come around in a complete circle from the days when men kept a silver tube in their top hats to enable them to catheterise themselves, circumventing their urethral strictures which were usually caused by a sexually transmitted disease such as gonorrhea or enlarged prostate glands (Home, 1797). Even as early as 30 BC Celsus recorded the value of this procedure in *Disquisation De Medicina*: 'sometimes we are compelled to draw off the urine by hand when it is not passed naturally. For this purpose bronze tubes are made.' The Chinese used the stems from an onion plant which were hollow tubes dried in a special way. Avicenna, a urologist in AD 980–1037, recommended catheterisation using a tube made of marine animal skins stuck together with a cheese glue (Cule, 1980). More recently Augustus Nelaton designed a rubber catheter following Goodyear's development of vulcanisation (1836) (Brown, 1975). Although a type similar to this is still available today the more commonly used catheter is manufactured in PVC.

The technique of intermittent self-catheterisation is used by both males and females who suffer some form of neurogenic bladder dysfunction due to spina bifida or paraplegia (Lapides *et al.*, 1972). Beneficial results have also been seen when it is used by women suffering from multiple sclerosis, who fail to empty their bladders completely due to a condition known as hypotonic bladder (Norton, 1986). The detrusor muscle fails to contract resulting in inefficient voiding and leaving a residual volume of urine. This can cause symptoms of frequency of micturition and dribbling incontinence. Age is no barrier to carrying out ISC. Children as young as 5 years old can be taught this procedure or in some cases the parents can learn to catheterise their babies. The elderly have also been successful in mastering this technique (Lapides *et al.*, 1975).

Reasons for ISC and the suitable client group

Neurogenic bladder

One of the most common indications for ISC is for those patients who have neurogenic voiding difficulties when there is damage to the neurological control mechanisms regulating normal bladder function. This can be caused by trauma or disease affecting the nervous system, such as spinal injury (Guttmann and Frankel, 1966) or multiple sclerosis. Incomplete bladder emptying can result in bladder infections (Slade and Gillespie, 1985), or if there is a high intravesical pressure there is a risk of damage to the upper urinary tract, due to reflux up the ureters to the kidneys. Incomplete emptying can lead to overflow incontinence with the patient presenting with frequency, passing small volumes or dribbling incontinence (Maes and Wyndaele, 1988). In patients with a neurogenic bladder there may be the added disadvantage of detrusor instability. This is frequently found in cases of multiple sclerosis and in the spinal injury patient. However detrusor instability can be helped with medication, such as anticholinergics (Thomas 1986).

Before teaching patients the technique of ISC it is vital that full investigations are carried out to establish the individual's problems. This can be done most successfully by urodynamic studies (see Chapter 3, Assessment of urinary incontinence).

Hypotonic bladder

A hypotonic bladder is one in which the detrusor muscle of the bladder does not produce a proper voiding contraction and may require abdominal pressure or manual expression to empty. Micturition is inefficient and a residual volume of urine can build up. The patient may not have any sensation despite the bladder being full resulting in a considerable volume being retained (500–2,000 ml). In these cases overflow incontinence can occur. This type of problem is found in those suffering from some lower spinal cord injury or in the neuropathy associated with diabetes (Herr, 1975; Perkash, 1975; Dionko *et al.*, 1983).

Overflow: incontinence due to obstruction

Incontinence due to obstruction is most commonly associated with prostatic hypertrophy in older men. It manifests itself with symptoms of frequency and straining to void and there may be postmicturition dribble. It can also be found in men and women who have a urethral stricture or stenosis following instrumental trauma, infection of the urethra or bad catheter management (Brocklehurst *et al.*, 1968; Brocklehurst, 1977).

One way of establishing the presence of an obstruction is to determine the patient's flow rate. This can be combined with an ultrasound scan of the bladder which will demonstrate the volume of residual urine and from this the degree of obstruction can be estimated. Another reason for urethral 'obstruction' is that of dyssynergia when the sphincter mechanism fails to relax during voiding. This can occur in neurological conditions such as multiple sclerosis (Murray *et al.*, 1984).

The elderly

Inefficient voiding leaving large residuals of urine becomes increasingly common with advancing age, and where medication or surgical procedures are not appropriate it can be an advantage to carry out intermittent catheterisation to maintain continence. This requires a radical change in the attitudes of the carers, as elderly patients with limited manual dexterity may find it impossible to do the procedure for themselves and it would fall to the nurse to carry this out for them. Older people who are voiding regularly need less frequent intermittent catheterisation since the residual urine accumulates gradually. Once a day or even on alternate days may be all that is necessary. Usually this is much more acceptable than an indwelling catheter with its inherent risk of urinary tract infection (Garibaldi *et al.*, 1974; Slade and Gillespie, 1985). Time and care must be given in explaining the reasons for and the technique of ISC to the elderly patient. It is important to note that if this procedure is being undertaken by a nurse in hospital it must be aseptic because of the risk of cross-infection (Guttmann and Frankel, 1966; Lapides *et al.*, 1975). The advantages are obvious since the patient is mobile, there is less risk of infection (Norton, 1986) and an antisocial problem remains private. The most important time to carry out this procedure is in the evening prior to sleep, as the patient would benefit from a less disturbed night often cause by frequent visits to the toilet (Hunt *et al.*, 1984).

Children

Intermittent catheterisation (ISC) in children with cord lesions was first advocated by Guttmann and Frankel in 1966 and was found to have good results. It was started in spina bifida children in Newcastle Royal Victoria Hospital in 1977 and is now widely used as a method of management in these and other children suffering from some form of congenital bladder dysfunction (Guttmann and Frankel, 1966; Scott and Deegan, 1982). Prior to starting this technique, a full investigation of the child's urinary tract is carried out, and will include an intravenous pyelogram and a cystometrogram.

This method of management (ISC) is carried out during the day and if it is done just before the child goes to bed it can result in a dry night. It is important to involve the child in all aspects of ISC as soon as possible, although individual problems can occur at different ages. Children must accept their genitalia as a normal part of their body and they require much encouragement to prepare them for managing their own future care. If the child cannot accept this procedure there must be consultation with the urologist and paediatrician to consider alternative forms of management relevant to the child's needs. In some cases where there is a small capacity bladder and leakage occurs due to detrusor instability it may be necessary to prescribe an anticholinergic such as Propantheline and Imipramine (Thomas, 1986). ISC has been found to improve the condition of the upper urinary tract (Scott and Deegan, 1982) and has given children great benefits in their social and educational independence. It enables them to lead a near normal life – they do not stand out from others as being different and in some cases frees them from the need for catheters, pads and appliances.

It is preferable to commence ISC prior to puberty as, at that time, children are experiencing so many emotional changes they may not be able to accept ISC as a method of management. There is, however, no written evidence to establish the optimum age of acceptance. In recent years some older children with ileal conduits have been undiverted back to using their own bladders as a reservoir and using ISC to maintain continence (Barrett *et al.*, 1984).

Urinary tract infections

It is assumed that emptying the bladder by ISC reduces the rate of urinary infection to below that associated with an indwelling urethral catheter (Guttmann and Frankel, 1966) (see Chapter 8, Use of indwelling catheters). However, it would be wrong to assume that there are no risks of urinary tract infection associated with ISC. Hunt *et al.* (1984) in their study of 46 patients who were taught ISC, found a decrease in their infection rates following its commencement. Forty-eight per cent of urine specimens showed pyuria and bacteriuria before they started ISC and 42 per cent following. More recently, Maes and Wyndaele (1988) in their review of 75 patients who continued to carry out ISC for a mean of five years and eight months (range one to twelve years) found 69 per cent of them had a chronic urine infection when they were first taught. Of these 75 patients, 41 per cent of them remained infected due to an underlying medical pathology (such as prostatism, pyelonephritis), 41 per cent had a sterile urine and 17 per cent had a recurrent symptomatic infection once or twice per year. Therefore, 59 per cent of this series of patients carrying out ISC had chronic bacteriuria. The prevalences of bacteriuria found by Hunt *et al.* (1984) and Maes and

Wyndaele (1988) are lower than that found in patients with long-term indwelling urethral catheters (Roe, 1989). ISC is, therefore, a more preferable approach to the management of incontinence because the risks of related pathologies associated with chronic bacteriuria (Carty *et al.*, 1981; Warren *et al.*, 1981) are reduced. However quite a high percentage of patients carrying out ISC do have a chronic bacteriuria and the prevention of cross-infection remains important.

Types of catheter and their use

There are various types of catheter available for ISC on the market today with most of them available on prescription (ACA, 1988) (Fig. 7.1). It is important to choose the right one for the individual's needs, for example a wheelchair-bound female may prefer to use a 40 cm tube to enable her to drain the urine directly down the toilet from her chair. The majority of catheters are made from PVC ranging in rigidity and some have a self-lubricating surface (Hellsten and Hjalmas, 1984). For female usage the length is approximately 22 cm and for males approximately 40 cm. When choosing a catheter, first ensure it meets a British Standard for manufacture (BS 1695). This confirms that the correct quality of material has been used. The catheter is a hollow tube with two eyelets at one end and a funnel opening at the other, and the

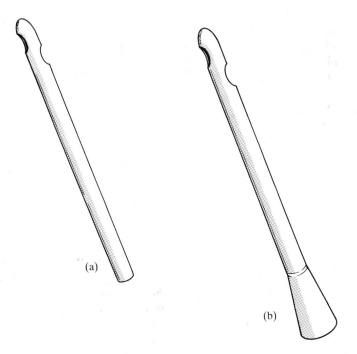

Fig. 7.1 Two types of catheter used for intermittent self-catheterisation: (a) Scott; (b) Nelaton.

circumference of the tube ranges from 6 Ch (charrière gauge) to 20 Ch. The most common sizes used in adult females are 10–12 Ch and in adult males 12–14 Ch. However for male patients with a history of urethral strictures sizes up to 18–20 Ch can be used (Lawrence and Macdonagh, 1988). The eyelets, through which the urine drains, must be smooth edged to prevent any trauma when the catheter is passed along the urethra which has a delicate sensitive lining and has a slight rotation. The funnel end is important as it enables patients who have poor eyesight to ensure that they insert the correct end, and to observe the colour of the urine, which is indicative of its concentration and important in establishing a correct fluid intake. Having a funnel also enables the patient to see if there is any blood or debris in the urine.

Cleaning

Each PVC catheter is sterile-wrapped, generally being used once only in hospital and more often by patients at home (Slade and Gillespie, 1985). The use of a sterilising fluid is not recommended as it can cause problems to the delicately balanced flora of the urethra (ibid.). To date no studies have investigated the effects of the reuse of a clean catheter versus single-use (sterile) catheters and their effects on urinary tract infection rates in the short- or long-term use of ISC. Reuse of intermittent catheters has not been investigated as a research project. Most studies were intended to see if patients could actually carry out ISC using a clean technique (Lápides *et al.*, 1972). Similarly, there has been no research to establish how long each catheter should be used. However, cleaning with soap and water after use and drying off with a clean tissue is felt to be adequate, although this remains to be empirically tested. The clean catheter can then be kept in a clean snap-topped plastic bag or container and carried around by the patient – some women even keep their catheter on the inside of their tights next to their pants! The self-lubricating type of catheter should be used once only as recommended by the manufacturer. This type of catheter has a hydrophilic layer which enables the surface to bind with water, so that the catheter surface is covered by a layer of water on coming into contact with the urethral mucosa. Manufacturers claim this results in less trauma to the urethral wall when the catheter is being inserted (Sullivan *et al.*, 1987).

Lubricants

The use of lubricants on the PVC catheter is optional. Most patients are taught to use a lubricant when first instructions are given, and the male is advised to use an analgesic lubricant. However many give this up as they become more confident in the technique. Use of analgesic lubricants in ISC appears to be a practice adapted from recommendations for general catheterisation (Lindan, 1969; Seal *et al.*, 1982).

If lubricants are used it is more advantageous to use individual sachets as this reduces the risk of a half open tube being left around risking contamination. However, if a tube is preferred, ensure a small amount is discarded first, prior to using it on a catheter. Despite a perfect technique, practice has shown that in some men infections have occurred because excessive amounts of lubricants have been used (Winder, personal observation). This leaves a residue in the urethra which on withdrawing the catheter, after the next insertion, is pushed up into the bladder. Unfortunately, there is no research to substantiate this statement. However, clinical observation has shown that those who use excessive amounts of gels continue to develop urinary tract infections despite having good techniques. On stopping use of the gels the urine infection appears to be reduced. If the catheter does not slide easily into the urethra and lubricants are not used it may be helpful to dip the catheter in clean water before insertion. Some patients complain the catheter is too hard and dipping it in hot water tends to soften the catheter slightly. However this is not recommended for use with children who have poor sensation because of the risk of scalding.

Storage

Catheters should be stored in a dry area, preferably in a bedroom in a flat position not close to hot radiators or pipes. This will prevent the outer packaging becoming torn which may result in damage to the catheter and a lack of sterility. Manufacturers will provide guidelines on storage if requested.

Disposal of used catheters in the community

It is advisable to wash the catheter thoroughly with soap and water after use, wrap in paper and tie in a plastic bag prior to disposal in a dustbin. People with infectious diseases such as HIV, AIDS are recommended to seek advice from Infection Control Officers in their individual areas, regarding the disposal of catheters and other appliances.

Catheters and appliances

As ISC has become accepted as a method of management many individual problems have presented themselves. Some women find it difficult to find the urethral orifice for themselves, either because of their disability, obesity or poor manual dexterity. Manufacturers have produced various types of appliances for overcoming these problems (Fig. 7.2).

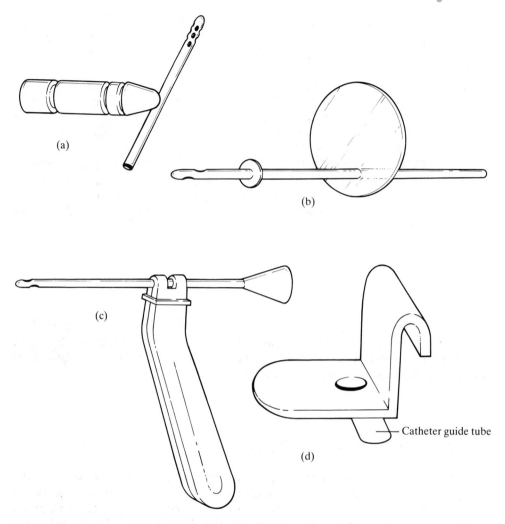

Fig. 7.2 Some different types of applicators used for intermittent self-catheterisation: (a) Porteus tube; (b) metal catheter with mirror; (c) catheter plus handle; (d) handle.

Teaching intermittent self-catheterisation

It is important to establish the individual's needs and type of bladder problem before teaching the technique of clean intermittent self-catheterisation, as each patient is different and may have varying requirements. It may be necessary to establish their voiding patterns, the volumes voided and the fluid intake as well as the residual urines they hold. This will give an assessment on which to base their care, especially if there are no urodynamic results to follow, and can be done with an accurate weekly fluid volume chart (Fig. 7.3).

Day	Time/Volume Daytime C = catheter	Night-time	Pads used in 24 hours
1	8am/50 C.700 W 12 am/100 C 80 4pm/100 8pm/75 C 80	2am/50 W C 900	2
2	739/100 C 600 12am/150 C 100 4pm/150 10pm/75 c 600 W	2 am/100 C 400	1
3	8am/50 C500 10am/100 12am/150 C300 4pm/100 6pm/100 11³⁰/150 C450	2am/200 C 350	0

Time/Volume passed normally

C = Urine drained from catheter

W = Wet periods

Night-time = When patient is in bed

Daytime = When patient is up

Fig. 7.3 Example of fluid output chart recording intermittent catheter drainage.

The residual urine must not be less than 100 ml to make the technique worthwhile teaching, and can only be established by emptying the bladder by catheter or using ultrasound techniques after voiding.

The medical and physical attributes required for ISC are the following:

1. Sufficient manual dexterity to enable them to manipulate a catheter.
2. Sufficient mental ability to understand the principles of the technique.
3. Acceptability and good motivation.
4. If a parent or partner is undertaking the catheterisation both partners must agree.
5. If female, the patient needs a reasonable agility to gain access to the urethra.

Before teaching ISC discussion should take place between the instructor and the patient, to explain why the patient needs to carry out the procedure and why this

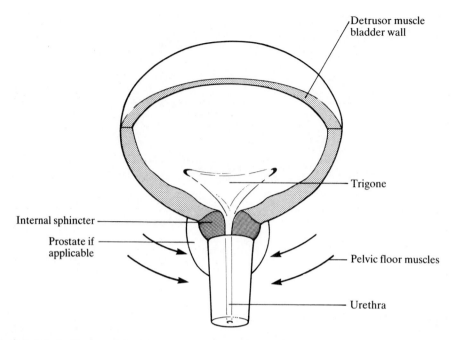

Fig. 7.4 A basic diagram of the bladder and urethra (male/female).

technique could be of benefit. Social events in the patients' daily lives also need to be taken into account. It may not be possible for a young mother to perform this technique in the morning when she has small children demanding attention prior to school. In the case of the handicapped person it may be beneficial to see them at home, to establish the best place to carry out this procedure. Bathrooms are not always accessible. Where applicable the sexual implications should be discussed, as it may be necessary to catheterise prior to intercourse. One of the main social aims of ISC is that the patient is able to have control of their bladder rather than their bladder ruining their daily lives.

Prior to demonstration, it is essential to explain simple basic anatomy to the patient (Fig. 7.4). Women may find the relationship of the urethra to the vagina difficult to understand and men need to be shown the angle to hold the penis in order to straighten out the 'loop' of the urethra. Always give the patient time to allay any fears and apprehensions he or she may have in carrying out this technique. There are many leaflets available for patients which will answer questions they may have when they are on their own. It is advisable that the 'teacher' should always keep a comprehensive record of the patient's learning needs and achievements. There may be a need for frequent visits in the beginning until the patient is confident with the procedure.

Some advantages of carrying out ISC include the following:

1. Patient retains independence.
2. Urinary tract infection is reduced.

3. Patient is in control of his or her own bladder.
4. The upper urinary tract is protected from reflux.
5. Normal sexual relations without incontinence may be maintained.
6. The need for aids and appliances is reduced.

Patients often have many questions they wish to ask, here are some examples of the most common questions with answers.

Q: How much should I drink?
A: 1.5–2 l of liquid in twenty-four hours, unless given other instructions. Remember, the urine should be a pale straw colour.

Q: What if I see blood in the urine?
A: You may see small flecks of blood, on the catheter tip or in the urine, do not worry. If bleeding continues contact the clinic or your GP.

Q: What if I feel unwell and hot?
A: Take a specimen of urine to your GP or clinic, you may have an infection.

Q: What if the urine becomes smelly or cloudy?
A: You may have a urine infection. Take a specimen of urine to your GP or clinic and drink extra fluids.

Q: What if the catheter will not go in?
A: Leave it for a while and try again later. Do not make yourself sore – if it still won't go in, contact GP or clinic.

Q: What if the catheter will not come out?
A: Relax, let go of the catheter. Leave for a few minutes and then cough, and gently remove the catheter.

Q: (females) What if I miss the urethra and go into the vagina?
A: Remove the catheter, wash it out and start again.

Q: Can I do any damage pushing the catheter in too far?
A: No – the catheter will curl up into the bladder.
   Females: push in 7.5 cm (approximately) or until urine flows.
   Males: push in until urine flows; length depends on individual male (15 cm approximately).

Some patients experience a 'thud', as if the bladder contracts down with a bang, when they start to drain their bladder. This may occur if the volume of urine is large. To avoid this problem patients could try kinking their catheter, thus restricting the flow, allowing the bladder to drain slowly.

Instructions for teaching the technique

- Wash hands and dry.
- Wash genitalia: females from front to back parting the labia; males carefully wash tip of penis and pull back the foreskin ensuring it is clean around the glans.

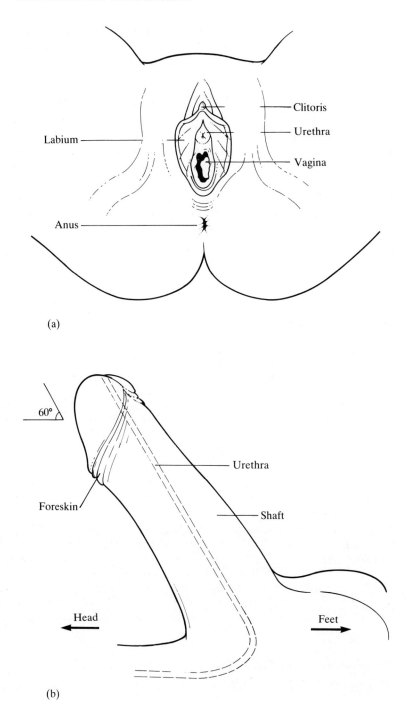

(a)

(b)

Fig. 7.5 (a) Position of urethral opening in the female; (b) angle of penis required to enable male catheterisation to take place.

- Adopt a suitable position: females lying with knees apart, sitting on a toilet or bidet, or standing with one leg on side of bath, or squatting against a wall, or sitting in an empty bath; males standing over a toilet, sitting on a toilet, sitting on a chair.

Females who use tampons occasionally find it difficult to catheterise themselves with the tampon *in situ*. Either remove the tampon or use extra lubricant during this time. Take extra care with personal hygiene. Urine can then drain into a toilet or suitable receptacle depending on position. Some disabled females prefer to sit on a bidet as the bowl is wider and they can get their hands into a more suitable position. The use of a mirror for ladies is optional, although it is useful to demonstrate to them their genitalia and position of the urethra prior to starting. Later, most women learn to insert the catheter by touch. Lubricants may be used initially to ease the passage of the catheter.

- Females should insert the catheter 5–7.5 cm inside the urethral orifice. The urethra usually slopes downwards from front to back (Fig. 7.5(a)).
- Males should hold the penis at an angle of 60° to horizontal with slight tension on the penis.
- When urine starts to flow stop insertion.
- When the flow stops, slowly withdraw the catheter so as to ensure all urine has been drained. In some cases it helps to bend forward, there may be a 'pocket' of urine as yet not drained. When all urine has drained the catheter should be removed, washed thoroughly and stored as previously described.

The nurse should always check that there is no urine infection prior to commencing the first teaching session and again when the patient returns two weeks later, or sooner if necessary. This may be achieved by asking the patient about any symptoms that have been experienced. If any are present, a urine sample may be sent for culture and sensitivity. On the first follow-up, it is important to observe the patient's technique to ensure no bad habits have developed. Some doctors prefer to give the patient antibiotic cover in these early stages, but in our experience this is not necessary.

The number of times the patient has to ISC is regulated by the problems of the individual. The residuals should be controlled below 400 ml. Some patients carry out ISC as often as two-hourly to enable them to be free from urinary incontinence, other patients who are in retention as well, carry out ISC three times per day.

Where there is detrusor instability it may be necessary to prescribe an anticholinergic medication (Thomas, 1986). Perfect management is to have no urinary loss between ISC, no residual volumes of urine higher than 400 ml and no urine infections.

Programme of teaching

A programme for teaching ISC has been recommended by Sheri and Barnes (1986) to be taught to patients either in hospital or the community. This programme is as follows:

1. Discussion with patients about their individual bladder problems and reasons for commencing self-catheterisation.
2. Observation of:
   (a) genitalia – explain position of urethra,
   (b) catheters – explain what they are made of and how to use them, and which end to insert,
   (c) hygiene – explain correct handwashing, i.e. cleaning between fingers.
3. Position: discuss the best, most comfortable and practical position to suit individual needs.
4. Catheter specimen of urine (CSU): send urine specimen to establish if there is any infection present on commencing ISC.
5. Observe technique: watch the patient actually carry out the procedure from preparation to catheterisation.
6. Records:
   GP notification for prescription,
   One catheter each time only,
   (let patient get used to technique first)
   Identity cards for the patients to keep,
   Follow up every two weeks,
   Observe technique,
   Teach about cleaning catheter (one PVC lasts approximately one week),
   Follow up at month, or as required.

Some problems with ISC

Catheter specimen of urine

Asymptomatic bacteriuria is quite common in patients using ISC as a long-term management technique (Lancet, 1979), but, unless the patient has vesico ureteric reflux or is very young this does not matter and should be left untreated.

A catheter specimen of urine (CSU) need only be sent if there are symptoms of infection such as hot flushes or frequency of micturition. Treating asymptomatic bacteriuria predisposes to the development of more serious infections (Slade and Gillespie, 1985). However, if there is a recurrent symptomatic urinary infection, always review the technique, using a new sterile catheter each time.

Support groups

Despite the increase in patients using ISC, they still feel they are the only ones undertaking this non-physiological technique and many complain that they feel isolated. The nurse can give support, but it is not the same as having a fellow sufferer to confide in. Although it may seem a sensible and safe practice to the medical profession, patients who confide in relatives can be given very disturbing advice, which can add strain and great apprehension for the anxious patient. In some health authorities patient support groups have been established, but a word of warning. It is helpful to have a well-informed nurse present at some of the formal meetings to offer sound and relevant advice and to contradict any misinformation.

Reasons why ISC is abandoned

ISC has often been abandoned due to poor patient compliance, and pregnancy. Some patients, especially the elderly, find the technique unacceptable although not necessarily difficult to perform. They have been brought up in an era when touching the genitalia is 'not nice'. If it distresses them greatly it is better to look for other forms of management. There may be psychological, social or physical problems occurring at the time that ISC is suggested and it may be advisable to wait until these have been sorted out before introducing the procedure. As previously stated, it is vital that there is patient commitment and acceptability for ISC to be a satisfactory method of management. Although the instructor can use firm persuasion, the patient should not be bullied into participating.

Pregnancy

It is safe to continue ISC during pregnancy. However, there are added points to be aware of, as follows:

1. The position used by the patient to insert the catheter may need to be reviewed as the abdominal size increases during pregnancy.
2. In the later stages of pregnancy the urethra can become more elongated and the catheter will need to be inserted a little further (7.5 cm approximately). Try using the male length catheter during this time as the patient may find this easier to manipulate and drainage will be more efficient.
3. Due to the normal effect of pregnancy, the weight of the baby on the bladder causes frequency and leakage in some mothers and pads may need to be worn at this time.
4. Any infection must be reported to the GP and always use a new catheter each time the procedure is carried out.
5. In some cases it may be necessary to abandon ISC during the later stages. Ensure that the patient's GP and obstetrician are aware of this and discuss it with them as problems arise. Obviously, it must be related to the individual's reasons for ISC originally.

Further uses and other considerations for ISC

Artificial valves

There are an increasing number of patients having an artificial valve surgically inserted as a means of controlling incontinence (Abrams and Warick 1990) (Fig. 7.6). When the valve is put in place it is not 'activated' and patients need to be taught to catheterise themselves prior to surgery so that they can carry out the technique for a short period while they await the activation of the valve.

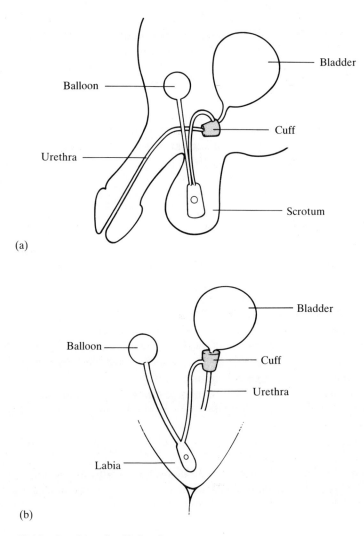

(a)

(b)

Fig. 7.6 The artificial valve: (a) male; (b) female.

Personal hygiene and handwashing

It is worthwhile explaining hygiene to patients as it is a personal skill which differs between individuals. Although all may say they wash, there are degrees of cleanliness that in some are lacking.

For hands, social handwashing is usually adequate for those doing ISC. Soap and water should be used after using the toilet and prior to procedure. In those who may have a high risk of infection it may be advisable to undertake a hygienic handwashing, using an antiseptic handwash preparation, although this recommendation would require empirical study for beneficial effects.

For meatal cleansing, both male and female have been advised to wash their genitalia twice a day with soap and water. If they carry out ISC it is not necessary to wash prior to catheterising, unless they are a high risk patient. If they need to cleanse the genitalia and a bathroom is not available, wet wipes can be used for this purpose.

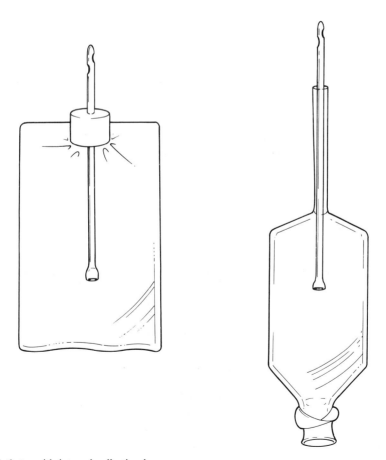

Fig. 7.7 Catheter with integral collection bag.

Travel

It is quite safe for patients to carry out this technique outside their home environment. Sadly many public toilets are not very clean and some lack hand basins. For this reason it is advisable to carry wet wipes, such as the ones used for babies or those available for general use. These can be used for cleaning the hands and genitalia prior to ISC. In these circumstances the catheter should be discarded after use as an added precaution.

When travelling abroad to areas where the water supply may be suspect, the patient should not reuse the catheter and must ensure that he or she has a sufficient supply of catheters which should be carried flat in a suitcase.

In most European countries catheters can be bought over the counter in pharmacies but it is always useful to check prior to departure where they can be obtained in case of emergency. The manufacturer of the catheter being used will be able to supply this information.

It may be useful for the patient to have a course of antibiotic tablets available in case an infection does develop. If the country visited has a hot climate, remind the patient to drink extra fluids and always ensure that the urine is a pale straw colour. Concentrated urine is an excellent medium for supporting bacterial growth (Asscher et al., 1966). When abroad, disabled clients may have difficulty in gaining access to a toilet – many use great initiative in developing containers for this sort of problem. A few companies have developed bags with integral catheter for this purpose (Fig. 7.7).

Summary

Intermittent self-catheterisation has met with considerable success and has replaced long-term indwelling catheters and, in certain groups of patients, urinary diversion. Patient management does require specialist knowledge and the decision to teach the patient or carer should not be taken lightly. Whether this is by a doctor or a nurse, they must be adequately trained in the assessment of bladder function and have a good understanding of the limitations of the technique. As yet, there has been little research on the long-term effects of ISC and in particular, nurses should investigate aspects of meatal cleansing, the use of lubricants and reuse of catheters.

In this chapter the present state of knowledge regarding ISC has been described. It is hoped that this will promote an awareness among nurses of the benefits gained by the patient and his or her family, and which will stimulate further research into the various aspects related to good practice.

References

Abrams, P. and Warick, D. (1990), 'The perineal artificial sphincter for acquired incontinence: a cut and dried solution?', *British Journal of Urology*, 66: 495–9.

ACA (1988), *Handbook of Continence and Toileting Aids*, London: Disabled Living Foundation.

Asscher, A.W., Sussman, H., Waters, W.E., Harvard Davies, R. and Chick, S. (1966), 'Urine as a medium for bacterial growth', *The Lancet*, Nov.: 1037–41.

Bakke, A. (1976), 'A valuable treatment regime, clean I.C.', Dept. of Surgery, Hackeland Hospital, University of Bergen, Norway (not published).

Barnes, S.H. (1986), 'The development of a comprehensive package for teaching self catheterisation', *Journal of Enterostomal Therapy*, 13: 238–41.

Barrett, D.M. and Furlow, W.L. (1984), 'Incontinence, intermittent self catheterisation and the artificial genitourinary sphincter', *Journal of Urology*, 132: 268–96.

Brocklehurst, J.C. (1977), 'The causes and management of incontinence in the elderly', *Nursing Mirror*, 144: 15.

Brocklehurst, J.C., Dillane, J.B., Griffiths, I. and Fry, J. (1968), 'The prevalence and symptoms of urinary infection in an aged population', *Gerontologica Clinica*, 10: 242–53.

Brown, G.I. (1975), *Introduction to Organic Chemistry*, London: Longman.

BSI 1695 Part 1 (1990), *Urological Catheters*, London: British Standards Institution.

Carty, M., Brocklehurst, J.C. and Carty, J. (1981), 'Bacteriuria and its correlates in old age', *Gerontology*, 27: 72–5.

Champion, V.L. (1976), 'Clean technique for intermittent self catheterisation', *Nursing Research*, 25(1): 13–18.

Cule, J. (1980), 'Forerunners of Foley', *Nursing Mirror*, 150(5): i–vi.

Deegan, S. (1985), 'Intermittent catheterisation for children', *Nursing Times*, 3 April: 72–4.

Dionko, A.C., Sondo, L.P., Hollander, J.B. and Lapides, J. (1983), 'Fate of patients started on clean intermittent self catheterisation therapy ten years ago', *Journal of Urology*, 129: 1120–2.

Fay, J. (1978), 'Intermittent non sterile catheterisation of children', *Nursing Mirror*, 14: xiii–xv.

Garibaldi, R.A., Burke, J.P., Dickman, M.L. and Smith, C.B. (1974), 'Factors predisposing to bacteriuria during indwelling urethral catheterisation', *New England Journal of Medicine*, 291(5): 215–19.

Guttmann, L. and Frankel, H. (1966), 'The value of intermittent catheterisation in early management of traumatic paraplegia and tetraplegia', *Paraplegia*, 4: 63–84.

Hellsten, S. and Hjalmas, K. (1984), 'The low friction catheter, a new device for urethral catheterisation', Conference Proceedings: International Conference Urologists, September 1984, Sweden.

Herr, W.H. (1975), 'Intermittent catheterisation in neurogenic bladder dysfunction', *Journal of Urology*, 113: 477–9.

Home, Ev. (1797), *Practical Observations on the Treatment of Strictures in the urethra and in the Oesophagus* (2nd edn), London: George Nicol.

Hunt, G., Whitaker, R. and Doyle, P. (1984), 'Intermittent self catheterisation in adults', *British Medical Journal*, 289: 467–8.

Kaye, K. and Van Blerk, P.J.P. (1981), 'Urinary continence in children suffering with neurogenic bladders', *British Journal of Urology*, 53: 241–5.

Lancet, The (1979), 'Clean intermittent catheterisation', 2: 448–9.

Lapides, J., Aanias, C., Dionko, A.C., Gould, F., Bette, S. and Lowe, B.S. (1975), 'Further observations of self catheterisation', *American Association of Genito Urinary Surgeons*, 67: 15–17.

Lapides, J., Dionko, A.C., Silber, S.J. and Lowe, B.S. (1972), 'Clean intermittent catheterisation in the treatment of urine tract disease', *Journal of Urology*, 107: 458–61.

Lawrence, W.T. and Macdonagh, R. (1988), 'The treatment of urethral stricture disease by internal urethrotomy followed by intermittent low friction self catheterisation', *Journal of Royal Society of Medicine*, 81: 136–9.

Lindan, R. (1969), 'The prevention of ascending catheter induced infections of the urinary tract', *Journal of Chronic Disease*, 22: 321–30.

Maes, D. and Wyndaele, J. (1988), 'Long term experience with intermittent self catheterisation', *Neurology and Urodynamics*, 73: 273–4.

Massey, J. and Abrams, P. (1988), 'Obstructed voiding in the female', *British Journal of Urology*, 61: 36–9.

Murray, K., Lewis, P., Blannin, J. and Shepherd, A. (1984), 'Clean intermittent self catheterisation in the management of adult lower urinary tract dysfunction', *British Journal of Urology*, 56: 379–80.

Norton, C. (1986), *Nursing for Continence*, Beaconsfield: Beaconsfield Publishers.

Pearman, J.W. (1976), 'Urological follow-up of 99 spinal cord injury patients managed by intermittent catheterisation', *British Journal of Urology*, 48: 297–310.

Perkash, I. (1975), 'Intermittent catheterisation and bladder rehabilitation in spinal cord injury patients', *Journal of Urology*, 114: 230–3.

Roe, B.H. (1989), 'Catheter care and patient teaching', unpublished PhD, University of Manchester.

Scott, J. and Deegan, S. (1982), 'Management of neuropathic urinary incontinence in children by intermittent catheterisation', *Archives of Disease in Childhood*, 57: 253–8.

Seal, D.V., Wood, S. and Barret, S. (1982), 'Evaluation of aseptic techniques and chlorhexidine on the rate of catheter associated urinary tract infections', *The Lancet*, 1: 89–91.

Sheri, H. and Barnes (1986), 'The development of a comprehensive instructional package for teaching intermittent self catheterisation', *Journal Enterostom Ther*, 13: 238–41.

Slade, N. and Gillespie, W. (1985), *The Urinary Tract and Catheter Infections and other problems*. Chichester: J. Wiley.

Sullivan, L., Carlsten, J., Bowald, S. and Nilsson, A. (1987), 'Effects of catheterisation and surface osmolarity on urethral epitheleum, an experimental study on dogs', International Medical Society of Paraplegia, Annual Scientific Meeting. Stoke Mandeville Hospital, UK, 13–16 May.

Thomas, D. (1986), *The Neurogenic Bladder*, Surgery Med. Education (International) Ltd, pp. 820–7.

Warren, J.W., Muncie, H.L., Berquist, E.J. and Hoopes, J.M. (1981), 'Sequelae and management of UTI in patients requiring chronic catheterisation', *Journal of Urology*, 125: 1–8.

Booklets for patients and staff in the use of intermittent self-catheterisation available from:

EMS   Unit 3, Stroud Industrial Estate, Stonehouse, Glos, GL10 2DG.
SIMPLA Cardiff Business Park, Cardiff, CF4 5WF.
BARD   Forest House, Brighton Road, Crawley, West Sussex, RH11 9SP.
LOFRIC Astra Meditec, P.O. Box 13, Stroud, Glos, GL5 3DL.

8 Use of indwelling catheters

BRENDA H. ROE

Introduction

Indwelling urethral catheters have been available since the 1920s. Prior to that, curled up reeds and palm leaves were the earliest known catheters and were used to alleviate retention (Wilson and Roe, 1986). This chapter focuses mainly on indwelling urethral catheters along with catheter care. It will present current research evidence relating to catheter care, in particular; selection of catheters and drainage systems, catheterisation, meatal cleansing, management of the drainage system, use of bladder washouts and catheter removal. It will also deal with the incidence and prevalence of catheterisation along with some aspects of patient education.

Use of catheters

It has been estimated that approximately 10–12 per cent of patients admitted to hospital will have a urethral catheter inserted (Kunin, 1979; Crow *et al.*, 1986). Catheters may be used to relieve anatomical or physiological obstruction of the urinary tract, to facilitate postoperative repair and to measure urine output. They may also be used for the management of urinary incontinence although alternative non-invasive techniques are now in widespread use (see Chapters 6 and 7), which should be considered before catheterisation is recommended. Catheterisation is often seen as the last resort in the management of incontinence. How long a patient needs or uses a catheter varies and can be anything from a few days to a number of years, generally being classified into short-term or long-term use.

The number of patients who use a catheter indefinitely to manage their incontinence or because of bladder outlet obstruction has not been well documented in the past. A recent study (Roe, 1989a) found 4 per cent (of 1,709) of community patients known to the District Nursing Services within one health district used a long-term catheter. This prevalence is less than half that expected in hospital populations (10–12 per cent) although community patients do have their catheters for longer periods of time – sometimes years. In a hospitals' survey, Crow *et al.* (1986) found 14 per cent of 294 patients were catheterised for incontinence and 18 per cent for outlet obstruction or retention. The majority of these patients had their catheters removed within fourteen days. In a recent community study of long-term catheter users, 16 patients (number in study = 36) had been catheterised for five years or more. The median use of catheters by patients was four years (Roe, 1986). There is now a trend for fewer patients to have an indwelling urethral catheter indefinitely, due to the implications of catheter use and alternative forms of drainage now being available.

Problems with catheter use

There are a number of problems associated with the use of indwelling urethral catheters, such as urinary tract infection and mechanical problems. Catheter-associated urinary tract infection has long been established and is the most researched area. Between 20 per cent and 44 per cent of patients catheterised in hospital develop bacteriuria (Seal et al., 1982; Crow et al., 1986). The risk of acquiring an infection increases with the number of days of catheterisation. Garibaldi et al. (1974) found that the average daily risk of acquiring an infection was 8.1 per cent with 50 per cent of patients infected after the tenth day. The long-term effects of such infections are difficult to establish, although they include prolonged hospital stay (Givens and Wenzel, 1980), renal pathology (Carty et al., 1981) and fatality (Platt et al., 1982). The focus of nursing practice for short-term catheterised patients is to prevent or delay onset of bacteriuria. Patients who are long-term catheterised will inevitably have bacteriuria (Slade and Gillespie, 1985; Roe, 1989a). However, this is no less important, and nursing practice should prevent further contamination and cross-infection.

The mechanical problems associated with catheter use are: blockage, leakage and discomfort from both the catheter and drainage system. Blockage of the catheter lumen results from encrustation with protein and salts (Bruce et al., 1974; Hukins et al., 1983). Leakage of urine from the bladder bypassing around the catheter not only causes patients distress and inconvenience but increases the demand on nursing time (Kennedy and Brocklehurst, 1982). Leakage may be due to encrustation of the catheter or the balloon irritating the bladder, resulting in spasm forcing the urine out. Discomfort has been attributed to urethral irritation, urethritis and stricture formation (Edwards et al., 1983), catheter material (Blannin and Hobden, 1980; Wilksch et al., 1983) and, more recently, a significant association has been found between catheter size and patients' feelings of pain and discomfort (Crow et al. 1986; Roe and Brocklehurst, 1987).

There are a number of problems associated with the use of indwelling urethral catheters, which is why a decision to use a catheter should not be taken lightly. The decision should include, therefore, when at all possible, the patient who is to use the catheter. Consideration of the patient's ability to manage the catheter should also be taken into account and include their physical abilities such as visual acuity, dexterity and mobility. Nursing practice has attempted to prevent, alleviate or minimise the problems of catheter use and comprises of catheter care, which should be based upon sound research evidence. The aim of this chapter is to present such evidence.

Catheter care

Catheter care may be defined as all those aspects of nursing practice that need to be considered when caring for a patient with an indwelling urethral catheter (Roe, 1985). Such aspects of nursing practice comprise: selection of the catheter to be used, along with the urine drainage system, the catheterisation procedure and meatal cleansing. Catheter care also consists of emptying and changing of the urine drainage bag, which requires knowledge of both the techniques used and their frequency. So, too, for collecting a specimen of urine. Irrigation or flushing of the bladder and catheter is sometimes required by patients, and knowledge of these techniques, and solutions used, is necessary; also the importance of removal of the catheter. Finally, there is a need to teach both patients and carers regarding all these aspects of catheter care so that they can manage their catheter and drainage systems both efficiently and safely.

Selection of catheter

Indwelling urethral catheters (Foley) are available in a variety of materials, sizes and lengths. Their design (Fig. 8.1), has changed little until recently. A collapsible catheter (the Bard conforming catheter) has now been developed for female patients (Brocklehurst *et al.*, 1988) and comprises of a section which is able to conform to the shape of the individual patient's urethra. Selection of a catheter depends upon the individual patient, the length of time catheterisation is required and what is envisaged being drained, for example blood clots will require a large-diameter catheter (Jenner, 1983).

Catheter materials

Catheters are available in a variety of materials, which can be grouped into short-term or long-term use, depending upon how long the patient is to be catheterised (Table 8.1). Catheters for short-term use are: plastic, latex and teflon-coated latex and are recommended for patients who will not be catheterised indefinitely.

Plastic or PVC catheters have little toxicity (Blacklock, 1986) and provide the widest internal diameter which remains unchanged, once *in situ*, due to their reduced absorption of water (Ryan-Wooley, 1987). However, they have been reported as causing bladder spasm, pain and leakage of urine, along with being stiff and inflexible (Blannin and Hobden, 1980). These catheters are used postoperatively and are stated by manufacturers to be suitable for up to fourteen days.

Latex catheters are more flexible and less expensive, but are prone to encrustation and blockage with urinary deposits (Blannin and Hobden, 1980). Latex absorbs water and body moisture, causing swelling of the catheter, which can lead to a reduced internal diameter and increased overall diameter (Ryan-Wooley, 1987). Chemicals within the latex have been found to leach out, causing urethral strictures and cytotoxic reactions (Wilksch *et al.*, 1983; Nacey *et al.*, 1985; Ruutu *et al.*, 1985). However, this

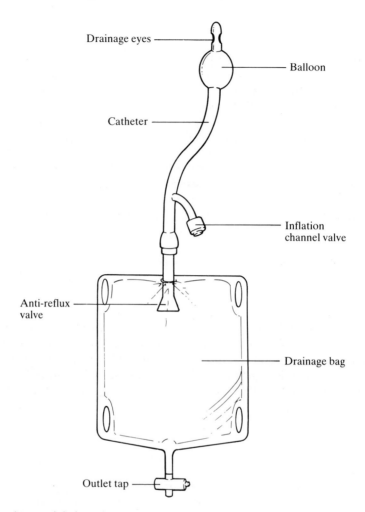

Drainage eyes

Balloon

Catheter

Inflation
channel valve

Anti-reflux
valve

Drainage bag

Outlet tap

Fig. 8.1 The catheter and drainage bag.

has resulted in a new British Standard (BS 1695), which ensures that all future latex catheters manufactured will adhere to a recommended level of safety. These catheters are for short-term use and recommended by manufacturers for up to fourteen days.

Teflon-coated catheters have a smoother finish as well as insulating the latex layers. The coat is intended to minimise trauma, irritation and encrustation (Blacklock, 1986). Teflon-coated catheters are recommended by manufacturers to be suitable for up to four weeks' use.

Long-term catheters are intended for patients who will go home with a catheter in for a longer period of time, or who may have to use one indefinitely. They comprise of silicone-coated or plastic-coated (hydrogel) latex catheters and pure silicone catheters. The purpose of the coatings is to provide a smoother surface, minimising

Table 8.1 Catheter materials grouped according to duration of catheterisation

Duration of catheterisation		Type of material
Short term	0–14 days	Latex
	0–14 days	Plastic
	0–28 days	Teflon elastomer coated latex
Long term	> 14 days	Silicone elastomer coated latex
		Hydrogel coated latex
		Silicone

trauma, urethral irritation and encrustation. A rough catheter surface has microscopic cracks where urinary deposits may build up, causing encrustation and blockage (Wilksch *et al.*, 1983).

Pure silicone catheters consist of an inert material which avoids tissue irritation (Nacey *et al.*, 1985) and damage. A recent comparative study of 18 long-term catheterised patients found silicone catheters encrusted less frequently than teflon-coated or latex catheters (Kunin *et al.*, 1987a). Cox *et al.* (1988), in an *in vitro* study, found no significant difference between silicone or hydrogel-coated catheters and their level of encrustation, both performing equally as well. Catheters for long-term use are recommended by manufacturers to be suitable for up to twelve weeks before requiring changing.

Catheter size and length

French terminology (charrière Ch) is used to size the external circumference of the catheter in millimetres, and is equal to about 3 times the external diameter. They are available in a range of sizes, from 8 Ch to 28 Ch. Postoperatively, a large catheter of 18 Ch or greater will be required to drain haematuria and blood clots following bladder or other urological surgery (Jenner, 1983; Ryan-Wooley, 1987). For drainage of normal urine, a much smaller catheter (12–16 Ch) may be used. Comparative studies of catheter size according to manufacturer conclude that small charrière, in particular 12 Ch, are adequate. A comparative study of flow rates through eight different sizes of catheter tubing (6–24 Ch) found that small charrières were suitable to transport the volumes of urine produced by the average human being over a twenty-four hour period (Edwards *et al.*, 1983). A more recent study compared thirty-four catheters of a variety of materials and sizes from ten manufacturers, and concluded that the size 12 Ch silicone catheter provided optimal drainage (Ebner *et al.*, 1985). Large size catheters have also been found to be associated with leakage of urine (Kennedy *et al.*, 1983). Significant associations have been found between large size catheters and discomfort or pain (Crow *et al.*, 1986; Roe and Brocklehurst, 1987). On the basis of these studies, a small size catheter for long-term use should be selected (12–16 Ch).

Two-way Foley catheters are the most commonly used, having two internal channels: one to drain the urine and the smaller to inflate the balloon with sterile water once it is in the bladder (Fig. 8.1). Balloon capacities range from 5 ml to 30 ml, with 50 ml available for specialist surgical operations. Balloon catheters of 30 ml capacity should not be used for long-term catheterisation as their design and intended use was to prevent haemorrhage following prostatectomy (Herman, 1973). Large balloon catheters have been stated to cause bladder spasm with leakage of urine (Blannin and Hobden, 1980). A recent study of 36 long-term catheterised patients in the community, found that 89 per cent of them stated they had leakage of urine, which some found embarrassing (Roe and Brocklehurst, 1987). As 58 per cent of patients had a 30 ml balloon catheter *in situ*, this may go some way to explaining such a high prevalence. The small size balloon (5–10 ml) should therefore be used for general drainage of urine, with the correct amount of water inserted, as specified by the manufacturer.

Two different length catheters are available. The traditional male length (41 cm) and the more recent female length (23 cm). Female length catheters have not been widely used (Crow *et al.*, 1986; Savage, 1986), which may be due to practitioners' lack of knowledge (Kennedy and Brocklehurst, 1982; Crummy, 1989), or problems with supply and demand. Female length catheters should be used for women, as the excess tubing of the traditional length is unnecessary. However, limitations to their use may be for women who are immobile, as they continually sit directly upon the shorter catheter. The new collapsible female length catheter (the Bard conforming catheter) (Brocklehurst *et al.*, 1988) is intended to be an improved design, with the intention that it will reduce discomfort, blockage and leakage by conforming to the elliptical shape of the female urethra, as shown by Pullen *et al.* (1982).

In summary, catheters with small charrière (12–16 Ch) and small balloons (5–10 ml) are recommended for patients who will use an indwelling urethral catheter to manage their incontinence. Materials for long-term use are recommended along with selection of a shorter length catheter for female patients. All information relating to the size, material and type of catheter inserted, including the manufacturer's batch number, should be documented in the nursing and medical notes, and the patient informed.

Selection of the urine drainage system

The range of urine drainage systems from which to choose has increased tremendously within recent years (Ryan-Wooley, 1987; ACA, 1988). In addition to conventional two-litre drainage bags, with and without a tap, there are a variety of smaller body and leg-worn bags along with connecting night drainage systems (ibid.). Two-litre drainage bags may be used postoperatively, or for patients catheterised for a short period of time. They may also be used for immobile patients on bed rest, or by

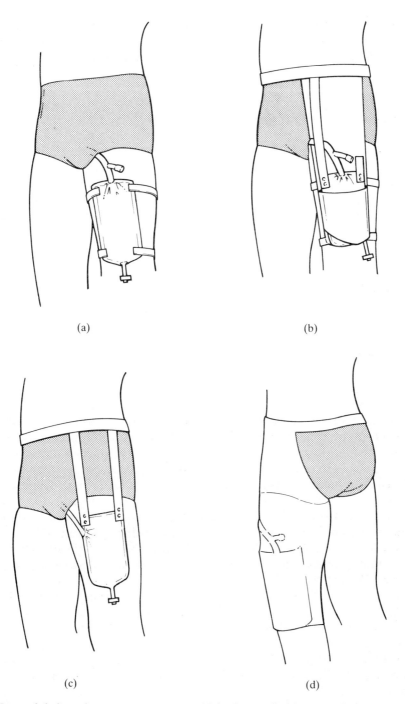

Fig. 8.2 Types of drainage bag suspensory systems: (a) leg bag used with straps; (b) leg bag used with holster; (c) leg bag used with a 'sporran' waistbelt; (d) leg bag worn inside a knicker pant.

patients in the community who are unable to empty their own bags (Roe, 1987). A drainage bag which incorporates a tap that avoids contamination of fingers with resultant risk of cross-infection and that is easy to use should be chosen (Kennedy, 1984a; Glenister, 1987; Roe *et al.*, 1988).

Leg bags and overnight link systems

Smaller capacity drainage bags, which can be worn on the leg, are now available. There is a range of capacities, from 120 ml for paediatrics and 350 ml to 1500 ml for adults, with a variety of supports: sporran waistbelts, leg holsters, knicker pants and leg straps (Roe, 1987) (Fig. 8.2). The leg bags connect to a 2-litre drainage bag for night time use, which prevents disconnection of the closed system and interrupted sleep in order to empty the leg bag (Kennedy, 1984a; Roe *et al.*, 1988). Drainage bags are available on prescription from general practitioners. It is important that patients choose the system they find most comfortable and easy to use when first catheterised, as they will learn to manage the system which is most suitable for them. An overnight link system that does not cause contamination of fingers with urine is also recommended (Kennedy, 1984a; Glenister, 1987; Roe *et al.*, 1988).

Catheterisation

Procedures for indwelling catheterisation are well documented and all state that techniques should be both aseptic and atraumatic (Lindan, 1969; Kunin, 1979; Seal *et al.*, 1982). A recent study of nursing procedures for catheter care found that the majority (98 per cent, number in study = 186) of districts had a documented procedure for catheterisation (Roe *et al.*, 1986). It has also been recommended that patients are given a thorough explanation of the catheterisation procedure (Smart and Ali, 1980), as adequate psychological preparation is an important factor in patient care (Boore, 1978). Jenner (1983) also confirms this and suggests that if the patient knows what is to happen, the risk of trauma through movement or tenseness is reduced, so reducing the risk of infection. Patients may also benefit by being shown the equipment to be used (see Chapter 11, Teaching patients and carers about continence). Details of the catheterisation procedure may be referred to in your local district policy or in the *Manual of Clinical Nursing Procedures* (Pritchard and David, 1988).

Use of antiseptic cleansing agents and local anaesthetic gel on initial insertion of the catheter has been found to reduce urinary tract infection rates in short-term catheterised patients, and have been widely recommended (Paterson *et al.*, 1960; Gillespie *et al.*, 1962; Roberts *et al.*, 1965; Seal *et al.*, 1982). The catheterisation technique is a vital factor in avoiding urinary tract infection. However, there is now a question about the effectiveness of antiseptics for patients who are long-term catheterised, particularly for recatheterisation (Stickler and Chawla, 1987) and does warrant further study. None the less, aseptic and atraumatic techniques are recommended for both short- and long-term catheterised patients.

Meatal cleansing

Urinary tract infection is one of the main problems of indwelling urethral catheters (Meers *et al.*, 1981; Crow *et al.*, 1986), with organisms gaining access at a number of sites, such as the catheter meatal junction and the drainage bag (Hart, 1985) (Fig. 8.3). Meatal cleansing refers to cleaning around the urethral meatus, where the catheter enters the body, and this has attempted to prevent onset of bacteriuria. A variety of practices to prevent entry of micro-organisms at the catheter meatal junction have been advocated, and include application of antibacterial cream (Viant *et al.*, 1971) and cleansing with antiseptic solutions (Walsh, 1980; Seal *et al.*, 1982). A large amount of this advice and recommendations for meatal cleansing have been based upon untested

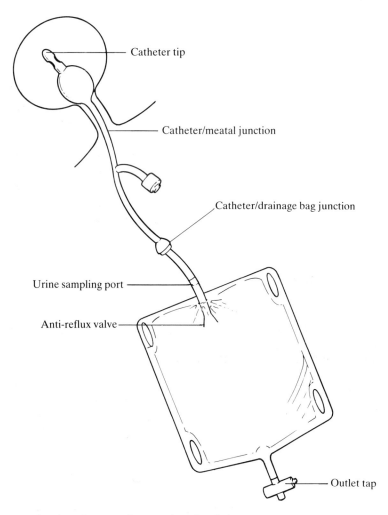

Fig. 8.3 Access points for micro-organisms on the urine drainage system.

practices. Both documented procedures and nursing practice reflect the confusion about meatal cleansing with soap and water and antiseptics being recommended and used by nurses (Crow *et al.*, 1986; Roe *et al.*, 1986).

Burke *et al.* (1981) found that meatal cleansing with soap and water, or povidone iodine solution, showed no beneficial effect on the rate of bacteriuria for short-term catheterised patients compared to untreated controls. They even suggested the mechanical action of cleansing may contribute to the onset of bacteriuria. Further research regarding meatal cleansing is warranted. However, on the basis of research evidence that is already available, recommendations may be made. Antiseptics do not appear to affect the acquisition of urinary tract infection (ibid.), and indeed are known to predispose to the emergence of multiresistant organisms (Walker and Lowes, 1985; Dance *et al.*, 1987). Therefore, personal hygiene, using soap and water and clean wash cloths, is advisable, particularly for people who use a catheter indefinitely and require some form of meatal care.

Bathing

Some authors have recommended that catheterised patients should shower rather than have a bath, in order to prevent bacteria entering the bladder (Seal *et al.*, 1982), while other, also untested, recommendations encourage bathing (Walsh, 1980). Interestingly, a prospective controlled study of catheterised patients bathing in water, with fluorescein dye added, found no evidence of uptake into their bladders (Degroot, 1979). Slade and Gillespie (1985) state that patients' comfort should dictate whether or not they shower or bathe, particularly when catheterised long term. This would seem a sensible recommendation, without sufficient evidence being available from which to base our practice.

Emptying of the drainage bag

Emptying of the drainage bag constitutes a potential break or disconnection of the closed system. As a large number of micro-organisms are present at the outlet tap, and may enter the drainage system when opened (Newman and Price, 1977; Glenister, 1987), techniques need to be used to minimise the risks of contamination and cross-infection.

Cross-infection may be transmitted by hands, due to poor hygiene (Maki *et al.*, 1972), which then results in further contamination of urine drainage bags (Newman and Price, 1977; Glenister, 1987). Contamination of the environment due to spillage of urine (Crow *et al.*, 1986; Glenister, 1987; Roe, 1989b) is also a hazard for cross-infection, as well as causing unpleasant smells in the ward or home. Use of unclean containers, contamination of taps, poor disposal of equipment and unsatisfactory hand washing have been reported for nurses (Crow *et al.*, 1986) and patients and carers (Roe, 1989b). Clearly, the risks of bag emptying and cross-infection are not appreciated.

Crow *et al.* (1986) recommend the use of disposable urinals when emptying drainage bags, which not only saves nursing time but reduces the risk of cross-infection. Disposable urinals are available in hospital; however, in the community this is not always feasible nor desirable, and so a patient specific receptacle, which is thoroughly cleaned with household detergent and hot water, has been recommended (Slade and Gillespie, 1985).

In summary, drainage bags should be emptied as infrequently as possible, with hand washing being carried out both before and after emptying. Alternatively, the wearing of disposable gloves has been recommended when dealing with body fluids in order to protect the nurse and prevent cross-infection (Mulhall *et al.*, 1988). The avoidance of spillage and contamination of fingers by urine is also advisable, along with the appropriate disposal of urine and equipment. When at all possible, a disposable urinal or receptacle should be used and unnecessary contact of the tap with other objects avoided.

Changing of the drainage bag

The frequency of urine drainage bag changing is arbitrary (Jenner, 1983), although recommendations have stated weekly (Reid *et al.*, 1982) and between five to seven days (DHSS, 1990). Large numbers of organisms have been found, both at the catheter drainage bag junction and inside the catheter tubing (Newman and Price, 1977), from which there is a risk of contamination each time the system is disconnected. Fortunately, with the overnight link drainage systems, the leg bag may remain *in situ* for a number of days and a large 2-litre bag attached to it for night-time use (Kennedy, 1984a; Ryan-Wooley, 1987; Roe *et al.*, 1988). This obviates the need for frequent disconnection of the leg bag from the catheter.

Hand washing, both before and after bag changing, is mandatory so as to avoid contamination and cross-infection (Lindsey *et al.*, 1976; Schaberg *et al.*, 1976). Admittedly, patients in their own home do not face as great a risk of infection as patients in a hospital environment, where widespread use of antibiotics produces a reservoir of resistant organisms (Hart, 1985). However, it is still a sensible practice, as patients may be cared for in institutions with other catheterised patients, and may also return to hospital, resuming an at-risk status. A recent recommendation has also included the wearing of disposable gloves when dealing with body fluids as a means of protection and avoidance of cross-infection (Mulhall *et al.*, 1988).

Use of a non-touch technique when applying a new bag avoids contamination from the environment. Contamination would also be avoided by the appropriate disposal of urine and the used drainage bag. In hospital, the drainage bag should be disposed of in the contaminated waste sacks. However, for the community patient, Department of Health directions are issued in the manufacturers' notes accompanying the drainage bags. They recommend that used bags be disposed of by a local authority collection scheme or emptied, cleaned and wrapped in layers of newspaper (or a sealed plastic bag) prior to placing in the dustbin.

Reuse of drainage bags

Disposal of used drainage bags in the hospital environment is mandatory, where risk of nosocomial infection is not only a hazard (Meers *et al.*, 1981; Crow *et al.*, 1986) but may also prove fatal (Platt *et al.*, 1983). However, in the community, practices vary with patients reusing drainage bags (Roe, 1989b). At present, there are no national guidelines regarding reuse of drainage bags. Hashisaki *et al.*, (1984) have managed successfully to decontaminate drainage bags for reuse. However, patients at home may have neither the solutions required nor the ability to do so. Until further evidence is available, the individual user or carer should decide to either dispose of their bags, or, as recommended by Slade and Gillespie (1985), wash them through with soap and water, then dry them thoroughly.

In summary, drainage bags should be changed using non-touch techniques, which avoid unnecessary contamination, with hand washing carried out, and/or use of disposable gloves, before and after bag changing. The appropriate disposal of urine, gloves and drainage bags should be ensured, both in hospital and community.

Use of bladder washouts

Bladder washouts may be performed to remove sediment and encrustations in patients' catheters which persistently block (Kennedy, 1984b; Slade and Gillespie, 1985; Burgener, 1987) and are prescribed both in hospital and the community. However, unless they are essential, bladder washouts should be avoided, due to the risk of introducing further infection each time the closed system is disrupted (Bielski, 1980; Blannin and Hobden, 1980; Burgener, 1987). However, for patients whose catheters persistently block, intermittent bladder washouts do have a part to play.

Use of antiseptic washout solutions for patients who have long-term catheters is questionable. Research has not found antiseptic solutions to be beneficial (Brocklehurst and Brocklehurst, 1978; Warren *et al.*, 1981; Slade and Gillespie, 1985). They do not prevent bacteriuria in long-term catheterised patients and may lead to the development and selection of resistant organisms (Walker and Lowes, 1985; Baillie, 1987). On this basis, Stickler and Chawla (1987) do not advocate the liberal use of antiseptics. In practice, this has not been appreciated, where use of chlorhexidine washouts for long-term catheterised patients has been commonplace (Roe, 1989c).

Difficulties arise in knowing which solutions to recommend. Prepacked sterile solutions are available that are easy to use (Kennedy, 1984b) and can be carried out by patients and carers. A weak citric acid solution (e.g. Suby G; Urotainer) may be useful in dealing with blockage of the catheter lumen due to encrustations.

A maintenance regime which suits the individual patient may lengthen their catheter life, thus reducing the need for recatheterisation. This recommendation does require further clinical testing but would seem a sensible practice to adopt. The weak citric acid solution with Magnesium Oxide (Suby G) was developed for the dissolution of phosphatic urinary calculi (Suby and Albright, 1943), but now may also be useful in increasing the acidity in urine, required to prevent bacterial growth and subsequent catheter encrustations (Griffith *et al.*, 1976; Griffith, 1978). Norberg *et al.* (1980) have also found that alkaline urine led to precipitation of urinary salts and catheter encrustations. A study of 50 elderly long-term catheterised patients found 48 per cent with blocked catheters excreted more alkaline urine, calcium and protein (Kunin *et al.*, 1987b). Problems such as encrustation, leakage of urine and reduced catheter life require frequent catheter change (Blannin and Hobden, 1980; Kennedy and Brocklehurst, 1982). Therefore, an intermittent washout with a weak acid solution may not only provide a mechanical flush, but alter the properties of the internal catheter environment, diminishing the effect of urease-producing bacteria and subsequent encrustation.

As yet, there is no tested clinical data available to dictate the frequency of performing bladder washouts. Therefore, a maintenance regime that suits the individual patient, which keeps their catheters patent, could be established.

Catheter removal

Little mention is made in the literature about the routine removal of catheters, except when there is a specific problem of non-deflation of the balloon (Moisey and Williams, 1980). Latex catheters absorb water and may increase their overall diameter (Ryan-Wooley, 1987). Barnes and Malone-Lee (1986) found all three types of catheter studied showed a substantial increase in shaft diameter with use, and emphasised the need for extreme care to avoid urethral trauma when removing catheters. This is an important aspect of nursing practice which has not always been appreciated, with less than half of district health authorities having a documented policy for catheter removal (Roe *et al.*, 1986). The catheter should only be removed once the balloon has been deflated using a sterile syringe (Pritchard and David, 1988).

Ross (1936) recommended that urethral catheters be clamped prior to removal in order to promote bladder conditioning. However this recommendation was not supported by any research evidence. It is still widely believed that clamping of catheters will improve bladder tone and sensation. To date no research has actually tested whether clamping of catheters for the long-term catheterised patient has any benefits (Roe, 1990). Although there is some evidence to suggest that clamping of catheters has been found useful in preventing postoperative neurogenic dysfunction (retention and bladder outlet retention) following short-term catheterisation of up to six days (Williamson, 1980; Oberst *et al.*, 1981).

However we do need to consider patients who have been catheterised for months or years as their bladders shrink and the bladder neck can become damaged (Kristiansen *et al.*, 1983). To try and regain bladder tone by clamping the catheter while it is still *in situ* does seem a false set of conditions, as the catheter is a foreign body and would not normally be present in the bladder. This would also prolong the chances of further damage and problems associated with the use of indwelling catheters which could be considered unethical. Greengold and Ouslander (1986) describe two case studies where patients achieved continence following removal of their long-term catheters by a programme of bladder re-education and intermittent self-catheterisation. This does seem a more sensible practice to adopt and warrants further investigation.

A more pertinent approach may be to prevent loss of bladder tone in the first place which may be achieved either by using the Conformable Catheter (Bard, Crawley) (see section above on selection of catheter) or a catheter valve (Lic Bivalve, Lic Ltd, Sunbury-on-Thames; Stabuli valve, Ortho Spectrum Ltd, Redhill) (Slade and Gillespie, 1985; Roe, 1990). Both these approaches could allow intermittent flow of urine rather than continuous drainage. Catheter valves have not been widely used but are intended to replace the use of drainage bags and may only be suitable for a selected group of patients. These initiatives do require further research to be carried out but may ensure that bladder tone is retained and prevent bladder shrinking in patients with long-term indwelling catheters.

Encrustation of the catheter is also a common problem (Bruce *et al.*, 1974) not just confined to the internal lumen, but including the tip and outer surfaces. A rough, crystallised surface may cause urethral trauma on removal and 42 per cent (number in study = 36) of community patients stated they found having their catheter removed painful (Roe and Brocklehurst, 1987). It may be suggested that the patient could remove his or her own catheter once the balloon has been deflated. As some patients are more susceptible than others to encrustation, this points to the need for increasing the catheter life by careful selection of the catheter material, use of bladder washouts and establishing the optimum time for catheter change for the individual patient.

Education of patients and carers

Teaching patients about catheter care has been recommended (Slade and Gillespie, 1985; Norton, 1986; Wilson and Roe, 1986), although, in practice, it has often been neglected. Patients have been found to lack knowledge of both their catheters' location and its function (Roe and Brocklehurst, 1987). Initial advice given to them for their catheter's care was not always based upon good practice, nor consistent between nurses (Roe, 1989c; 1989d). This is not only confusing for patients, but does not equip them or their carers to manage the catheter and urine drainage system efficiently.

The importance of teaching patients and carers for the promotion of continence is dealt with in greater depth in Chapter 11; therefore only brief mention is made here regarding education of patients and carers about catheter care. Teaching is important, and patients need to know where their catheter is, what it is for, and what to do should problems occur. Norton (1986) has acknowledged the effect of catheterisation on a patient's sexuality and recommends it be discussed with them. In reality, Roe and Brocklehurst (1987) found no health professional had voluntarily discussed sex with patients (number in study = 36) since being catheterised, despite information regarding sexuality and sexual intercourse being available (SPOD).

Further information required, by users and carers, is the importance of an increased fluid intake to flush the bladder and maintain a dilute urine (Asscher, 1966; Smart and Ali, 1980; Blannin, 1982), as well as the avoidance of constipation, which results in poor drainage (Slade and Gillespie, 1985). Patients also need to know how to: manage the urine drainage system, empty and change the bags, where to obtain supplies, and how to dispose of them, also who to contact if they need help and the signs and symptoms of urinary tract infection, such as pyrexia, fever, loin pain (Slade and Gillespie, 1985). Knowledge is required for the intelligent management of the urine drainage system so as to minimise risk of contamination by micro-organisms, as well as the minimisation of other associated mechanical problems.

An understanding of the catheter as a prosthesis and its function would lead not only to better acceptance, but would enable intelligent management of the urine drainage system, so diminishing the effect of some management problems. This would be a positive contribution to a patient's care.

Summary

Nursing practice for catheter care should be based upon sound scientific evidence. Catheter care comprises all aspects of practice which need to be considered when caring for a patient with an indwelling urethral catheter. Further fundamental research does need to be carried out to elucidate certain aspects of practice; however, evidence already available should be implemented. Fewer patients are receiving long-term indwelling urethral catheters, as alternative means for managing urinary incontinence are preferred (see Chapters 6 and 7). Therefore it is important not only that their care is based upon good practice, but also that they and their carers are taught how to manage their catheters and urine drainage systems efficiently and safely.

References

ACA (1988), *Directory of Continence and Toileting Aids*, London: Disabled Living Foundation.

Asscher, A.W., Sussman, H., Waters, W.E., Harvard Davis, R. and Chick, S. (1966), 'Urine as a medium for bacterial growth', *The Lancet*, Nov.: 1037–41.

Baillie, L. (1987), 'Chlorhexidine resistance among bacteria isolated from urine of catheterised patients', *Journal of Hospital Infection*, 10: 83–6.

Barnes, K.E. and Malone-Lee, J. (1986), 'Long term catheter management: minimising the problem of premature replacement due to balloon deflation', *Journal of Advanced Nursing*, 11: 303–7.

Bielski, M. (1980), 'Preventing infection in the catheterised patient', *The Nursing Clinics of North America*, 4: 703–13.

Blacklock, N.J. (1986), 'Catheters and urethral strictures', *British Journal of Urology*, 58: 475–8.

Blannin, J.P. and Hobden, J. (1980), 'The catheter of choice', *Nursing Times*, 76: 2092–3.

Boore, J.R.P. (1978), *Prescription for Recovery*, London: Royal College of Nursing.

Brocklehurst, J.C. and Brocklehurst, S. (1978), 'The management of indwelling catheters', *British Journal of Urology*, 50: 102–5.

Brocklehurst, J.C., Hickey, D.S., Davies, I., Kennedy, A.P. and Morris, J.A. (1988), 'A new urethral catheter', *British Medical Journal*, 296: 1691–3.

Bruce, A.W., Sira, S.S., Clark, A.F. and Awad, S.A. (1974), 'The problem of catheter encrustation', *Canadian Medical Association Journal*, 111: 238–41.

Burgener, S. (1987), 'Justification of closed intermittent urinary catheter irrigation/instillation: a review of current research and practice', *Journal of Advanced Nursing*, 12: 229–34.

Burke, J.P., Garibaldi, R.A., Britt, M.R., Jacobson, J.A., Conti, M. and Alling, D.W. (1981), 'Prevention of catheter associated urinary tract infections', *The American Journal of Medicine*, 70: 655–8.

Carty, M., Brocklehurst, J.C. and Carty, J. (1981), 'Bacteriuria and its correlates in old age', *Gerontology*, 27: 72–5.

Cox, A.J., Hukins, W.L. and Sutton, T.M. (1988), 'Comparison of in-vitro encrustation on silicone and hydrogel coated latex catheters', *British Journal of Urology*, 61: 156–61.

Crow, R.A., Chapman, R.G., Roe, B.H. and Wilson, J.A. (1986), *A Study of Patients with an Indwelling Urethral Catheter and related Nursing Practice*, Nursing Practice Research Unit, University of Surrey.

Crummy, V. (1989), 'Ignorance can hurt', *Nursing Times*, 85(21): 66–70.

Dance, D.A.B., Pearson, A.D., Seal, D.V. and Lowes, J.A. (1987), 'A hospital outbreak caused by a chlorhexidine and antibiotic resistant Proteus mirabilis', *Journal of Hospital Infection*, 10: 10–16.

Degroot, J.E. (1979), 'Entrance of H_2O into the bladder during sitz bath in elderly catheterized and non-catheterized females', *Investigative Urology*, 17(3): 207–8.

DHSS (1990), Drug tariff, March. Stanmore, London.

Ebner, A., Madersbacher, H., Schober, F. and Marbeger, H. (1985), 'Hydrodynamic properties of Foley catheters and its clinical relevance', in *Proceedings of International Continence Society*, 15th meeting, London, 217–18.

Edwards, L.E., Lock, R., Powell, C. and Jones, P. (1983), 'Post-catheterisation urethral strictures: a clinical and experimental study', *British Journal of Urology*, 55: 53–6.

Garibaldi, R.A., Burke, J.P., Dickman, M.L. and Smith, C.B. (1974), 'Factors predisposing to bacteriuria during indwelling urethral catheterization', *The New England Journal of Medicine*, 291(5): 215–19.

Gillespie, W.A., Lennon, G.G., Linton, K.B. and Slade, N. (1962), 'Prevention of catheter infection of urine in female patients', *British Medical Journal*, ii: 13–16.

Givens, C.D. and Wenzel, R.P. (1980), 'Catheter-associated urine tract infections in surgical patients: a controlled study on the excess morbidity and costs', *The Journal of Urology*, 124: 646–7.

Glenister, H. (1987), 'The passage of infection', *Nursing Times*, 83(22): 68–73.

Greengold, B.A. and Ouslander, J.G. (1986), 'Bladder retraining program for elderly patients with post indwelling catheterisation', *Journal of Gerontological Nursing*, 2(6): 31–5.

Griffith, D.P. (1978), 'Struvite stones', *Kidney International*, 13: 372–82.

Griffith, D.P., Musher, O.N. and Itin, C. (1976), 'Urease, the primary cause of infection induced urinary stones', *Investigative Urology*, 13(5): 346–50.

Hart, J.A. (1985), 'The urethral catheter: a review of its implications in urinary tract infection', *International Journal of Nursing Studies*, 22(1): 57–70.

Hashisaki, P., Swenson, J., Mooney, B., Epstein, B. and Bowcutt, C. (1984), 'Decontamination of urinary bags for rehabilitation patients', *Archives of Physical and Medical Rehabilitation*, 65: 474–6.

Herman, J.R. (1973), *Urology: A view through the Rectrospectroscope*, London: Harper & Row.

Hukins, D.W.L., Hickey, D.S. and Kennedy, A.P. (1983), 'Catheter encrustation by struvite', *British Journal of Urology*, 55: 304–05.

Jenner, E.A. (1983), 'Prevention of catheter association UTI', *Nursing Supplement* (2nd Series), 13 May: 1–3.

Kennedy, A.P. (1984a), 'Drainage system on trial', *Nursing Mirror*, 158(7): 19–20.

Kennedy, A.P. (1984b), 'A trial of a new bladder wash out system', *Nursing Times*, 80(46): 48–51.

Kennedy, A.P. and Brocklehurst, J.C. (1982), 'The nursing management of patients with long term indwelling catheters', *Journal of Advanced Nursing*, 7: 411–17.

Kennedy, A.P., Brocklehurst, J.C. and Lye, M.D.W. (1983), 'Factors related to the problems of long term catheterisation', *Journal of Advanced Nursing*, 8(3): 207–12.

Kristiansen, P., Pompeius, R. and Wadtrom, L.B. (1983), 'Long-term urethral catheter drainage and bladder capacity', *Neurology and Urodynamics*, 2: 135–43.

Kunin, C.M. (1979), *Detection, Prevention and Management of Urinary Tract Infections* (3rd edn), Philadelphia: Lea & Febiger.

Kunin, C.M., Chin, Q.F. and Chambers, S. (1987a), 'Formation of encrustations on indwelling urinary catheters in the elderly: a comparison of different types of catheter materials in blockers and non-blockers', *The Journal of Urology*, 138: 899–902.

Kunin, C.M., Chin, Q.F. and Chambers, S. (1987b), 'Indwelling urinary catheters in the elderly', *The American Journal of Medicine*, 82: 405–11.

Lindan, R. (1969), 'The prevention of ascending catheter induced infections of the urinary tract', *Journal of Chronic Diseases*, 22: 321–30.

Lindsey, J.A., Martin, W.T., Sonnenwirth, A.C. and Bennett, J.V. (1976), 'An outbreak of nosocomial proteus rettgeri urinary tract infection', *American Journal of Epidemiology*, 103: 261–9.

Maki, D.G., Hennekens, C.H. and Bennett, J.V. (1972), 'Prevention of catheter associated UTI: an additional measure', *Journal of the American Medical Association*, 221(11): 1270–1.

Meers, P.D., Ayliffe, G.A.J., Emmerson, A.M., Leigh, D.A., Mayon-White, R.T., Mackintosh, C.A. and Stronge, T.L. (1981), 'Report on the national survey of infection in hospitals: 1981', *Journal of Hospital Infection*, 2(Suppl): 25–8.

Moisey, C.U. and Williams, L.A. (1980), 'Self retained balloon catheters: a safe method for removal', *British Journal of Urology*, 52: 67.

Mulhall, A., Chapman, R. and Crow, R. (1988), 'Emptying urinary drainage bags', *Nursing Times*, 84(4): 65–6.

Nacey, J.N., Tulloch, A.G.S. and Ferguson, A.F. (1985), 'Catheter induced urethritis: a comparison between latex and silicone catheters in a prospective clinical trial', *British Journal of Urology*, 57: 325–8.

Newman, E. and Price, M. (1977), 'Bacteriuria in patients with spinal cord lesions: its relationship to urinary drainage appliances', *Archives of Physical and Medical Rehabilitation*, 58: 427–30.

Norberg, A., Norberg, B., Lundbeck, K. and Parkhede, U. (1980), 'Urinary pH and the indwelling catheter', *Upsala Journal of Medical Science*, 85: 143–50.

Norton, C. (1986), *Nursing for Continence*, Beaconsfield: Beaconsfield Publishers.

Oberst, M.T., Graham, D., Geller, N.L., Stearns, M.W. and Tiernan, E. (1981), 'Catheter management programs and post operative dysfunction', *Research in Nursing and Health*, 4: 175–81.

Paterson, M.L., Barr, W. and Macdonald, S. (1960), 'Urinary infection after colporrhaphy: its incidence, causation and prevention', *Journal of Obstetrics and Gynaecology*, 67: 394–401.

Platt, R., Polk, B.F., Murdock, B. and Rosner, B. (1983), 'Reduction of mortality associated with nosocomial urinary tract infection', *New England Journal of Medicine*, 307: 637–42.

Pritchard, A.P. and David, J.A. (1988), *The Royal Marsden Manual of Clinical Nursing Procedures*, London: Harper & Row.

Pullan, B.R., Phillips, J. and Hickey, D.S. (1982), 'Urethral lumen cross sectional shape, radiological determination and relationship to function', *British Journal of Urology*, 54: 399–407.

Reid, R.I., Pead, P.J., Webster, O. and Maskell, R. (1982), 'Comparison of urine bag changing regimens in elderly catheterised patients', *The Lancet*, October, 754–6.

Roberts, J.B.M., Linton, K.B., Pollard, B.R., Mitchell, J.P. and Gillespie, W.A. (1965), 'Long Term Catheter Drainage in the Male', *British Journal of Urology*, 37: 63–72.

Roe, B. (1985), 'Catheter care: an overview', *International Journal of Nursing Studies*, 22: 45–56.

Roe, B.H. (1986), 'Patients' perceptions of their catheters and study of urine drainage systems', Unpublished MSc thesis, University of Manchester.

Roe, B.H. (1987), 'Aspects of catheter care', *Geriatric Nursing and Home Care*, 7(8): 21–3.

Roe, B.H. (1989a), 'Catheters in the community', *Nursing Times*, 85(36): 43.

Roe, B.H. (1989b), 'Catheter care and patient teaching', Unpublished PhD thesis, University of Manchester.

Roe, B.H. (1989c), 'Use of bladder washouts: a study of nurses' recommendations', *Journal of Advanced Nursing*, 14: 494–500.

Roe, B.H. (1989d), 'Study of information given by nurses for catheter care to patients', *Journal of Advanced Nursing*, 14(3): 203–11.

Roe, B.H. (1990), 'Do we need to clamp catheters?', *Nursing Times*, 86(43): 66–7.

Roe, B.H., Chapman, R.G. and Crow, R.A. (1986), *A study of the procedures for Catheter Care recommended by district health authorities and schools of nursing*, Nursing Practice Research Unit, University of Surrey.

Roe, B.H. and Brocklehurst, J.C. (1987), 'Study of patients with indwelling catheters', *Journal of Advanced Nursing*, 12: 713–18.

Roe, B.H., Reid, F.J., Brocklehurst, J.C. (1988), 'Comparison of four urine drainage systems', *Journal of Advanced Nursing*, 13: 374–82.

Ross, J.C. (1936), 'Some observations on the indwelling catheter', *Practitioner*, 136: 638–44.

Ruutu, M., Alfhan, O., Talja, M. and Anderson, L.C. (1985), 'Cytotoxicity of latex urinary catheters', *British Journal of Urology*, 57: 82–7.

Ryan-Wooley, B. (1987), *Aids for the Management of Incontinence*, London: King's Fund.

Savage, S.P. (1986), 'The female length catheter', Unpublished, Bachelor of Nursing Honours degree, University of Manchester.

Schaberg, D.R., Weinstein, R.A. and Stamm, W.E. (1976), 'Epidemics of nosocomial urinary tract infection caused by multiple resistant gram negative bacilli: epidemiology and control', *Journal of Infectious Diseases*, 133: 363–6.

Seal, D.V., Wood, S., Barret, S., Bartlett, D.I., Coton, J., Cuthbert, E.H., Ebbs, A., Gregory, J.B., Pearson, A.D., Read, J.M., Sowden, M.H. and Suckling, W.G. (1982), 'Evaluation of aseptic techniques and chlorhexidine on the rate of catheter associated UTI', *The Lancet*, 1: 89–90.

Slade, N. and Gillespie, W.A. (1985), *The Urinary Tract and the Catheter: infection and other problems*, Chichester: Wiley.

Smart, M. and Ali, N. (1980), 'Long term indwelling catheters: questions nurses ask', *Nursing Times Community Outlook*, 10 April: 107–11.

SPOD, Association for the Sexual and Personal Relationships of the Disabled, 286 Camden Road, London N7 0BJ; tel: 071-607 8851.

Stickler, D.J. and Chawla, J.C. (1987), 'The role of antiseptics in the management of patients with long term indwelling bladder catheters', *Journal of Hospital Infection*, 10: 219–28.

Suby, H.I. and Albright, F. (1943), 'Dissolution of phosphatic urinary calculi by the retrograde introduction of a citrate solution containing magnesium', *The New England Journal of Medicine*, 228(3): 81–91.

Viant, A.C., Linton, K.B. and Gillespie, W.A. (1971), 'Improved method for preventing movement of indwelling catheters in female patients', *The Lancet*, 1: 736–7.

Walker, E.M. and Lowes, J.A. (1985), 'An investigation into in vitro methods for the detection of chlorhexidine resistance', *Journal of Hospital Infection*, 6: 389–97.

Walsh, R. (1980), 'Urethral catheterisation', *Nursing*, Oct.: 792–4.

Warren, J.W., Muncie, H.L., Berquist, E.J. and Hoopes, J.M. (1981), 'Sequelae and management of UTI in the patient requiring chronic catheterisation', *Journal of Urology*, 125: 1–8.

Wilksch, J., Vernon-Roberts, B., Garrett, R. and Smith, K. (1983), 'The role of catheter surface morphology and extractable cytotoxic material in tissue reactions to urethral catheters', *British Journal of Urology*, 55: 48–52.

Williamson, M.L. (1980), 'Reducing post catheterisation bladder dysfunction by reconditioning', *Nursing Research*, 31(1): 28–30.

Wilson, J. and Roe, B. (1986), 'Nursing management of catheterised patients', in Tierney, A. (ed.) *Clinical Nursing Practice*, Edinburgh: Churchill Livingstone.

9   Faecal incontinence

JAMES A. BARRETT

Introduction

Faecal incontinence is an unpleasant problem which has been the subject of many research studies in the last thirty years. These have lead to a better understanding of the problem though many questions remain unanswered. In this chapter the main topics discussed are the normal physiology of continence, defaecation and the causes and management of constipation and faecal incontinence.

Prevalence

Faecal incontinence is a problem that is often concealed for long periods or may be described as diarrhoea (Read *et al.*, 1979; Leigh and Turnberg, 1982). It may affect patients of any age but is most prevalent among the elderly. The prevalence of faecal incontinence is less than 1 per cent in the community (Thomas *et al.*, 1985), approximately 10 per cent in residential homes (Clarke *et al.*, 1979; Tobin and Brocklehurst, 1986) and 25–35 per cent in geriatric long-stay wards (Clarke *et al.*, 1979; Capewell *et al.*, 1986). In the elderly it is nearly always associated with urinary incontinence (Brocklehurst *et al.*, 1977). Its development is poorly tolerated by carers and frequently leads to the breakdown of community care (Sanford, 1975).

Anatomy of the colon, rectum and anus

The colonic and rectal wall contains two layers of smooth muscle (circular and longitudinal) and two nerve plexuses (myenteric and submucous) which are important for normal propulsive and non-propulsive motility. The myenteric plexus is an important part of the enteric nervous system which has been described as the 'gut brain' and in which many neurotransmitters have been identified. The precise role of the enteric nervous system has yet to be fully elucidated.

The anatomy of the anus and pelvic floor is shown in Fig. 9.1. The internal anal sphincter is under the control of the autonomic nervous system and is supplied by both excitatory and inhibitory fibres. The external anal sphincter and levator ani muscles

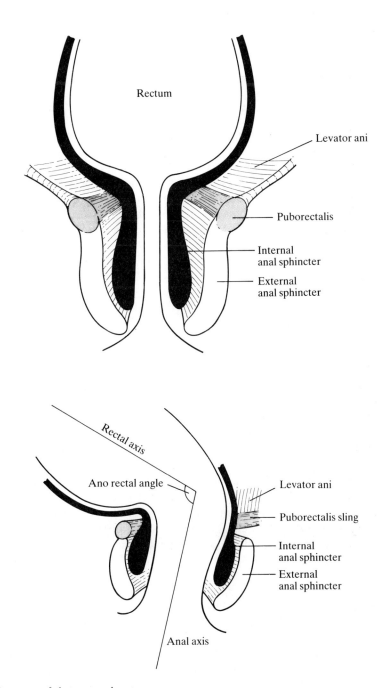

Fig. 9.1 Anatomy of the anus and rectum.

are supplied by the pudendal nerve. The puborectalis muscle has a separate innervation from S3 and S4 nerve roots.

Maintenance of continence

The following mechanisms contribute towards the maintenance of continence;

1. The internal anal sphincter maintains anal resting pressure above rectal pressure and thus prevents faecal leakage (Read *et al.*, 1983).
2. The external anal sphincter makes little contribution to resting pressure (Frenckner and Euler, 1975). Its main contribution to continence lies in its reflex activity in response to sudden rectal distension or increased intra-abdominal pressure on standing or coughing. Voluntary contraction of the external sphincter may also prevent leakage from occurring when there is an urgent desire to defaecate until either the desire wanes or a toilet is found.
3. The anorectal angle is normally 60–105°. Continence may be lost when this angle exceeds 110° (Hardcastle and Parks, 1970).
4. The other mechanisms that play a role in the maintenance of continence include:
   (a) anal sensation (Rogers *et al.*, 1988);
   (b) the slit shape of the anal canal;
   (c) anal cushions: these are vascular projections that aid closure of the anal canal (Gibbons *et al.*, 1986). Interruption of this mechanism in the treatment of haemorrhoids may lead to incontinence (Bennett *et al.*, 1963).

Defaecation

Faecal material is presented to the rectum for defaecation by a series of colonic mass movements often termed the gastrocolic reflex (Christensen, 1971). The main stimuli for these movements are physical activity (Holdstock *et al.*, 1970) and the ingestion of food (Holdstock and Misiewicz, 1970; Duthie, 1978).

Faeces in the rectum increases the ano-rectal angle and causes relaxation of the anal sphincters (recto-anal inhibitory reflex). This reflex requires the myenteric plexus to be intact for the coordination of colonic and rectal motility.

Bowel habit

The normal frequency of defaecation varies between three times per day and three times per week (Connell *et al.*, 1965; Rendtorff and Kashigarian, 1966; Milne and Williamson, 1972) and does not appear to change with age (Connell *et al.*, 1965). Laxative use is, however, increased in the elderly (Milne and Williamson, 1972; Duthie, 1978) many of whom dread becoming constipated probably because they grew up at a time when auto-intoxication from the colon was considered to be the cause of a large number of medical ailments (Lane, 1915) and was treated by colectomy.

Faecal incontinence

Causes of faecal incontinence

The causes of faecal incontinence can be classified as the following:

1. Colorectal disease/diarrhoea.
2. Ano-rectal incontinence (idiopathic faecal incontinence).
3. Faecal impaction.
4. Neurological:
   (a) dementia,
   (b) unconsciousness,
   (c) behavioural.

5. Immobility.

Faecal incontinence in most elderly patients is due to a combination of these causes.

Faecal incontinence secondary to colorectal disease/diarrhoea

Faecal incontinence may be the presenting feature of rectal or colonic disease, especially if it is associated with diarrhoea. The following causes should always be considered: infective diarrhoea; carcinoma of the rectum or colon; proctitis or colitis (due to ischaemia or inflammatory bowel disease); diverticular disease; and drugs especially laxatives.

Ano-rectal incontinence (idiopathic faecal incontinence)

External sphincter weakness
The main abnormality in ano-rectal incontinence is weakness of the anal sphincter and pelvic floor muscles (Porter, 1962; Read *et al.*, 1979; Kiff and Swash, 1984a; Snooks *et al.*, 1985a) which may be due to surgical or traumatic division of the anal sphincters but most cases were, until recently, considered idiopathic. Most patients with ano-rectal incontinence are either young or middle aged females (sex ratio 8 female to 1 male).

Histological (Parks *et al.*, 1977; Beersiek *et al.*, 1979) and electromyelogram (EMG) studies (Neill *et al.*, 1981; Bartolo *et al.*, 1983b; Bartolo *et al.*, 1983c; Kiff and Swash, 1984b; Snooks *et al.*, 1985a) of these younger incontinent patients have demonstrated denervation atrophy of the external anal sphincter and puborectalis muscles. There is also evidence that they have a pudendal neuropathy (Kiff and Swash, 1984a; Kiff and Swash 1984b; Snooks *et al.*, 1985a) and a neuropathy affecting the innervation of puborectalis (Snooks *et al.*, 1985a).

Stretch injury during childbirth or as a result of chronic straining at stool (Kiff *et al.*, 1984; Snooks *et al.*, 1985b) have been identified as causes of pudendal neuropathy. Forceps delivery (Snooks *et al.*, 1985c) and high birth weight (Snooks *et al.*, 1984) increase the risk of pudendal nerve damage. This is, however, reversible in 60 per cent of cases (Snooks *et al.*, 1984). Many of these patients also have perineal descent (Read *et al.*, 1984; Snooks *et al.*, 1985c) but the presence of incontinence is not related to the degree of descent (Bartolo *et al.*, 1983a).

A number of changes in ano-rectal function occur with increasing age which may account for the increased risk of faecal incontinence in the elderly.

The strength of contraction of the external anal sphincter muscle decreases with age (Read *et al.*, 1979; Matheson and Keighley, 1981; Bannister *et al.*, 1987b; Laurberg and Swash, 1989). This appears to be due to denervation (Neill and Swash, 1980; Percy *et al.*, 1982; Bartolo *et al.*, 1983b) and also occurs in many other muscles in old age (Grimby and Saltin, 1983).

Reflex contraction of the external sphincter in response to rectal distension is also absent in many elderly individuals (Barrett *et al.*, 1989). It is also deficient in many patients with spinal cord disease (Frenckner, 1975; Wheatley *et al.*, 1977). Loss of this protective mechanism may contribute towards the increased incidence of faecal incontinence in the elderly.

Distal pudendal neuropathy does not appear to account for the age related weakness (Barrett *et al.*, 1989). This is more likely to be due to a central conduction delay possibly due to age related loss of anterior horn cells from the spinal cord or motor nerve fibres from the proximal innervation of the external sphincter (Duncan, 1934; Gardner, 1940).

The presence of faecal incontinence in the elderly does not, however, appear to be related to the degree of external sphincter weakness (Barrett *et al.*, 1989) though the age related external sphincter weakness may render elderly patients liable to the development of faecal incontinence. External sphincter pressures even in the continent elderly (Barrett *et al.*, 1989) are similar to those recorded in younger faecally incontinent patients (Kiff and Swash, 1984a).

Internal sphincter weakness
The effect of age on the internal anal sphincter is not entirely clear. Some studies have reported an age related reduction in anal resting pressure (internal sphincter pressure) (Read *et al.*, 1979; Bannister *et al.*, 1987b; McHugh and Diamant, 1987) but this has not been confirmed in other studies (Matheson and Keighley, 1981; Loening-Baucke and Anuras, 1984; Barrett *et al.*, 1989; Laurberg and Swash, 1989).

Resting pressure is, however, significantly reduced in faecally incontinent patients, both young (Porter, 1962; Read *et al.*, 1979; Kiff and Swash, 1984a; Snooks *et al.*, 1985a) and old (Barrett *et al.*, 1989) and has been found to be one of the main factors leading to faecal incontinence in geriatric patients (Barrett, 1988).

The suggestion that faecally impacted patients are incontinent due to stretch or reflex inhibition of the anal sphincter muscles (Tobin, 1987) has recently been disproved. Normal anal resting pressures have been found in elderly faecally impacted patients (Read *et al.*, 1985; Read and Abouzekry, 1986; Barrett *et al.*, 1989) in whom the recto-anal inhibitory reflex can also be elicited.

Anal sensory impairment

Anal sensation is often impaired in younger incontinent patients (Roe *et al.*, 1986b; Miller *et al.*, 1987; Rogers *et al.*, 1988) and has also been found to be impaired in old age (Barrett *et al.*, 1989) with a greater degree of sensory loss among elderly incontinent patients.

Loss of anal sensation, however, does not necessarily result in faecal incontinence as Read and Read (1982) have demonstrated that continence can be maintained when the anal canal is anaesthetised with lignocaine gel. This suggests that continence is lost only when a number of coexistent abnormalities are present.

Constipation

This is the commonest cause of faecal incontinence in the elderly and often a contributory factor in urinary incontinence in this age group. It is therefore important to consider constipation in detail.

Constipation is a term used to indicate either the infrequent passage of stool (two or fewer stools passed per week) or excessive straining on attempted defaecation. In the elderly it may be the presenting symptom of colonic disease (Table 9.1). Laxatives, while used in the treatment of constipation, may also contribute towards it by producing dehydration, hypokalaemia or even myenteric plexus degeneration (Smith, 1968).

Diagnosis

The methods used to diagnose constipation in the elderly have been evaluated by Donald *et al.* (1985) who found that less than half of their patients who complained of constipation were truly constipated. Straining at stool was the only symptom they found to be associated with radiological evidence of colonic faecal loading. They also confirmed that the presence of some faeces in the rectum is not necessarily abnormal (Goligher and Hughes, 1951).

The term faecal impaction is used by many physicians to describe faecal loading of the rectum and/or colon with hard stool usually in patients with a history of chronic constipation. Many elderly patients would however be excluded by this definition as they develop massive faecal loading with soft or liquid stool (Barrett, 1988a). Impaction with rock hard stool tends to occur less frequently in the disabled elderly. Faecal impaction may therefore be better defined as faecal loading of the rectum and/or colon with a large amount of stool of any consistency. Frequently this occurs as a result of an immobilising illness, for example stroke, in the absence of a history of chronic constipation.

The presentation may be atypical as many patients may continue to have a bowel action every day or even spurious diarrhoea or may present with incontinence of urine, faeces or both.

Some patients have high faecal loading, i.e. colonic, in the absence of rectal loading. Detection of this may require an abdominal radiograph (Smith and Lewis, 1990) but this should not be used routinely as it is generally unnecessary.

Table 9.1 Causes of constipation

General factors:
  Immobility
  Dehydration
  Inadequate diet
  Anorectal abnormalities

Drugs:
  Opiates
  Anticholinergic agents
  Antidepressants
  Diuretics
  Aluminium containing antacids
  Laxatives

Gut lesions:
  Intestinal obstructions:
  — carcinoma
  — other causes
  Aganglionosis:
  — Hirschsprung's disease
  — laxative induced
  Idiopathic megacolon

Neurological:
  Paraplegia

Endocrine
  Hypothyroidism

Psychiatric:
  Depression
  Dementia

Metabolic:
  Hypercalcaemia
  Hypokalaemia

Pathophysiology

Most of the information currently available on the pathophysiological changes in idiopathic constipation is derived from studies performed on young women with severe chronic constipation, supplemented by a few recent studies of elderly constipated patients.

The physiological changes that may contribute towards the development of constipation and/or faecal impaction in the elderly include deficient colonic propulsion, defaecatory difficulty and impaired rectal sensation.

Colonic propulsion

Immobility is an important contributory factor towards the development of both constipation (Donald *et al.*, 1985) and faecal incontinence in the elderly (Barrett 1988b; Barrett *et al.*, 1989). The mechanism is likely to be a reduction in colonic mass movements but no specific studies have been performed to confirm this. A significant reduction in these movements has, however, been demonstrated in young constipated patients (Bassotti, 1987).

Reduced appetite and food intake may also reduce colonic propulsive motility. Evidence from studies performed on younger patients suggests that the usual postprandial increase in rectosigmoid motility is less marked in constipated patients than in normal individuals (Roe *et al.*, 1986a).

Whole gut transit time has been measured by serial abdominal radiographs following the ingestion of 20 radio-opaque markers in a series of studies. Using this method Hinton *et al.* (1969) found that 54 of their 55 normal subjects passed 80 per cent of the markers within five days which they considered to be the upper limit of normal. These results are consistent with those of workers using other methods (Cummings *et al.*, 1976) but only apply to a Euro-American culture. Shorter transit times have been reported in Africans which Burkitt *et al.* (1972) suggest is due to their higher dietary fibre intake.

Whole gut transit time does not appear to change with age (Eastwood, 1972) but markedly prolonged transit times have been demonstrated in constipated long-stay geriatric patients (Brocklehurst *et al.*, 1969; Eastwood, 1972; Brocklehurst *et al.*, 1983). In one of these studies all of the patients had 80 per cent transit times in excess of five days and 30 per cent still had markers *in situ* fourteen days after ingestion (Brocklehurst *et al.*, 1983). They clearly suffer with slow transit constipation as do many younger constipated patients. Other patients have normal transit constipation (Preston, 1985).

Preston and Lennard-Jones (1985a) in a study of 28 chronically constipated patients, all of whom had taken laxatives for many years, demonstrated differences between slow transit and normal transit patients. In simulated defaecation studies slow transit patients were unable to expel a water filled balloon from the rectum, their colonic motility traces were normal but they tended to be rather flat. In contrast patients with normal transit constipation were able to expel a rectal balloon and were found to have increased colonic activity which Preston and Lennard-Jones suggested may contribute towards the production of small hard stools and pain in these patients.

A myenteric plexus abnormality has been proposed as a possible cause of slow transit constipation as evidence of myenteric plexus degeneration has been found in colectomy specimens excised from patients with intractable chronic constipation (Preston, 1983; Krishnamurphy *et al.*, 1985).

Preston and Lennard-Jones (1985b) assessed the myenteric plexus in patients with slow transit constipation by recording the colonic motility response to the direct colonic instillation of the stimulant laxative bisacodyl which acts on the myenteric plexus. This produced progressive peristaltic waves in 11 patients but in their other 7 patients no response was obtained which was though to indicate a myenteric plexus abnormality.

Patients with slow transit constipation therefore appear to be a heterogeneous population. Primary myenteric plexus degeneration may be the cause of their constipation (Preston and Lennard-Jones, 1985b) but alternatively it may be present secondary to prolonged use of laxatives (Smith, 1968; Preston, 1983). Myenteric plexus degeneration may also occur as a secondary phenomenon as it has been seen after section of the pelvic nerves (Devroede and Lamarche, 1974) and in patients with spinal cord injuries (Devroede *et al.*, 1979). Myenteric plexus degeneration may contribute towards constipation in the elderly and/or disabled but this has not been investigated.

The main sites at which gut transit appears to be delayed in constipated geriatric patients are the pelvic colon and rectum (Brocklehurst *et al.*, 1983). Although mechanical obstruction by impacted faecal masses in the rectum may be the cause of this delay, other mechanisms may be in operation.

Recent studies performed on young constipated women have shown that rectal distension is associated with a reduction in their small bowel motility and transit (Youle and Read, 1984; Kellow *et al.*, 1987). Oro-caecal transit is also prolonged in these patients (Bannister *et al.*, 1986). This appears to be due to a small bowel abnormality as their gastric emptying times are normal and emptying the colon and rectum does not correct the transit delay. This delay in colonic and small bowel transit could possibly be due to a generalised abnormality within the enteric nervous system.

Defaecatory difficulty

The main purpose of propulsive colonic motility is to present faeces to the rectum for defaecation. Defaecatory abnormalities have been demonstrated in young women with severe slow transit constipation. Many are unable to expel simulated stools from the rectum (Barnes and Lennard-Jones 1985; Preston and Lennard-Jones, 1985a; Read *et al.*, 1986). They also experience difficulty expelling barium or saline (Turnbull *et al.*, 1986) and may have obstructed defaecation (Martelli *et al.*, 1978; Bartolo *et al.*, 1983a; Preston *et al.*, 1984).

Normally during defaecation the internal and external anal sphincter and puborectalis muscles relax to allow the passage of stool. Many young constipated patients exhibit a paradoxical increase in EMG activity in these muscles during attempted defaecation which obstructs defaecation (Preston and Lennard-Jones, 1985a; Womack *et al.*, 1985; Kuipers *et al.*, 1986; Read *et al.*, 1986; Roe *et al.*, 1986a; Turnbull *et al.*, 1986). The term 'anismus' has been used to describe this phenomena.

It has also been suggested that failure of the internal sphincter to relax as in Hirshsprung's disease (Lawson and Nixon, 1967) could cause defaecatory difficulty. A normal recto-anal inhibitory reflex in response to rectal distension has, however, been demonstrated in both elderly impacted patients (Read and Abouzekry, 1986) and in young chronically constipated patients (Bannister *et al.*, 1986; Read *et al.*, 1986).

Other mechanical causes of obstructed defaecation have been revealed by defaecatory proctography studies of young patients with intractable constipation (Bartolo *et al.*, 1985; Roe *et al.*, 1986a; Hansen *et al.*, 1987). Roe *et al.*, (1986a) found that 46 per cent of these patients had a rectal intussusception, 12 per cent had an anterior rectal wall prolapse, 10 per cent rectocoele alone, and accentuation of puborectalis impression was seen in 7 per cent. Failure of the ano-rectal angle to open on defaecatory straining has also been demonstrated in these patients (Preston *et al.*, 1984; Read *et al.*, 1986; Roe *et al.*, 1986a; Womack *et al.*, 1986). In elderly impacted patients, however, although the angle is obtuse at rest it appears to increase on straining (Read and Abouzekry, 1986).

The character of the stool may also cause defaecatory difficulty as even normal individuals find it more difficult to expel small hard stools (Bannister *et al.*, 1987a). Simulated defaecation studies performed on healthy elderly subjects have revealed that although they are able to voluntarily expel a simulated soft stool (50 ml balloon) (Read *et al.*, 1985) they require longer to achieve this than younger subjects (Bannister *et al.*, 1987b).

Read *et al.* (1985) in a study of elderly impacted patients, all of whom were impacted with hard stool and had been constipated for at least five years, found that nearly all were able to expel a simulated soft stool but experienced difficulty expelling a simulated hard stool (small solid sphere). Only 32 per cent of their patients successfully expelled the simulated hard stool compared with 63 per cent of the control group. This difference, however, did not reach significance.

The degree of defaecatory difficulty demonstrated by Read *et al.* (1985) is less than might be expected as many elderly patients experience defaecatory difficulty even when stool is soft (personal observations). This appears to be most severe among confused patients who were not included in Read *et al*'s (1985) study group.

Normally during defaecation intra-rectal pressure increases and there is a reduction in anal pressure. This produces a pressure gradient which facilitates expulsion of faeces. The increase in intra-rectal pressure may be produced by rectal smooth muscle contraction, contraction of the abdominal muscles and diaphragm, or a combination of both.

There appears to be a reduction in rectal motility in old age. Read *et al.* (1985) were able to elicit regular rectal contractions in response to rectal distension in only 10 per cent of normal elderly people compared with 71 per cent of a group of young healthy subjects who underwent a similar examination in another study (ibid.). Only 14 per cent of Read *et al.*'s elderly impacted patients and 36 per cent of their younger constipated patients exhibited these contractions. Read *et al.* (1985) also found that the volume of distension required to produce a steady state rectal pressure of 25 cm H_2O was higher in impacted patients. This suggests an increase in rectal compliance in these patients possibly due to a megarectum.

Varma *et al.* (1988) recently reported the results of their measurements of rectal compliance in a group of constipated old people compared with an elderly control group. No difference was detected between the two groups but the authors suggest that there are two distinct groups of elderly constipated patients; one group of patients with high compliance (megarectum presumably associated with a myenteric plexus abnormality); and another group with a hypertonic rectal motility response. Although the division of patients into these two groups is rather arbitrary it suggests that there is a heterogeneous mixture of motility disorders contributing towards the development of constipation and faecal impaction in the elderly.

In patients in whom rectal motility is deficient one would expect greater dependence to be placed on the ability to voluntarily increase intra-abdominal pressure to produce an increase in intra-rectal pressure for defaecation to proceed. Young constipated patients retain the ability to voluntarily increase intra-rectal pressure (Barnes and Lennard-Jones, 1985). In some elderly patients weakness of the abdominal musculature due to either age related changes in the muscles (probably secondary to denervation) or disuse particularly in immobile patients could limit this ability but this has not been studied.

Rectal sensation

Loss of awareness of the call to stool may also contribute towards the development of constipation. Impaired rectal sensation of distension has been demonstrated in patients with chronic constipation (Read *et al.*, 1986) and in elderly impacted patients (Read *et al.*, 1985; Varma *et al.*, 1988).

Faecal incontinence secondary to faecal impaction

Faecal soiling in impacted patients is more common when soft stool is present. Many of these incontinent patients leak before they experience a call to stool (Barrett *et al.*, 1990) probably due to anal sphincter relaxation before the onset of rectal sensation (Buser and Miner, 1986) and absence of the reflex external sphincter contraction in response to rectal distension (Wald and Tunuguntla, 1984). Rectal sensation, though impaired in elderly impacted patients (Read and Abouzekry, 1986, Read *et al.*, 1985; Varma *et al.*, 1988) does not appear to account for their incontinence (Barrett 1988b; Rogers *et al.*, 1988; Ferguson *et al.*, 1989). Anal sphincter weakness and loss of the ano-rectal angle (Read and Abouzekry, 1986) appear to be contributory factors.

Faecal incontinence may also be produced by the treatment of faecal impaction. Immobile patients tend to be slow to respond to the call to stool which therefore renders them liable to incontinence when they are given laxatives, especially when a potent preparation is administered.

Neurological causes of faecal incontinence

Impaired consciousness

Faecal incontinence is common in stroke patients (Brocklehurst *et al.*, 1985) in whom the level of consciousness is the most important factor determining whether continence is maintained.

Dementia

Many demented patients are incontinent of faeces. This may be due to confusion and loss of awareness of the 'call to stool' but other explanations have been sought.

Rectal motility is normally under inhibitory cerebral control (Garry, 1933; Denny-Brown and Robertson, 1935; Langworthy and Rosenberg, 1939a; 1939b). This control is absent in many patients with dementia who exhibit uninhibited rectal contractions

(Brocklehurst, 1951; Barrett *et al.*, 1990) similar to the uninhibited detrusor contractions that may cause urinary incontinence (Brocklehurst and Dillane, 1966). These contractions are sufficient to expel a simulated soft stool (Brocklehurst, 1951; Barrett *et al.*, 1990) but not a simulated firm stool (Barrett *et al.*, 1990). Although faecal incontinence occurs when rectal pressure exceeds anal pressure (Read *et al.*, 1983) the pressure differential may need to be greater for a solid stool to pass.

Behavioural

Patients with psychiatric illnesses frequently suffer from behavioural disturbances which may result in defaecation in inappropriate places. In severe cases this may be associated with faecal smearing and/or coprophagia. Frontal lobe pathology with consequent loss of social skills probably accounts for this disturbed behaviour. These patients tend to resist treatment and pose a major care problem in local authority homes and psycho-geriatric units.

Assessment of the faecally incontinent patient

A careful history should be taken and this should include an enquiry about the following:

- Onset of constipation.
- Defaecation history:
  - frequency of defaecation,
  - stool consistency,
  - straining,
  - rectal sensation (call to stool),
  - ano-rectal discomfort,
  - prolapse.
- Rectal bleeding.
- Incontinence (urinary and/or faecal).
- Fluid and dietary intake.
- Medications especially constipating drugs and laxatives.
- Mobility.
- Mental status assessment.

Patients with severe constipation should be asked the following question: 'Some people with this problem use their fingers to assist the bowels to empty. Have you ever needed to do this?'

Physical examination of the constipated and/or faecally incontinent patient should include the following:

1. General assessment of mobility and hydration.
2. Abdominal examination: this should include careful palpation to detect the presence of any abdominal masses especially in the sigmoid colon.

3. Rectal examination for observation for the presence of:
   (a) perineal descent;
   (b) faecal soiling;
   (c) haemorrhoids;
   (d) anal lesions, e.g. fissure;
   (e) anal scars, e.g. previous surgery;
   (f) gaping anus.

Perineal descent is a sign of pelvic floor muscle weakness. It can be considered present if the anus is at the level of or below the level of the ischial tuberosities of the pelvic either at rest or on attempted straining. The latter may also reveal the presence of rectal prolapse.

Palpation should test for the following:

● Anal resting tone.
● Ability to squeeze anus tightly shut. (Good assessment of pelvic floor.)
● Faecal loading. (Note stool consistency.)
● Rectal lesions, e.g. carcinoma, polyp.

Investigations may include the following;

● Abdominal radiograph. (Not necessary when rectum is loaded with faeces. Reserve for when there is a suggestive history of constipation but an empty rectum as there may be high faecal impaction.)
● Biochemical profile – especially serum potassium, calcium.
● Full blood count – especially haemoglobin.
● Faecal occult bloods – when microscopic blood loss is suspected.
● Thyroid function tests.
● Sigmoidoscopy, barium enema, colonoscopy when colorectal lesion(s) is suspected.

Faecal incontinence may induce profound psychological changes in individual patients. The extent of this, however, has not yet been formally investigated.

Treatment of faecal incontinence

Treatment of faecal impaction and constipation

The main cause of faecal incontinence in geriatric patients is faecal impaction, even in patients with dementia. The initial aim in the treatment of these patients is to empty the rectum and colon. Laxatives, for example, lactulose or stool softeners, such as docusate (dioctyl sodium sulphasuccinate) are often prescribed as first line treatment. This tends to be unsuccessful because many of these impacted and incontinent patients are impacted with very soft stool. Further softening tends to increase the frequency of incontinent episodes.

The preferred treatment for these patients is to empty the rectum from below by administering an enema each day until the faecal mass is cleared. Phosphate enemas are the most commonly used. They contain 10 per cent sodium acid phosphate and 8 per cent sodium phosphate in a total volume of 128 ml. Sodium acid phosphate is poorly absorbed from the rectum. Its osmotic activity increases the water content of the stool. The rectal distension that follows probably induces defaecation by stimulating rectal motility. Phosphate enemas are occasionally ineffective, usually because the enema is not retained. In these patients a better result may be achieved with use of a microenema or suppository. Microenemas (e.g. Micralax, SKF) contain agents which allow water to penetrate into and soften faeces and then stimulate defaecation, usually within five to fifteen minutes.

Some patients, however, require manual removal of faeces especially if they are impacted with very hard faeces. For patients with an atonic rectum this is often the only treatment available. This problem is particularly prevalent among patients with severe spinal cord lesions in whom the stimulatory nerve supply to the rectum (parasympathetic from the S3, 4, 5 nerve roots) is deficient.

More drastic treatments to produce bowel clearance in one procedure have also been described. Whole gut irrigation (Smith et al., 1978), involved the infusion of 2.5–3 litres per hour of isotonic saline via a nasogastric tube. Irrigation continued until the effluent emerging was clear. This procedure has now been abandoned as it may cause water and sodium retention (sometimes fatal) in the elderly. The risk of electrolyte disturbance and water retention is reduced by substituting mannitol for saline in the above regimen (Palmer and Khan, 1979; Davis et al., 1980). A further modification of this preparation has been made with the substitution of polyethylene glycol for mannitol to produce 'Golytely' (Davis et al., 1980). Puxty and Fox (1986) suggest this is a well tolerated effective treatment for faecal impaction in geriatric patients.

An alternative preparation that may be used is Picolax (Nordic Pharmaceuticals, Feltham, Middlesex). This is a mixture of sodium picosulphate (a stimulant laxative) with citric acid and magnesium oxide (which form magnesium citrate in solution). Magnesium citrate is a poorly absorbed osmotic laxative which produces a semi-fluid or watery evacuation after three to six hours. Sodium picosulphate exerts its effect ten to fourteen hours after administration.

Picolax is currently used by many radiologists as bowel preparation prior to barium enema examination. It has been shown to produce an excellent bowel clearance and is better tolerated than mannitol as it causes less nausea and vomiting (Foord et al., 1983). It has not, however, been compared with Golytely.

My own observations of the use of Picolax in geriatric patients with severe faecal impaction confirm that it is a potent laxative. Its effect is unfortunately difficult to control. Very severe faecal incontinence may be produced in the twenty-four hours after administration. This can, however, be successfully contained by a faecal collection device (Hollister Ltd, Reading).

Picolax or Golytely should be reserved for the treatment of faecal impaction in patients who are resistant to conventional treatment, i.e. enemas (personal observations). When Picolax is used the starting dose should be just a quarter of the manufacturer's recommended dose, i.e. half a sachet as a single dose. If this is ineffective the dose can then be increased. Sodium picosulphate alone may be equally effective especially in patients with soft stool (starting dose 5 mg as a single dose).

The clearance of faecal masses from severely impacted patients does not necessarily shorten their whole gut transit time (Brocklehurst *et al.*, 1983). Many of these patients have a continuing tendency to constipation possibly due to the presence of a defaecatory abnormality. The next step in their management should be to keep the rectum empty by preventing the recurrence of constipation. A number of treatments have been tried including increased dietary fibre.

The results of a number of studies on the effect of wheat bran in constipated patients were recently analysed by Muller-Lissner (1988). He demonstrated that bran is only partially effective in restoring stool weight and gastrointestinal transit time of constipated patients to normal. An association has also been shown between high dietary fibre intake and colonic faecal loading in immobile elderly patients (Donald *et al.*, 1985). It is therefore not advisable to recommend increased dietary fibre as routine for constipated elderly patients as this may add to the constipation that already exists and it may also increase their risk of faecal incontinence (Ardron and Main, 1990). An alternative approach is to use a laxative. The choice of a laxative should always be guided by the character of the stool and the patient's ability to defaecate.

An osmotic laxative, e.g. lactulose, is indicated for patients with hard stool. Lactulose, a synthetic disaccharide, is not digested or absorbed by the small intestine. It exerts its osmotic effect in the small bowel and is metabolised in the colon to short chain organic acids which are absorbed. The osmotic effect therefore does not continue throughout the colon. Lactulose significantly increases faecal weight, volume, water, and bowel movements (Bass and Dennis, 1981) and acts within two days. It is effective in the treatment of constipation (Wesselius-DeCasparis *et al.*, 1968) but it is expensive and many patients dislike the taste.

Faecal softeners, e.g. docusate sodium, act by lowering the surface tension of faeces and allowing the penetration of water. Docusate may also have a weak stimulatory effect but it is a poor laxative (Goodman *et al.*, 1976).

For patients with soft or formed stool a stimulant laxative is required. The most commonly used are senna (Senokot), sodium picosulphate, and bisacodyl. Senna is an anthracine laxative which is hydrolysed, probably by bacteria in the colon (Hardcastle and Wilkins, 1970). Its derivatives are absorbed in the colon where they have a direct stimulatory effect on the myenteric plexus. Most patients respond to between 15 and 60 mg daily (Marcus and Heaton, 1986). The laxative effect of sodium picosulphate is similar to senna (MacLennan and Pooler, 1975). Bisacodyl exerts its stimulant effect directly on the myenteric plexus (Hardcastle and Mann, 1968). It is not absorbed from the gut. It may be given orally or by suppository. Defaecation usually occurs 35 to 75 minutes after the insertion of a suppository (Deiling *et al.*, 1959) or ten to twelve hours after an oral dose. Stimulant laxatives should be given at night to avoid faecal incontinence (Harvard and Hughes-Roberts, 1962). Liquid paraffin, once a popular laxative, should not be used as it may cause lipoid pneumonia if inhaled.

Laxatives are often administered to geriatric patients to prevent recurrent constipation. Brocklehurst *et al.* (1983), however, found in a study of long-stay geriatric patients that Lactulose and Dorbanex (now withdrawn by Riker Laboratories) did not prevent constipation recurring, although they were better than no treatment. It appears therefore that many of these patients require regular emptying of the bowel from below. This may be achieved by using either enemas (preferably miniature enemas) or suppositories (glycerine or bisacodyl).

Treatment of diarrhoea

Diarrhoea is often associated with faecal incontinence. While the cause is sought and treated antidiarrhoeal agents should be administered to alter stool consistency. This alone should cure the faecal incontinence but the application of a faecal collection device in the initial stages can considerably improve the management of this problem. Traditionally codeine phosphate has been used for the treatment of diarrhoea. It stimulates opiate receptors to produce an increase in non-propulsive intestinal motility without increasing propulsive motility. Gastrointestinal transit is thus prolonged.

Additional information is available about the action of a new antidiarrhoeal agent loperamide and its effect on continence mechanisms. Loperamide is a synthetic opiate which is devoid of central nervous system side-effects (Galambos et al., 1976). It has been shown to increase intestinal motility in humans (Schiller et al., 1984; Kachel et al., 1986). It was also found in an animal study to have a direct effect on the internal sphincter mediated by the activation of opiate receptors (Rattan and Culver, 1987). It also inhibits the normal internal sphincter relaxation that follows rectal distension (ibid.). In a clinical study, Read et al. (1982) found that loperamide increased anal resting pressure and improved the ability of patients with chronic diarrhoea and faecal incontinence to retain saline in the rectum. Loperamide therefore appears to improve the anal sphincter's ability to retain liquid stool. It would appear therefore that constipating drugs, and in particular loperamide, may prevent faecal incontinence by mechanisms other than just changing stool consistency.

Treatment of the faecally incontinent demented patient

Severely demented patients with faecal incontinence are usually unaware of the presence of faeces in the rectum and the need to defaecate and their incontinence is secondary to faecal impaction. This should be treated as described above. Patients however who continue to have a tendency to faecal incontinence and or constipation should have a regimen of planned defaecation implemented. Defaecation may be stimulated by the use of an enema one to three times per week though this is usually twice weekly. To prevent leakage between these enemas a constipating drug (loperamide or codeine phosphate) may be needed.

Patients with severe dementing illness who have behavioural abnormalities, however, are usually not amenable to treatment by the above methods as they tend to resist the introduction of any rectal preparations. Planned defaecation in these patients can, however, be induced by use of a potent laxative given once per week. Picolax can usually be relied upon to clear the bowel but patients need to be carefully supervised on 'Picolax day' as otherwise they are prone to severe faecal incontinence in the twenty-four hours after its administration. Sodium picosulphate alone can be substituted in patients in whom stool is soft in consistency. A once weekly treatment is usually sufficient as these patients typically have slow transit constipation and therefore tend to accumulate faeces over the next seven days by which time a further bowel clearance will be required to prevent faecal soiling during everyday activities.

Treatment of ano-rectal incontinence

The principles for treating patients with ano-rectal incontinence are similar to those described above. Maintaining firm stool will cure the majority of cases. Resistant cases may need further treatment. It is unlikely that this will be indicated for many elderly people apart from the occasional elderly woman in good health with an isolated ano-rectal abnormality.

Biofeedback, electrical stimulation and post-anal repair have all been used in the treatment of ano-rectal incontinence. Some favourable results have been achieved with biofeedback techniques (Cerulli *et al.*, 1979; Macleod, 1987) and with electrical stimulation of the pelvic floor muscles (Caldwell, 1963; Hopkinson and Lightwood, 1966; Matheson and Keighley, 1981) though this has not been reproduced elsewhere (Collins *et al.*, 1969). Eutrophic electrical stimulatory techniques are currently being assessed. There have been some encouraging preliminary reports.

The operation of post-anal repair was first performed by Parks (Parks, 1967). It appears to be a moderately successful method of restoring continence to patients with ano-rectal incontinence particularly in patients aged 50–69 years (Henry and Simson, 1985). The results in older patients are not as good probably because of the multifactorial nature of their problem. Yoshioka *et al.* (1988) have recently confirmed that 60–70 per cent of patients with otherwise intractable faecal incontinence gain substantial benefit from post-anal repair. They were able to identify factors which were associated with a poor operative result. These included very low anal resting and squeeze pressures, a severe degree of perineal descent and a short anal canal. Surgery does not appear to affect any of these parameters apart from anal canal length (Yoshioka *et al.*, 1988; Scheur *et al.*, 1989). Modification of the original surgical technique is currently being assessed.

Surgery has also been used in the management of severe intractable constipation usually by total colectomy. Other surgical procedures have been investigated but no satisfactory alternative has yet been found. There does, however, appear to be hope for spinal injured patients with severe constipation as a recent study has demonstrated that the implantation of an intradural sacral anterior nerve root stimulator can reduce the need for assisted defaecation, e.g. manual evacuation, and in approximately 50 per cent defaecation can be induced by the stimulator (MacDonagh *et al.*, 1990).

Summary

Tobin and Brocklehurst (1986) in a study of the treatment of faecal incontinence in the elderly have demonstrated that the simple therapeutic measures described in this chapter are effective. Complete restoration of faecal continence was achieved in 87 per cent of their treatment group who complied with the treatment compared with 32 per cent spontaneous resolution among their control group.

This chapter has presented information on the causes of faecal incontinence and its treatment. Faecal incontinence should be regarded as a curable and preventable problem. It must not be accepted as inevitable.

References

Ardron, M.E. and Main, A.N.H. (1990), 'Management of constipation', *British Medical Journal*, 300: 1400.

Bannister, J.J., Abouzekry, L. and Read, N.W. (1987b), 'Effect of aging on anorectal function', *Gut*, 28: 353–7.

Bannister, J.J., Davison, P., Timms, J.M., Gibbons, C. and Read, N.W. (1987a), 'Effect of stool size and consistency on defaecation', *Gut*, 28: 1246–50.

Bannister, J.J., Timms, J.M., Barfield, L.J., Donnelly, T.C. and Read, N.W. (1986), 'Physiological studies in young women with chronic constipation', *International Journal of Colorectal Disease*, 1: 175–82.

Barnes, P.R.H. and Lennard-Jones, J.E. (1985), 'Balloon expulsion from the rectum in constipation of different types', *Gut*, 26: 1049–52.

Barrett, J.A. (1988a), 'Effect of wheat bran on stool size', *British Medical Journal*, 296: 1127–8.

Barrett, J.A. (1988b), 'A study of the pathophysiology of faecal incontinence among geriatric patients', MD Thesis, University of Liverpool.

Barrett, J.A., Brocklehurst, J.C., Kiff, E.S. and Ferguson, G. (1989), 'Anal function in geriatric patients with faecal incontinence', *Gut*, 30: 1244–51.

Barrett, J.A., Brocklehurst, J.C., Kiff, E.S., Ferguson, F. and Faragher, E.B. (1990), 'Rectal motility studies in geriatric patients with faecal incontinence', *Age and Ageing*, 19: 311–17.

Barrett, J.A., Faragher, E.B., Kiff, E.S., Ferguson, G. and Brocklehurst, J.C. (1988), 'Why are geriatric patients incontinent of faeces?', *Clinical Science*, 75(Suppl 19): 10 pp.

Bartolo, D.C.C., Jarratt, J.A. and Read, N.W. (1983b), 'The use of conventional electromyography to assess external sphincter neuropathy in man', *Journal of Neurology Neurosurgery and Psychiatry*, 46: 115–18.

Bartolo, D.C.C., Jarratt, J.A., Read, M.G., Donnelly, T.C. and Read, N.W. (1983c), 'The role of partial denervation of the puborectalis muscle in idiopathic faecal incontinence', *British Journal of Surgery*, 70: 664–7.

Bartolo, D.C.C., Read, N.W., Jarratt, J.A., Read, M.G., Donnelly, T.C. and Johnson, A.G. (1983a), 'Differences in anal sphincter function and clinical presentation in patients with pelvic floor descent', *Gastroenterology*, 85: 68–75.

Bartolo, D.C.C., Roe, A.M., Virjee, J. and Mortensen, N.J.McC. (1985), 'Evacuation proctography in obstructed defaecation and rectal intussusception', *British Journal of Surgery*, 72(Suppl): S111–16.

Bass, P. and Dennis, S. (1981), 'The laxative effects of lactulose in normal and constipated subjects', *Journal of Clinical Gastroenterology*, 3(Suppl 1): 23–8.

Bassotti, G., Gaburri, M., Imbimbo, B., Pelli, M.A. and Morelli, A. (1987), 'Colonic mass movements in health and in constipation', *Gastroenterology*, 92: 1310.

Beersiek, F., Parks, A.G. and Swash, M. (1979), 'Pathogenesis of ano-rectal incontinence: a histometric study of the anal sphincter musculature', *Journal of Neurological Science*, 42: 111–27.

Bennett, R.C., Friedman, M.H.W. and Goligher, J.C. (1963), 'Late results of haemorrhoidectomy by ligature and excision', *British Medical Journal*, 2: 216–19.

Brocklehurst, J.C. (1951), *Incontinence in old age*, Edinburgh: Livingstone.

Brocklehurst, J.C., Andrews, K., Richards, B. and Laycock, P.J. (1985), 'Incidence and correlates of incontinence in stroke patients', *Journal of the American Geriatrics Society*, 33: 540–2.

Brocklehurst, J.C., Bee, P., Jones, D. and Palmer, M.K. (1977), 'Bacteriuria in geriatric hospital patients: its correlates and management', *Age and Ageing*, 6: 240–5.

Brocklehurst, J.C. and Dillane, J.B. (1966), 'Studies of the female bladder in old age', *Gerontologia Clinica*, 8: 306–19.

Brocklehurst, J.C. and Khan, M.Y. (1969), 'A study of faecal stasis in old age and the use of 'Dorbanex' in its prevention', *Gerontologia Clinica*, 11: 293–300.

Brocklehurst, J.C., Kirkland, J.L., Martin, J. and Ashford, J. (1983), 'Constipation in long-stay elderly patients: its treatment and prevention by lactulose, poloxalkol-dihydroxyanthroquinolone and phosphate enemas', *Gerontology*, 29: 181–4.

Burkitt, D.P., Walker, A.R.P. and Painter, N.S. (1972), 'Effect of dietary fibre on stools and transit-times, and its role in the causation of disease', *The Lancet*, ii: 1408–11.

Buser, W.D. and Miner, P.B. (1986), 'Delayed rectal sensation with faecal incontinence: successful treatment using anorectal manometry', *Gastroenterology*, 91: 1186–91.

Caldwell, K.P.S. (1963), 'The electrical control of sphincter incompetence', *The Lancet*, ii: 174–5.

Capewell, A.E., Primrose, W.R. and MacIntyre, C. (1986), 'Nursing dependency in registered nursing homes and long term care geriatric wards in Edinburgh', *British Medical Journal*, 292: 1719–21.

Cerulli, M.A., Nikoomanesh, P. and Schuster, M.M. (1979), 'Progress in biofeedback conditioning for faecal incontinence', *Gastroenterology*, 76: 742–6.

Christensen, J. (1971), 'The controls of gastrointestinal movements: some old and new views', *New England Journal of Medicine*, 285: 85–98.

Clarke, M., Hughes, A.O., Dodd, K.J., Palmer, R.L., Brandon, S., Holden, A.N. and Pearce, D. (1979), 'The elderly in residential care: patterns of disability', *Health Trends*, 11: 17–20.

Collins, C.D., Brown, B.H. and Duthie, H.L. (1969), 'An assessment of intraluminal electrical stimulation for anal incontinence', *British Journal of Surgery*, 56: 542–6.

Connell, A.M., Hilton, C., Irvine, G., Lennard-Jones, J.E. and Misiewicz, J.J. (1965), 'Variation of bowel habit in two population samples', *British Medical Journal*, 2: 1095–9.

Cummings, J.H., Jenkins, D.J.A. and Wiggins, H.S. (1976), 'Measurement of the mean transit time of dietary residue through the human gut', *Gut*, 17: 210–18.

Davis, G.R., Santa Ana, C.A., Morawski, S.G. and Fordtran, J.S. (1980), 'Development of a lavage solution associated with minimal water and electrolyte absorption or secretion', *Gastroenterology*, 78: 991–5.

Deiling, D.A., Fischer, R.A. and Fernandez, O. (1959), 'The therapeutic usefulness of Dulcolax', *American Journal of Digestive Diseases*, 4: 311.

Denny-Brown, D.E. and Robertson, E.G. (1935), 'An investigation of the nervous control of defaecation', *Brain*, 58: 256–310.

Devroede, G., Arhan, P., Duguay, C., Tetreault, L., Akanry, M. and Percy, B. (1979), 'Traumatic constipation', *Gastroenterology*, 77: 1258–67.

Devroede, G. and Lamarche, J. (1974), 'Functional importance of extrinsic parasympathetic innervation of the distal colon and rectum in man', *Gastroenterology*, 66: 273–80.

Donald, I.P., Smith, R.G., Cruikshank, J.G., Elton, R.A. and Stoddart, M.E. (1985), 'A study of constipation in the elderly living at home', *Gerontology*, 31: 112–18.

Duncan, D. (1934), 'A determination of the number of nerve fibres in the 8th thoracic and largest lumbar ventral roots of the albino rat', *Journal of Comparative Neurology*, 59: 47–60.

Duthie, H.L. (1978), 'Colonic response to eating', *Gastroenterology*, 75: 527–9.

Eastwood, H.D.H. (1972), 'Bowel transit studies in the elderly: radioopaque markers in the investigation of constipation', *Gerontologia Clinica*, 14: 154–9.

Ferguson, G.H., Redford, J., Barrett, J.A. and Kiff, E.S. (1989), 'The appreciation of rectal distension in faecal incontinence', *Diseases of the Colon and Rectum*, 32: 964–7.

Foord, K.D., Morcos, S.K. and Ward, P. (1983), 'A comparison of Mannitol and Magnesium Citrate preparations for double-contrast barium enema', *Clinical Radiology*, 34: 309–12.

Frenckner, B. (1975), 'Function of the anal sphincters in spinal man', *Gut*, 16: 638–44.

Frenckner, B. and Euler, C.V. (1975), 'Influence of pudendal nerve block on the function of the anal sphincter in man', *Gut*, 16: 482–9.

Galambos, J.T., Hersh, T., Schroder, S. and Wenger, J. (1976), 'Loperamide a new antidiarrheal agent in the treatment of chronic diarrhea', *Gastroenterology*, 70: 1026–9.

Gardner, E. (1940), 'Decrease in human neurones with age', *Anatomical Record*, 77: 529–36.

Garry, R.C. (1933), 'The nervous control of the caudal region of the large bowel in the cat', *Journal of Physiology*, 77: 422–31.

Gibbons, C.P., Trowbridge, E.A., Bannister, J.J. and Read, N.W. (1986), 'Role of anal cushions in maintaining continence', *The Lancet*, i: 886–8.

Goligher, J.C. and Hughes, E.S.R. (1951), 'Sensibility of the rectum and colon: its role in the mechanism of anal continence', *The Lancet*, i: 543–8.

Goodman, J., Pang, J. and Bessman, A.N. (1976), 'Dioctyl sodium sulphasuccinate: an ineffective prophylactic laxative', *Journal of Chronic Diseases*, 29: 59–63.

Grimby, G. and Saltin, B. (1983), 'Mini-review: the ageing muscle', *Clinical Physiology*, 3: 209–18.

Hansen, F.C., Ensor, R., Marcum, S. and Schuster, M.M. (1987), 'Diagnostic and physiologic usefulness of the videoproctogram', *Gastroenterology*, 92: 1425.

Hardcastle, J.D. and Mann, C.V. (1968), 'Study of large bowel peristalsis', *Gut*, 9: 512–20.

Hardcastle, J.D. and Parks, A.G. (1970), 'A study of anal incontinence and some principles of surgical treatment', *Proceedings of the Royal Society of Medicine*, 63: 116–18.

Hardcastle, J.D. and Wilkins, J.L. (1970), 'The action of sennosides and related compounds on human colon and rectum', *Gut*, 11: 1038–42.

Harvard, L.R.C. and Hughes-Roberts, H.E. (1962), 'The treatment of constipation in mental hospitals', *Gut*, 3: 85–90.

Henry, M.M. and Simson, J.N.L. (1985), 'Results of postanal repair: a retrospective study', *British Journal of Surgery*, 72(Suppl): S17–19.

Hinton, J.M., Lennard-Jones, J.E. and Young, A.C. (1969), 'A new method for studying gut transit times using radioopaque markers', *Gut*, 10: 842–7.

Holdstock, D.J. and Misiewicz, J.J. (1970), 'Factors controlling colonic motility: colonic pressures and transit after meals in patients with total gastrectomy, pernicious anaemia or duodenal ulcer', *Gut*, 11: 100–10.

Holdstock, D.J., Misiewicz, J.J., Smith, T. and Rowlands, E.N. (1970), 'Propulsion (mass movements) in the human colon and its relationship to meals and somatic activity', *Gut*, 11: 91–99.

Hopkinson, B.R. and Lightwood, R. (1966), 'Electrical treatment of anal incontinence', *The Lancet*, i: 297–8.

Kachel, G., Ruppin, H., Hagel, J., Barina, W., Meinhardt, M. and Domschke, W. (1986), 'Human intestinal motor activity and transport: effects of a synthetic opiate', *Gastroenterology*, 90: 85–93.

Kellow, J.E., Gill, R.C. and Wingate, D.L. (1987), 'Modulation of human upper gastrointestinal motility by rectal distension', *Gut*, 28: 864–8.

Kiff, E.S., Barnes, P.R.H. and Swash, M. (1984), 'Evidence of pudendal neuropathy in patients with perineal descent and chronic straining at stool', *Gut*, 25: 1279–82.

Kiff, E.S. and Swash, M. (1984a), 'Slowed conduction in the pudendal nerves in idiopathic (neurogenic) faecal incontinence', *British Journal of Surgery*, 71: 614–16.

Kiff, E.S. and Swash, M. (1984b), 'Normal proximal and delayed distal conduction in the pudendal nerves of patients with idiopathic (neurogenic) faecal incontinence', *Journal of Neurology Neurosurgery and Psychiatry*, 47: 820–3.

Krishnamurphy, S., Schniffer, M.D., Rohrmann, C.A. and Ope, C.E. (1985), 'Severe idiopathic constipation is associated with a distinctive abnormality of the colonic myenteric plexus', *Gastroenterology*, 88: 26–34.

Kuipers, H.C., Bleijeuberg, G. and Morree, H.D.E. (1986), 'The spastic pelvic floor syndrome: large bowel outlet obstruction caused by pelvic floor dysfunction: a radiological study', *International Journal of Colorectal Disease*, 1: 44–8.

Lane, W.A. (1915), *The operative treatment of chronic intestinal stasis*, London: James Nesbit.

Langworthy, O.R. and Rosenberg, S.J. (1939a), 'Abnormalities of rectal tone and contraction in paraplegia and hemiplegia', *American Journal of Digestive Diseases*, 6: 455–8.

Langworthy, O.R. and Rosenberg, S.J. (1939b), 'The control by the central nervous system of the rectal smooth muscle', *Journal of Neurology*, 2: 356.

Laurberg, S. and Swash, M. (1989), 'Effects of ageing on the anorectal sphincters and their innervation', *Diseases of the Colon and Rectum*, 32: 737–42.

Lawson, J.N. and Nixon, H.H. (1967), 'Anal canal pressures in the diagnosis of Hirschsprung's disease', *Journal of Paediatric Surgery*, 2: 544–52.

Leigh, R.J. and Turnberg, L.A. (1982), 'Faecal incontinence: the unvoiced symptom', *The Lancet*, i: 1349–51.

Loening-Baucke, V. and Anuras, S. (1984), 'Anorectal manometry in healthy elderly subjects', *Journal of American Geriatrics Society*, 32: 636–9.

MacDonagh, R.P., Sun, W.M., Smallwood, R., Forster, D. and Read, N.W. (1990), 'Control of defaecation in patients with spinal injuries by stimulation of sacral anterior nerve roots', *British Medical Journal*, 300: 1494–7.

McHugh, S.M. and Diamant, N.E. (1987), 'Effect of age, gender, and parity on anal canal pressures', *Digestive Diseases and Science*, 32: 726–36.

MacLennan, W.J. and Pooler, A.F.W.M. (1975), 'A comparison of sodium picosulphate (Laxoberal) with standardised senna (Senokot) in geriatric patients', *Current Medical Research and Opinion*, 2: 641–7.

Macleod, J.H. (1987), 'Management of anal incontinence by biofeedback', *Gastroenterology*, 93: 291–4.

Marcus, S.N. and Heaton, K.W. (1987), 'Irritable bowel-type symptoms in spontaneous and induced constipation', *Gut*, 28(2): 156–9.

Martelli, H., Devroede, G., Arhan, P., Duguay, C., Dornic, C. and Faverdin, C. (1978), 'Mechanism of idiopathic constipation: outlet obstruction', *Gastroenterology*, 75: 623–31.

Matheson, D.M. and Keighley, M.R.B. (1981), 'Manometric evaluation of rectal prolapse and faecal incontinence', *Gut*, 22: 126–9.

Miller, R., Bartolo, D.C.C., Cervero, F. and Mortensen, N.J.McC. (1987), 'Anorectal temperature sensation: a comparison of normal and incontinent patients', *British Journal of Surgery*, 74: 511–15.

Milne, J.S. and Williamson, J. (1972), 'Bowel habit in older people', *Gerontologia Clinica*, 14: 56–60.

Muller-Lissner, S.A. (1988), 'Effect of wheat bran on weight of stool and gastrointestinal transit time: a meta analysis', *British Medical Journal*, 296: 615–17.

Neill, M.E., Parks, A.G. and Swash, M. (1981), 'Physiological studies of the anal sphincter musculature in faecal incontinence and rectal prolapse', *British Journal of Surgery*, 68: 531–6.

Neill, M.E. and Swash, M. (1980), 'Increased motor unit fibre density in the external anal sphincter in ano-rectal incontinence: a single fibre EMG study', *Journal of Neurology Neurosurgery and Psychiatry*, 43: 343–7.

Palmer, K.R. and Khan, A.N. (1979), 'Oral mannitol: a simple and effective bowel preparation for barium enema', *British Medical Journal*, 2: 1038.

Parks, A.G. (1967), 'Post-anal perineorrhaphy for rectal prolapse', *Proceedings of the Royal Society of Medicine*, 60: 920–1.

Parks, A.G., Swash, M. and Urich, H. (1977), 'Sphincter denervation in anorectal incontinence and rectal prolapse', *Gut*, 18: 656–65.

Percy, J.P., Neill, M.E., Kandiah, T.K. and Swash, M. (1982), 'A neurogenic factor in faecal incontinence in the elderly', *Age and Ageing*, 11: 175–9.

Porter, N.H. (1962), 'A physiological study of the pelvic floor in rectal prolapse', *Annals of the Royal College of Surgeons of England*, 31: 379–404.

Preston, D.M. (1985), 'Arbuthnot Lane's disease: chronic intestinal stasis', *British Journal of Surgery*, 72(Suppl): S8–10.

Preston, D.M., Butler, M.G., Smith, B. and Lennard-Jones, J.E. (1983), 'Neuropathology of slow transit constipation', *Gut*, 24: A997.

Preston, D.M., Lennard-Jones, J.E. and Thomas, B.M. (1984), 'The balloon proctogram', *British Journal of Surgery*, 71: 29–32.

Preston, D.M. and Lennard-Jones, J.E. (1985a), 'Anismus in chronic constipation', *Digestive Disease and Science*, 30: 413–18.

Preston, D.M. and Lennard-Jones, J.E. (1985b), 'Pelvic colon motility and response to intraluminal bisacodyl in slow transit constipation', *Digestive Disease and Science*, 30: 289–94.

Puxty, J.A.H. and Fox, R.A. (1986), 'Golytely: a new approach to faecal impaction in old age', *Age and Ageing*, 15: 182–4.

Rattan, S. and Culver, P.J. (1987), 'Influence of loperamide on the internal anal sphincter in the oppossum', *Gastroenterology*, 93: 121–8.

Read, N.W. and Abouzekry, L. (1986), 'Why do patients with faecal impaction have faecal incontinence?', *Gut*, 27: 283–7.

Read, N.W. Abouzekry, L., Read, M.G., Howell, P., Ottewell, D. and Donnelly, T.C. (1985), 'Anorectal function in elderly patients with faecal impaction', *Gastroenterology*, 89: 959–66.

Read, N.W., Bartolo, D.C.C. and Read, M.G. (1984), 'Differences in anal function in patients with incontinence to solids and in patients with incontinence to liquids', *British Journal of Surgery*, 71: 39–42.

Read, N.W., Harford, W.V., Schmulen, A.C., Read, M.G., Santa Ana, C.A. and Fordtran, J.S. (1979), 'A clinical study of patients with faecal incontinence and diarrhoea', *Gastroenterology*, 76: 747–56.

Read, N.W., Haynes, W.G., Bartolo, D.C.C., Hall, J., Read, M.G., Donnelly, T.C. and

Johnson, A.G. (1983), 'Use of anorectal manometry during rectal infusion of saline to investigate sphincter function in incontinent patients', *Gastroenterology*, 85: 105–13.

Read, M.G. and Read, N.W. (1982), 'Role of anorectal sensation in preserving continence', *Gut*, 23: 345–7.

Read, M., Read, N.W., Barber, D.C. and Duthie, H.L. (1982), 'Effects of loperamide on anal sphincter function in patients complaining of chronic diarrhoea with faecal incontinence and urgency', *Digestive Diseases and Science*, 27: 807–14.

Read, N.W., Timms, J.M., Barfield, L.J., Donnelly, T.C. and Bannister, J.J. (1986), 'Impairment of defaecation in young women with severe constipation', *Gastroenterology*, 90: 53–60.

Rendtorff, R.C. and Kashigarian, M. (1966), 'Stool patterns of healthy adult males', *Diseases of the Colon and Rectum*, 10: 222–8.

Robinson, J.M. (1984), 'Evaluation of methods for assessment of bladder and urethral function', in Brocklehurst, J.C. (ed.), *Urology in the elderly*, Edinburgh: Churchill Livingstone, pp. 19–54.

Roe, A.M., Bartolo, D.C.C. and Mortensen, N.J.McC. (1986a), 'Diagnosis and surgical management of intractable constipation', *British Journal of Surgery*, 73: 854–61.

Roe, A.M., Bartolo, D.C.C. and Mortensen, N.J.McC. (1986b), 'New method for assessment of anal sensation in various anorectal disorders', *British Journal of Surgery*, 73: 310–12.

Rogers, J., Henry, M.M. and Misiewicz, J.J. (1988), 'Combined sensory and motor deficit in primary neuropathic faecal incontinence', *Gut*, 29: 5–9.

Sanford, J.R.A. (1975), 'Tolerance of debility in elderly dependents by supporters at home: its significance for hospital practice', *British Medical Journal*, 3: 471–3.

Scheuer, M., Kuijpers, H.C. and Jacobs, P.P. (1989), 'Postanal repair restores anatomy rather than function', *Diseases of the Colon and Rectum*, 32: 960–3.

Schiller, L.R., Santa Ana, C.A., Morawski, S.G. and Fordtran, J.S. (1984), 'Mechanism of the anti diarrheal effect of loperamide', *Gastroenterology*, 86: 1475–80.

Smith, B. (1968), 'Effect of irritant purgatives on the myenteric plexus in man and the mouse', *Gut*, 9: 139–43.

Smith, R.G., Currie, J.E.J. and Walls, A.D.F. (1978), 'Whole gut irrigation: a new treatment for constipation', *British Medical Journal*, 2: 396–7.

Smith, R.G. and Lewis, S. (1990), 'The relationship between digital rectal examination and abdominal radiographs in elderly patients', *Age and Ageing*, 19: 142–3.

Snooks, S.J., Barnes, P.R.H., Swash, M. and Henry, M.M. (1985b), 'Damage to the innervation of the pelvic floor musculature in chronic constipation', *Gastroenterology*, 89: 977–81.

Snooks, S.J., Henry, M.M. and Swash, M. (1985a), 'Anorectal incontinence and rectal prolapse: differential assessment of the innervation to puborectalis and external anal sphincter muscles', *Gut*, 26: 470–6.

Snooks, S.J., Henry, M.M. and Swash, M. (1985c), 'Faecal incontinence due to external anal sphincter division in childbirth is associated with damage to the innervation of the pelvic floor musculature: a double pathology', *British Journal of Obstetrics and Gynaecology*, 92: 824–8.

Snooks, S.J., Setchell, M., Swash, M. and Henry, M.M. (1984), 'Injury to the innervation of the pelvic floor musculature in childbirth', *The Lancet*, ii: 546–50.

Thomas, T.M., Egan, M. and Meade, T.W. (1985), 'Prevalence and implications of faecal (and double) incontinence', *British Journal of Surgery*, 72(Suppl): S141.

Tobin, G.W. (1987), 'Incontinence in the elderly', *Practitioner*, 231: 843–7.

Tobin, G.W. and Brocklehurst, J.C. (1986), 'Faecal incontinence in residential homes for the elderly: prevalence, aetiology and management', *Age and Ageing*, 15: 41–6.

Turnbull, G.K., Lennard-Jones, J.E. and Bartram, C.I. (1986), 'Failure of rectal expulsion as a cause of constipation: why fibre and laxatives sometimes fail', *The Lancet*, 1: 767–9.

Tytgat, G.N. and Huibregtse, K. (1975), 'Loperamide and ileostomy output: placebo controlled double-blind crossover study', *The Lancet*, ii: 667.

Varma, J.S., Bradnock, J., Smith, R.G. and Smith, A.N. (1988), 'Constipation in the elderly: a physiologic study', *Diseases of the Colon and Rectum*, 31: 111–15.

Wald, A. and Tunuguntla, A.K. (1984), 'Anorectal sensorimotor dysfunction in faecal incontinence and diabetes mellitus: modification with biofeedback therapy', *New England Journal of Medicine*, 310: 1282–7.

Wesselius-DeCasparis, A., Braadbaart, S., Van den Bergh-Bohlken, G.E. and Micica, M. (1968), 'Treatment of chronic constipation with "lactulose" syrup: results of a double blind study', *Gut*, 9: 84–6.

Wheatley, I.C., Hardy, K.J. and Dent, J. (1977), 'Anal pressure studies in spinal patients', *Gut*, 18: 488–90.

Womack, N.R., Morrison, J.F.B. and Williams, N.S. (1986), 'The role of pelvic floor denervation in the aetiology of idiopathic faecal incontinence', *British Journal of Surgery*, 73: 404–7.

Womack, N.R., Williams, N.S., Holmfield, J.H.M., Morrison, J.F.B. and Simpkins, K.C. (1985), 'New method for the dynamic assessment of anorectal function in constipation', *British Journal of Surgery*, 72: 994–8.

Yoshioka, K., Hyland, G. and Keighley, M.R.B. (1988), 'Physiological changes after postanal repair and parameters predicting outcome', *British Journal of Surgery*, 75: 1220.

Youle, M.S. and Read, N.W. (1984), 'Effect of painless rectal distension on gastrointestinal transit of solid meal', *Digestive Disease and Science*, 29: 902–6.

10 Setting up a continence advisory service

KATHLEEN E.M. BAKER AND BRENDA H. ROE

Introduction

The scope and extent of continence advisory services differ from one district health authority to another. The service may encompass only one unit or a whole health authority. The formulation of services are also influenced by the unit which funds the post. The age groups seen by the adviser are also dependent on local policy. Many services have developed in response to the increase on the budget that continence problems have made. These four factors have made many continence advisers' roles unique and have affected the setting up of services.

The *Working for Patients* (Department of Health, 1989a) and *Caring for People* (Department of Health, 1989b) White Papers, now the National Health Service and Community Care Act (1990), will also have an effect on existing and future services. Both White Papers make reference to the efficient and effective utilisation of resources. In some health districts this may be viewed from a purely budgetary angle and the effect on the continence services will have to be evaluated. Quality of services is also an integral part of the papers and little research has been completed on the effect of continence services to prove or disprove their value.

History of the services

In 1974 the Disabled Living Foundation appointed an incontinence adviser, offering a nationwide service. At that time there were no nurse specialists involved in continence care. In 1977 Dame Phyllis Friend, Chief Nursing Officer at the Department of Health, recommended that health authorities recognise the need for a nurse to act as a reference point on the subject of incontinence. The recommendation suggested that this function be incorporated within the role of an existing Nursing Officer's post. The recommendations were directed at improving standards of care for those suffering from incontinence.

The response of the health authorities was slow. At the inaugural meeting of the Association of Continence Advisers in September 1980, only one of the six founder members was in a post entitled Incontinence Adviser. The other members were either involved in research or had a specific interest in the subject of incontinence.

At this time, the products available to clients with incontinence were limited and many were reusable. Consequently, the health authorities did not view incontinence as a major budgetary expenditure. It was only when the manufacturing companies developed their ranges and disposable products became readily available that many health authorities appointed continence advisers (see Chapter 6, Aids and appliances for incontinence). Further support was given to the appointment of continence advisers by the findings of the King's Fund Working Party (1983) which identified the lack of education of both doctors and nurses regarding continence.

A combination of the King's Fund recommendations and the increased number of products began to have an influence on the health authorities. During the early 1980s many health authorities began to appoint continence advisers. At first, many of the continence advisers found themselves acting as 'pad and pant' nurses, supplying products from the boot of their cars. Many were district nurses with a part-time role of continence adviser within their job descriptions. Those with enlightened nurse managers were able to develop the role to a full-time post. Slowly the role became that of a clinical nurse specialist. The nurse gave advice to clients, carers, health care professionals, voluntary groups and organisations. The introduction at this time of the English National Board Course (ENB 978) provided the introduction to the promotion of continence for all nurses. The course has assisted in developing a more positive attitude to continence problems. The ENB course is only an introduction and its remit did not include the setting up of a continence advisory service. Nurses newly appointed to continence advisory posts will find that very little has been written on this subject.

The Association of Continence Advisers (1985) produced a leaflet outlining the elements of a job description for a continence adviser. In this leaflet reference is made to the four main areas of any nurse specialist post. This is a good starting point for any adviser, each element forming objectives for a service.

Starting a service

The setting up of a service will require cooperation and collaboration with many services, such as the nurse and health care professional education divisions, support service managers, finance, etc. The newly appointed adviser will need to seek the help of these professionals in establishing a service.

A baseline of the health authorities' clients who are known to have a continence problem should be identified. This can be accomplished by identifying the buying patterns for all continence products and their points of issue. The supplies manager has access to this information. The linen usage will also indicate areas with known continence problems and the linen supplies/laundry manager is usually able to supply this information.

The cost of these physical resources can be obtained from the finance manager. The number of clients with a known/identified continence problem can be compared with the financial and physical resources committed by the health authority. Thomas *et al.*

(1980) conducted a postal survey which showed that 5 per cent of the population will have regular urinary incontinence. Roe (1990) stated that one health authority in the United Kingdom was aware of 4,312 clients with a problem. When this figure is compared with the Thomas *et al.* study, it could be expected that there were 7,000 clients not known to the service. Comparison of known clients with possible potential need within a health authority will also form part of the baseline.

Roe (1990) describes component parts of a continence service as: practice, management, education and research. These four areas are described in detail in the following sections. The findings of the baseline can be utilised in the formation of objectives for a continence service.

Objectives for a service should be realistic and attainable. In 1983 Badger *et al.*, when evaluating a new continence service, stated that it was difficult to measure outcomes. Both *Working for Patients* (Department of Health, 1989a) and *Caring for People* (Department of Health, 1989b) White Papers refer to objectives and outcomes as quality measures for services. The emphasis of both these papers on quality will need to be included with the objectives in a service specification.

The involvement of all managers affected by the introduction of the service should be sought. The active involvement of Social Services and voluntary and statutory organisations is imperative for the success of the service. Customer involvement, through such organisations, will provide feedback on the effectiveness of the service. This involvement can be through a multidisciplinary working group, nursing practice group, or a continence promotion group.

Practice

A continence advisory service should not only set standards for practice, but provide a resource, reference and educational service to all nurses and carers. Unfortunately, incontinence has always been a taboo subject and many negative attitudes prevail. The improvement in practice should be a prime objective of all services. Identifying the attitudes to incontinence within a health authority will enable the adviser to target areas for continence education. This can be achieved with questionnaires on staff knowledge of continence problems or by informal discussion. The adviser should identify any existing continence policies (if available) – these may require updating or rewriting. The involvement of the multidisciplinary group in these tasks should enable acceptance of continence policies. The emphasis of the continence policy should be on the promotion of continence and not on the more negative aspect of management of incontinence.

The individual assessment of a client's incontinence forms a fundamental basis of any continence service. Raising the profile of continence to the same priority as any other individual need is the key to an effective service for all clients (see Chapter 3, Assessment of urinary incontinence). How incontinence is to be assessed, and by whom it should be completed, requires inclusion in the continence policy.

An operational policy for the service needs to be agreed with all managers and circulated to all personnel involved in continence care. This policy should include the following points:

1. Method of referral to the service, including whether written or verbal referrals are acceptable. Which personnel, clients and carers referrals are accepted from and any criteria for their acceptance, such as adults only, children with handicapping conditions only, over 65 years of age, etc.
2. Continence clinics: sites and frequency of clinics; which member of staff runs the clinic; who is seen at the clinic.
3. Home/domiciliary visits: whether offered and to whom available.
4. Areas of responsibility of the continence service, e.g. hospitals only, community only, client groups seen, etc.
5. Role of the manufacturing companies, e.g. whether seen by individual service managers, or the continence service, amount and type of involvement in the continence policy if any, etc.
6. Management of product trials and evaluations, e.g. whether conducted solely by the continence service, monitored by the service or individual units having responsibility.
7. Budget holders for continence products, e.g. whether the continence service has this responsibility or named managers, names of personnel who have to give permission for alteration or extension of product lines.
8. Clinical policies, procedures, standards, e.g. who is responsible for those relating to continence and sphere of responsibility.
9. Continence education programmes, e.g. who is responsible for sessions and when will they be conducted, who is eligible to attend and how they are nominated, etc.
10. Research responsibilities of the service, e.g. the type of research the service will be involved in and the contact person, etc.

To ensure that all personnel are aware of the operational and continence policy, the adviser will need to meet with all staff in order to explain it and answer any questions. This task can prove daunting if the service covers a whole health district and only one adviser is in post. The 'link nurse' system has been successfully used by several continence services, to improve communication and client care.

Hall *et al.* (1988) adopted this approach by utilising the skills and interest of other nurses in teaching continence care. These link nurses had extended education and imparted their knowledge to others. Several continence services have adopted this approach to the dissemination of knowledge, throughout a health district. These nurses will require additional training in continence promotion and the management of incontinence to be able to fulfil this role. The link nurses can teach the use of individual assessment and how to interpret the findings. Once an assessment form has been developed it needs to be tested for its reliability and validity. To date, no studies have tested the reliability and validity of continence assessment forms. Once an acceptable form has been developed its use needs to be agreed with the local policy/procedure committee for district wide implementation.

Management

The management of a continence service will often be seen within the performance review structures, based on the achievement of the service objectives. These objectives require careful formulation. Although many health authorities view continence problems from a financial aspect, care needs to be exercised when including financial reductions in the service objectives.

Ramsbottom (1982) showed that continence promotion intervention was not always the most cost effective option. Although the products used may decrease, nursing intervention time may increase costs. As the service becomes more widely known the demand should increase. This may have a direct effect on the number of clients treated and the resultant costs of those not previously known. Objectives should be formulated around the four areas of clinical speciality, practice, management, education and research. Examples of possible first year objectives are given in Table 10.1.

The operational policy and service objectives form the initial building blocks of the service. White (1982) described the functions of a continence advisory service in the

Table 10.1 Possible first-year objectives for a continence advisory service

Area	Objective	Influence/support
Clinical	1. Establish individual continence assessment for all clients.	(a) Post basic education department. (b) Nurse manager's support.
	2. Extend product range to encompass all types of incontinence.	(a) Commodity/continence advisory group. (b) Budget holder's agreement.
Education	1. Develop continence workshop programme for all areas.	(a) Liaise with nurse education to produce.
	2. Conduct continence workshops in all areas.	(b) Nurse managers to nominate key staff to attend.
Management	1. Develop system to monitor continence expenditure in all areas.	(a) Liaise with finance to produce monthly reports to continence budget holders.
	2. Identify number and type of products used monthly in each area.	(b) Liaise with supplies and distribute to budget holders.
Research	1. Identify area of research.	(a) Agree with line manager.
	2. Conduct literature search.	(b) Gain access to suitable library.

Northern Region. These functions would nowadays be described as service objectives or operational policy. King (1979) described a plan to assist nurses to look at continence problems from a more positive angle. The elements of this plan could be incorporated into service objectives. The education of nurses and the involvement of nurse managers are essential elements of this plan. Stewart (1985) referred to continence advisers as people designated to make policies and manage budgets. Again, this emphasises the need for operational and service objectives.

The involvement of the multidisciplinary team in the setting of operational and service objectives is important. Continence promotion and management requires a multidisciplinary approach and the care of clients will require input from several services. Tattersall (1985) suggested possible members of an assessment team and included health care professionals and the client and family. The following professions can contribute to continence policies: occupational therapists, physiotherapists, school nurses, health visitors, social services personnel, carers' support groups, doctors (hospital or community), district nurses and environmental health officers.

Following the *Working for Patients* (Department of Health, 1989a) and *Caring for People* (Department of Health, 1989b) White Papers the emphasis on continence services will be expected to have a more business-like approach. Continence services are expected to prepare mission statements describing the main purpose and direction of the service. An example of a mission statement is:

> The Continence Service will provide individual assessment, for all clients with a continence problem. This assessment will be offered to any individual referred to the service. This will be followed by a planned intervention, offering a package of care, for that client based upon the promotion of continence and effective management of intractable incontinence.

A service specification will also be included into the business plan. This should include: manpower in post and their grades, area of care covered by the service, availability to other purchasers and costs per head or block contract for the continence service.

Standards of care and quality

The *Working for Patients* (Department of Health, 1989a) and *Caring for People* (Department of Health, 1989b) White Papers require the continence service to be part of an overall quality assurance programme. This will also need to be included in the business plan by incorporating measurable outcomes of the quality of the service. The three main elements of measuring any service involve quality, quantity and cost, and are seen as key objectives.

The Department of Health Nursing Division's document *A Strategy for Nursing* (1989) directs all nurses to key targets in the following areas: practice, manpower, education, leadership and management. All standards should reflect these targets and the four component parts of the continence service – practice, management, education and research. All continence advisers will need to produce standards of care for the continence service.

A nursing standard

A definition of a nursing standard is a professionally agreed level of performance, appropriate to the population addressed. It is achievable, desirable, observable and measurable. This means a method whereby the customer is able to see what should be received and to what degree that care should be given. It is this element of quality and customer satisfaction that the two White Papers (Department of Health, 1989a,b) and Health Service Act (1990) refer to for the future health care services.

The White Papers see the future of the National Health Service (NHS) as a free market and customer satisfaction as paramount. This will not only govern where money is allocated, but which continence service the customer or purchasers requests care from. Therefore, the continence standards must reflect the services offered and identify their quality. Audit is a necessary component of any quality assurance programme and therefore the standards must be measurable. Wherever possible these standards should be based upon identified research evidence. When formulating standards of continence care it is important that they do not appear as policies or procedures. They must be viewed as a statement of the service's outcomes of care.

How are standards set?
Many health authorities have core standards. If continence standards have already been formulated, decide whether the service's operational policy and objectives will enhance or improve them. Where there are no local standards they will need to be formulated. Donabedian (1966; 1980) outlined the following approach to standard setting and incorporates three areas involving structure, process and outcome.

The structure
This area should describe what is required to meet the standard, e.g. equipment, staff knowledge and level of skill required, etc. A standard for continence assessment could read as: 'All qualified nurses are able to complete a continence assessment and have local access to suitable products as required by the client.'

The process
The process part of the standard is the action that staff should take. The framework of the nursing process is a good example and basis from which to start, e.g. assessment, planning, implementation and evaluation. A process for continence assessment may therefore read: 'The qualified nurse will complete a continence assessment, using the locally recognised form (continence assessment form), and then plan the intervention or referral for that client.'

The outcome

This describes how the care will affect the client. It must be achievable and measurable. For example, if the client has intractable double incontinence at night-time only, the following may be written: 'The client will receive a product to contain effectively and efficiently the continence problem, that is suitable for their lifestyle. The client will receive a follow-up visit one week later to assess the effectiveness of the product. The client will be asked to complete a product satisfaction questionnaire.'

Education

The success of the service is dependent upon the knowledge, skills and attitudes of all nurses. Without their commitment and motivation the service will not be efficient and effective. Green and Blannin (1983) outlined a curriculum for the promotion and management of continence designed to teach nurses new concepts, skills and attitudes. Holding *ad hoc* talks, with purely voluntary attendance, is a recipe for an empty room. A great deal has to be said for a captive audience. Interested staff should be nominated by their manager for attendance at educational programmes and where possible this should be recognised as part of their professional development and continuing education. Identifying nurses' current knowledge of continence is essential when setting up a continence advisory service and prior to arranging any teaching programmes. This may be achieved by a questionnaire or more informally by group discussion.

A suggested teaching plan is outlined in Table 10.2. The overall aim of the session would be to introduce the course members to the attitudes of society regarding incontinence.

There should be no more than five objectives per session and course members informed of them prior to the class. The objectives should reflect the knowledge to be

Table 10.2 Suggested teaching plan for a nurses' education session on the continence advisory service

Course members:	Teaching environment:
Numbers	Room size
Current knowledge	Seating available
	Parking facilities
	Beverages/meals
	Toilets
Length of session	Audio-visual aids
Teaching method:	Evaluation method:
Lesson	Written evaluation
Discussion	Verbal evaluation
Experiential learning	Handouts

gained from the session. For example, at the end of the session the course member should be able to do the following:

1. State three negatives attitudes to incontinence found in society today.
2. Discuss the Victorian attitudes still prevalent today.
3. List the colloquial expressions for micturition.

The words used in the objectives must be measurable, for example 'list' or 'discuss' are measurable, but 'know' or 'understand' are hard to measure. All educational programmes should be evaluated and the evaluations distributed to line managers and course members. The comments from the evaluations should then be incorporated when planning the next course.

Developing a resource centre
All continence services should be a resource for staff and clients. A comprehensive range of products should be on view regardless of whether they are available within that health authority. Leaflets, educational booklets and product information should be on display and sufficient copies available for distribution or collection. The White Papers *Working for Patients* (Department of Health, 1989a) and *Caring for People* (Department of Health, 1989b) both refer to the need to increase the information given to clients. Leaflets about the continence service with contact addresses and telephone numbers should be available to all.

The educational role of the service needs to encompass clients and carers as well as staff (see Chapter 11, Teaching patients and carers about continence). Teaching programmes should also be implemented to prevent continence problems, e.g. courses for school nurses and health visitors to target teenagers, young mothers and fathers and infants. Collaboration with continuing education centres within a health authority is advisable. If the service undertakes courses it is best to plan compatible training times with the department responsible for continuing education.

An essential part of the development of the service is also to identify the training needs of individual continence advisers, which should then be agreed with their line manager. These needs can be identified from the service objectives, in conjunction with the four components of the continence adviser's role: practice, management, education and research. In the business climate of the National Health Service not all professional development needs will be met by traditional nursing courses. Therefore, courses at further and higher education establishments may be more applicable, e.g. marketing diplomas, or management, teaching and research qualifications.

Research

Finally, research is one of the key areas of the continence adviser's role. To date, other than the Badger *et al.* (1983) study, no research has been carried out to evaluate a continence advisory service. There is certainly much expertise among continence advisers and the majority of them are involved in some element of enquiry or data collection in their everyday role. This frequently takes the form of product evaluation. The results of these evaluations often remain in one health authority or region.

They are not published, because the advisers know they are not based on a sound research methodology. This lack of information, to other health authorities and colleagues, results in practices and product purchases still being based on untested recommendations.

Manufacturers of incontinence products are in the business of profit otherwise they do not survive. Therefore, no product samples issued for trialing are free and the use of samples will be calculated in the end product price. Therefore it is pointless in carrying out product trials that will not produce meaningful information. It is essential, therefore, that products for incontinence should be thoroughly tested in controlled trials before they are more widely used in practice. The results of such trials would be worth publishing and reduce the tendency to reinvent the wheel and indiscriminate use of untested products. This would also return the most costly commodity of all, which is the time of the continence adviser to devote to other areas of priority (see Chapter 6, Aids and appliances for incontinence).

The vast number of product developments, short product purchase agreement times, and the workload of continence advisers, all contribute to a lack of their being able to carry out research. Also, many of them may not have received any initial training for undertaking a research project. Nurses know that their practice must be based on research evidence (Briggs, 1972) and continence advisers find themselves on a never-ending treadmill of product trial and evaluation, not research. Newly appointed continence advisers must be wary of this trap. If they have not undertaken any research then they should find someone within the health authority who has, or attend a research appreciation course.

There is a great need to evaluate clinical nursing practice and this is a challenge for all clinical nurse specialists. Continence advisers are certainly not the only nurse specialists who do not conduct research. One of the main reasons for this may, in some areas, rest with their management. The research element of the nurse specialist role is still not fully appreciated. There is a need to exert pressure for this vital element to be recognised. All nurse specialists should contribute either directly or indirectly to research into clinical nursing practice. This will help to further develop and improve nursing, in particular the promotion of continence and management of incontinence. Continence advisers must share their knowledge, not only through research but through their everyday role. If they are unable to conduct research then they may act as facilitators for others to do so. Many undergraduate and postgraduate nurses may be interested in carrying out research into the promotion of continence and management of incontinence.

Summary

In summary, this chapter on setting up a continence service, has focused on the four main components of a clinical nurse speciality, namely, practice, management, education and research. The importance of establishing service objectives and an operational policy are outlined with examples given. Quality assurance measures are introduced in the form of standard setting. The emphasis on education for formal and informal carers is outlined. Professional development for the continence adviser has also been recommended in line with their stated service objectives. Finally the role of the continence adviser in utilising, conducting and facilitating the much needed research into clinical nursing practices, for the promotion and management of continence has been discussed and recommendations made. The continued development of continence services following on from the last decade and into the next, remains an exciting challenge keeping in step with the wider changes in health care delivery.

References

Association of Continence Advisers (1985), *Guidelines*, London: Association of Continence Advisers.

Badger, F.J., Drummond, M.F. and Isaacs, B. (1983), 'Some issues in the clinical, social and economic evaluation of new nursing services', *Journal of Advanced Nursing*, 8: 487–94.

Briggs, A. (1972), *Report of the Committee on Nursing*, London: HMSO.

Department of Health (1989a), *Working for Patients*, London: HMSO.

Department of Health (1989b), *Caring for People*, London: HMSO.

Department of Health Nursing Division (1989), *A Strategy for Nursing*, London: Department of Health.

Donabedian, A. (1966), 'Evaluating the quality of medical care', *Milbank Memorial Fund Quarterly*, 4(2): 166–203.

Donabedian, A. (1980), *The Definition of Quality and Approaches in Assessment: Explorations in quality assessment and monitoring*, vol. 1, the Health Administration Press.

Green, J. and Blannin, J. (1983), 'Promoting continence', *Nursing Times*, 30 February.

Hall, C., Castleden, C.M. and Grove, G.J. (1988), 'Fifty-six continence advisers, the peripatetic teacher', *British Medical Journal*, 297: 6657, 1181.

King, M.R. (1979), 'A study of incontinence in a psychiatric hospital', *Nursing Times*, July: 1133–5.

King's Fund Working Party (1983), *Action on Incontinence*, London: King's Fund, p. 43.

National Health Service and Community Care Act (1990), London: HMSO.

Ramsbottom, F. (1982), 'Is advice really cheap?', *Journal of Community Nursing*, 5(11): 9–16.

Roe, B.H. (1990), 'Development of continence advisory services in the United Kingdom', *Scandinavian Journal of Caring Sciences*, 4(2): 51–4.

Stewart, M. (1985), 'Preparing for the future', *Nursing Times*, April: 62–3.

Tattersall, A. (1985), 'Getting the whole picture', *Nursing Times*, April: 55–8.

Thomas, T.M., Plymatt, K.R., Blannin, J. and Meade, T.W. (1980), 'Prevalence of urinary incontinence', *British Medical Journal*, 281: 1243–5.

White, H. (1982), 'Setting up an advisory service', *Journal of District Nursing*, 1(3): 4–6.

11 Teaching patients and carers about continence

BRENDA H. ROE

Introduction

Teaching is recognised as an important aspect of nursing practice for the promotion of continence and management of incontinence. Despite recognition of this role, few research studies in nursing have looked at the effectiveness of teaching and incontinence. As previous chapters have shown, the main thrust in recent years has been to change attitudes, both professional and public, in relation to continence and to establish successful treatments. This chapter presents current research evidence in relation to teaching patients and carers about continence and incontinence. It will present, first of all, details about how people learn, and describe the teaching methods available to be used. This will be followed by a discussion of the role of the nurse in relation to patient education and a review of studies which have involved behavioural strategies for the promotion of continence. The chapter is completed by research which has dealt with teaching the management of appliances used for incontinence.

Theories of learning

Learning has been traditionally categorised into three areas which relate to cognitive, affective and psychomotor skills (Bloom, 1956; Krathwohl *et al.*, 1965; Redman, 1984; Coutts and Hardy, 1985). Cognitive learning refers to the process of thinking or of acquiring information and working with it. For example, acquiring knowledge of the causes of incontinence. Affective learning incorporates the values, attitudes or beliefs which can create change and has important motivational influences. Finally, psychomotor skill learning is the acquisition of a motor skill; such as learning how to go to the toilet or how to change a urine drainage bag. Such skills are learned and perfected through frequent reinforcement and practice. The majority of teaching by continence advisers, nurses and medical personnel has been to change both the professional and public's attitude to incontinence: not to treat incontinence as a taboo subject or accept it as a consequence of ageing or being female (Wells, 1984). As all the previous chapters have shown, incontinence is a symptom, for which the underlying cause should be sought and appropriate treatment or management instigated.

Learning has been said to take place at different levels and times, with people acquiring and using knowledge in different ways (Coutts and Hardy, 1985). An individual's style of learning also helps to determine the teaching approach adopted which will achieve a positive outcome. Learning in a number of areas may be required at the same time or before learning can take place. For example, cognitive processes are also involved in most adult psychomotor learning. An understanding of the relevance of a skill needs to be developed along with how to carry out the skill movements. The next section describes the teaching methods available and their suitability for the types of learning. Verbal reinforcement and praise have also been found to be useful in health teaching (ibid.). A number of key factors: motivation, memory, age and environment, may affect learning and need to be taken into account when teaching both patients and carers.

Motivation

Coutts and Hardy (1985) state that motivation is a crucial factor which influences learning. Two kinds of motivation have been described: intrinsic, where behaviour continues without reward or reinforcement, and extrinsic, which requires re-inforcement. For example, in hospital, reinforcement with bladder training may be provided by nurses. The patient complies and may rarely have an opportunity to create his or her own motivation. Once home, the reinforcement is no longer there, and without an established intrinsic motivation, the behaviour, that is bladder training, may discontinue. In order to ensure intrinsic and extrinsic motivation is achieved, Webb (1983) has suggested that teaching should not just consist of one-way information giving, but should be two-way, by involving the patient. The author also stated that motivation is greatest when learning is seen to help overcome a problem without fear of failure, the relationship between the patient and nurse being based upon respect and sharing.

Memory

Both memory and learning are interrelated. Memory depends upon being able to store and retrieve information, either to short- or long-term memory. A person's ability to store and retrieve information varies, and may be enhanced by reinforcement and repetition, which has a practical application and is important when selecting the methods of teaching (Coutts and Hardy, 1985).

Age

Physiological changes which relate to ageing need to be borne in mind when teaching people. Most important are the visual and auditory changes of ageing which affect people's ability to see and hear information (Culbert and Kos, 1971). Written materials should be of a large typeface, particularly for people with poor vision. Also, the teacher should speak slowly and audibly. Further age changes which need to be borne in mind are the decline in short-term memory and attention. Culbert and Kos (1971) recommend repetition be used to compensate and to be aware when concentration has been lost. Concepts are best taught with a combination of methods: written and audio-visual materials and learning of skills through demonstration and illustration.

Psychological factors

Motivation to learn may also be influenced by a number of psychological factors. The crisis of illness is perhaps not the best time to learn and a period of adaptation is required to come to terms with life's events and changes in self-image. Until this is achieved, the patient is poorly motivated and unable to learn (Culbert and Kos, 1971; Kelly, 1987). Once adaptation has commenced, learning of knowledge and skills can take place. Mild anxiety and awareness of a need to learn can be highly motivating factors (Culbert and Kos, 1971). The higher the educational level of the patient the more aware they are of the need for information and they both express this need and obtain information to assist in coping with their condition (Pender, 1974). Adequate explanation and information given prior to certain procedures has a positive influence on postoperative conditions (Boore, 1978), recovery and level of anxiety (Hayward, 1978; Wilson-Barnett, 1978). However, White *et al.* (1980) studied patients with cardiovascular disease and found learning took place once patients were at home rather than in hospital. The authors felt this was due to postoperative pain and fear inhibiting their learning. Therefore, it is important to establish the optimum time for learning which is dependent upon patients' motivation and individual circumstances.

Environment

Where learning takes place is another important factor. As already mentioned, White *et al.* (1980) found the majority of patients' learning took place once discharged in the community, despite the hospitals' formal approach to teaching. A number of studies have reported a lack of information prior to discharge from hospital regarding care at home (Wilson-Barnett, 1981; Kelly, 1987; Roe and Brocklehurst, 1987). Indeed, planning for discharge has been found to be inadequate (Wilson-Barnett, 1981; Waters, 1987). Waters's (1987) exploratory study into discharge planning in four geriatric wards found it was not a priority for ward nurses and doctors. She concluded that the present methods of communicating with patients in hospitals needs to be supplemented with written information.

Teaching patients has been recommended to be commenced prior to discharge and continued in the community (Carter, 1981; Webb, 1983; Roe, 1989a). Where possible, carers should also be included. They need to be advised about follow-up appointments, further treatments, have adequate supplies of drugs, charts and/or appliances along with information of how to obtain more, and their appropriate disposal. They also need to know who to contact should there be a problem (Carter, 1981; Webb, 1983). All of this advice may be supported with written information (Webb, 1983; Waters, 1987; Roe, 1989a).

Compliance

Teaching has been found to positively affect patients' compliance with recommendations (Haynes *et al.*, 1976; Youssef, 1983). Having knowledge has been found to positively influence compliance, while some situations, e.g. cold weather, colds and 'flu, have been found to have a negative influence on compliance (Tirrel and Hart, 1980). Wong and Wong (1985) studied prevalence of postoperative exercises and found greater compliance by those who had received pre-operative teaching. They concluded that a designed educational programme not only increases knowledge but enhances the patient's desire to comply. Therefore, teaching patients and carers not only increases knowledge but the likelihood of compliance, which can only be of benefit to the person with incontinence. However, a number of studies have reported non-compliance with bladder training regimens at follow-up which result from the extrinsic motivation or reinforcement being removed (Frewen, 1980; Pengelly and Booth, 1980; Burgio *et al.*, 1985).

To summarise, all of the above factors, such as motivation, age, memory, psychological factors and environment, relate to learning taking place, and these need to be borne in mind when teaching patients and carers. They all point to the importance of assessing patients, planning and implementing teaching, along with its evaluation.

Methods of teaching

There are many teaching strategies available, suitable for teaching individuals or groups of people. This section will look at what is available and identify their suitability for each type of learning and the target groups, along with their advantages and disadvantages. Wilson and Desruisseaux (1983) stress the importance of focusing on the learner and including them when adopting the teaching method, the emphasis therefore being on the individual. However, for research purposes, in order to be able to test a particular educational method or programme it is necessary for it to be standardised and administered to all people (White *et al.*, 1980; Gregor, 1981; Roe, 1990a; 1990b). However, in practice the method most suited to meeting the individual's learning should be adopted. Wilson and Desruisseaux (1983) have a wealth of experience in teaching stoma care to patients and carers and stress the importance of setting the right climate for learning along with assessing the individual, planning the teaching and evaluating learning.

Cognitive learning

Teaching methods available to bring about cognitive learning or increase people's knowledge include discussion, printed aids (e.g. booklets), visual aids (e.g. prints), audio-visual aids (e.g. videos) and lectures. Discussion, visual/audio-visual aids and lectures are suitable for teaching individuals or groups of people. However, printed aids such as booklets are only suited to teaching individuals, e.g. patients and/or carers.

The advantages of discussion are that it may be both individualised and informing, allowing response to individual cues. Clarification of points is possible and permits the teacher flexibility. However, the main disadvantage is that it may be time-consuming. Use of printed aids such as booklets offer consistent information and knowledge that allows the learner to control the timing and encourages self-directed learning. They also provide continued learning and promote questioning by individuals. However, the main disadvantages of printed aids are that they may be misunderstood if not accompanied by discussion; also people need to be able to read (Visser, 1980).

The advantages of using visual or audio visual aids are that they can pass on knowledge to the learner, provide consistent information, promote understanding of body form and changes in its function. They also enforce learning by using sight and hearing and instigate questions from learners. Their main disadvantage is that they may be confusing because of too much detail being given all at once. Lectures conserve the teacher's time and are particularly suited to large groups; however their formality may threaten learners and can minimise discussion.

Further information on teaching methods for cognitive learning may be obtained from Wilson and Desruisseaux (1983) and Redman (1984).

Affective learning

This learning relates to feelings, attitudes and changing values. Teaching methods or skills available to bring about such changes include: listening, discussion, encouragement of individuals' verbal expressions and exploration and counselling. Listening and discussion can be used for individual or small group learning whereas counselling and verbal expression/exploration are more suited to the individual. Their main advantages are that they can form a relationship based upon caring, security and trust and promote people's coping and adaptation. The main disadvantage is that the teacher or nurse is uncomfortable confronting her own attitudes and feelings towards elimination or sexuality. Again, further suggested reading is Wilson and Desruisseaux (1983) and Redman (1984).

Psychomotor skills

Finally, the teaching methods used for psychomotor skills include verbal description and explanation, written instructions and diagrams, photographs, demonstrations, repetitive practice and re-evaluation. Learning of psychomotor skills is best suited to individual learning along with one other carer. The advantage of verbal description is that it encourages understanding of the skill. Demonstration in a logical sequence will avoid confusion, while repetition of the skill by the learner promotes achievement and their independence. There are no reported disadvantages for any of the teaching methods available when learning psychomotor skills (Wilson and Desruisseaux, 1983; Redman, 1984).

There is a wide range of teaching methods which will bring about learning. Some methods are more suited to teaching individuals and groups. A combination of methods should be selected, particularly when learning needs to be achieved in all three areas, i.e. cognitive, affective and psychomotor skills.

Role of the nurse

Within the last decade the nurse's role in patient teaching has gained in importance and recognition (Cohen, 1981; Close, 1988; Wilson-Barnett, 1988; Luker and Caress, 1989) with a developed body of research evidence being available (Wilson-Barnett, 1989). Patient teaching has been recently defined as the process of increasing patients' or clients' understanding about their state of health/disease, treatment and rehabilitation, by giving specific information in a planned and structured way (ibid.).

An early study in the United States of the scope of teaching carried out by nurses, and their preparation, found both confusion and a marked lack of preparation for patient teaching (Pohl, 1965). Indeed, even today some researchers feel that current education of nurses does not equip them to be competent patient teachers (Luker and Caress, 1989). Factors attributed to teaching not occurring have been lack of time, heavy workload, understaffing and lack of knowledge or necessary skills (Pohl, 1965; Winslow, 1976; Syred, 1981).

Despite nurses being uniquely placed to teach patients and carers (Syred, 1981) they sometimes fail to appreciate the necessity of patient teaching and underestimate the contribution they have to make (Luker and Box, 1986; Lafferty and Salter, 1987). Although one study in particular found nurses discussed nursing care and treatment significantly more often with patients than physicians (Pender, 1974). With increasing numbers of patients being cared for in the community (Anderson, 1987) in particular by lay carers (Goodman, 1986; Luker and Perkins, 1987), nurses clearly have a role in supporting and teaching aspects of health promotion and self-care, particularly in relation to the promotion of continence and management of incontinence (Norton, 1986).

Nurses are in a prime position to initiate and carry out teaching behavioural strategies for the promotion of continence, such as bladder training (Rooney, 1989) or pelvic floor exercises (Norton, 1986; Mandelstam, 1984). So, too, for the management of incontinence appliances. This not only ensures that appliances are fitted appropriately and managed efficiently but helps to promote patients' acceptance and independence. To date, despite recommendations for nurses' involvement in teaching for the promotion of continence and management of incontinence, little research has evaluated the method of teaching used. Most research based and non-research based publications have concentrated on changing professional and public attitudes (Swaffield, 1981) and proving treatments are successful in eradicating or improving incontinence (Cardozo *et al.*, 1978; Frewen, 1980; Castleden *et al.*, 1985). The literature rarely mentions non-compliance or evaluates the actual methods of teaching. However, as nursing research into incontinence develops, these issues will hopefully be investigated.

Nursing literature is unanimous in the fact that nurses have a responsibility to commence and continue teaching patients and carers about health education and self-care, in particular incontinence, both in hospital and the community (Wilson-Barnett, 1983; Redman, 1984; Coutts and Hardy, 1985; Norton, 1986). Clearly, this has implications for the content of nurse education and nursing practice. In order to be able to teach patients, nurses must be familiar with the theories of learning and the different methods of teaching.

Luker and Caress (1989) contend that it is not feasible for all nurses to carry out patient education as they neither have the knowledge nor the teaching skills required. They suggest that this should be the role of the clinical nurse specialist. However, in relation to incontinence, often districts have only one continence adviser who could not possibly see all patients or client groups. Therefore it is essential that they act in an advisory capacity and support nurses in their teaching of patients and carers about continence.

The following sections review the current research evidence for teaching behavioural strategies for the promotion of continence and management of appliances for incontinence.

Teaching behavioural strategies for the promotion of continence

Norton (1983) has cited nurses as the principal teachers in relation to continence and those strategies involving training. Indeed, such strategies can offer an effective and relatively inexpensive method for re-establishing continence (Whitehead *et al.*, 1984). Restoring continence is the optimal goal rather than simply managing incontinence and can not only improve people's quality of life but prevent institutional care. These strategies comprise bladder training, pelvic floor exercises, behaviour modification and biofeedback (which have been dealt with in Chapters 4 and 5). The purpose of this chapter is not to describe the strategies already covered but to review the research evidence in relation to the teaching methods used.

Pelvic floor re-education

Much of the literature has expounded the benefits of teaching pelvic floor exercises to reduce stress incontinence (Kegel, 1948; Shepherd and Montgomery, 1984; Laycock, 1987), although some authors have found pelvic floor exercises along with regular exercise to be more beneficial (Gordon and Logue, 1985). How this teaching is carried out is not always clearly documented, nor is it demonstrated that each patient has received exactly the same information. Norton (1983) has recommended the pelvic floor is described, two fingers are inserted into the patient and they are instructed to squeeze their pelvic floor muscles. Laycock (1987) taught patients to contract the pelvic floor muscles and instructed them to practise contractions. These were evaluated by digital examination by the instructor and by self-digital evaluation. Castleden *et al.* (1984) had patients use a perineometer to confirm they were practising the right exercises. However, no difference in improved continence outcome was found between the two groups of physiotherapy alone or physiotherapy plus perineometer. All of the studies demonstrate improvement in stress incontinence following initiation of pelvic floor exercises. However, it is not clear whether verbal instructions were the same for all patients or if the patients understood them or would have benefited from alternative teaching, nor was there any follow up to measure long-term compliance.

Physiotherapy using electrical stimulation has been shown to be effective as exercise in strengthening the pelvic floor muscles and controlling incontinence (Dougall, 1985; Plevnik *et al.*, 1986; Laycock, 1989). Despite a favourable treatment outcome, client learning does not necessarily take place, and repeated short courses of stimulation may be required.

Plevnik (1985) has carried out a small study using a set of nine graded cones inserted one at a time into the vagina as a means of exercising the pelvic floor muscles and increasing their strength by biofeedback (n = 10). Laycock (1987) has maintained that the procedure teaches patients the appropriate muscles to contract, which is often the greatest hurdle in pelvic floor re-education. However, biofeedback does not ensure learning has taken place nor whether there is long-term compliance. The research in all these studies is primarily designed to measure a treatment outcome with no clear presentation of the teaching method used or its evaluation.

Bladder re-education

A standard definition for the approaches used in bladder re-education has not been developed. Its broad usage for a variety of regimens not only causes confusion but also makes comparison of research studies difficult (Hadley, 1986; Rooney, 1989). Four logical and useful categories have been developed: bladder training, habit retraining, timed voiding and prompted voiding (Hadley, 1986) (see Chapter 4, Bladder re-education for the promotion of continence). A number of studies have found bladder training regimens to be of use particularly for urgency, unstable detrusor and incontinence with no apparent cause, and advocate their use (Frewen, 1978; Pengelly and Booth, 1980; Jarvis, 1981; Svigos and Matthews, 1977; Castleden *et al.*, 1985). However, due to there being many inherent differences in the subjects chosen, research designs and methods, it is difficult to compare findings. Some have included bladder training, use of drugs and differing environments (Jarvis, 1981; Castleden *et al.*, 1985), making outcome variables difficult to isolate and cannot therefore attribute the beneficial effects to the behavioural manipulation. Indeed, Meyhoff *et al.* (1983), in a small cross-over study including 19 females with urge incontinence, found a placebo medication resulted in decreased micturition and incontinent episodes. This study used patients' own assessment of micturition and incontinent episodes which may have been unreliable. Frazer *et al.* (1989) have found discrepancies between 84 females' subjective assessment of their incontinence and concurrent objective assessment using a two-hour pad-weighing test. This questions the reliability of studies which rely solely on patients' subjective outcomes (Pengelly and Booth, 1980). Often the type of incontinence has not been defined, nor a control group used (Hadley, 1986).

Looking specifically at the teaching methods used, they are not often detailed in studies with the word 'instruct' provided as the sole description of what took place. Teaching methods are not usually described or evaluated (Svigos and Matthews, 1977; Jarvis, 1981). Frewen (1978) and Pengelly and Booth (1980) have provided written information to their clients along with verbal instruction when teaching bladder training, and have also acknowledged non-compliance with reasons given to support why this occurred. They recommend that cognitive understanding is required for training to be successful with social conditions and their environments having a part to play. As already stated, studies have predominantly looked at treatment outcomes for incontinence rather than evaluating the teaching methods used. Rigorous adherence and documentation of the teaching methods used, measures of their validity, and long-term follow-up of patients would be useful.

Biofeedback

Biofeedback is a form of behaviour therapy used to teach patients how to control bladder contractions and contraction/relaxation of the sphincters (Whitehead *et al.*, 1984). Biofeedback is useful in learning motor skills whereby the patient has repeated practice and learns by success and failure. Electronic equipment may be used to provide visual and auditory information from physiological changes which can help the patient learn how to control the responses. Biofeedback has the advantage of avoiding surgery or the use of drugs. It can also help to give patients a better understanding of bladder function. However, it is labour intensive with failure to attend sessions being a repeated problem.

Cardozo *et al.* (1978) and Burgio *et al.* (1985) have both used biofeedback, using cystometry and bladder training regimens. Thirty-two female patients with detrusor instability underwent cystometric biofeedback as part of their treatment; 50 per cent cured and improved their incontinence and 50 per cent failed to respond or did not have objective improvement (Cardozo *et al.*, 1978). The authors stated that for patients to benefit they need to be highly motivated and reasonably intelligent. It is unclear what actual teaching the patients received. Burgio *et al.* (1985) included 39 elderly outpatients with stress incontinence, detrusor motor instability and urge incontinence without instability, who underwent cystometric biofeedback and habit retraining. Teaching took the form of audio and visual feedback from cystometry, verbal instruction and reinforcement, along with repeated practice. Patients with detrusor motor instability and patients with urge incontinence improved their continence after teaching, which still remained after twelve months' follow-up. However, for patients with incontinence (number in study = 19) only 10 had improved continence at twelve month follow-up, while 9 patients reported regression after termination and did not continue with the home programme. Regression was mainly due to non-compliance. Therefore, despite some success, once again it can be stated that biofeedback does not necessarily ensure learning takes place nor therefore compliance with bladder training strategies. This points to the need for continued reinforcement. Hadley (1986) stated that it is important to determine whether biofeedback alone, or in conjunction with bladder training strategies, is more successful than bladder training alone. Obviously, biofeedback requires additional instruments and personnel, whose purchase and time need to be justified. It must also be borne in mind that some patients' incontinence is transient, with Yarnell and St Leger (1979) finding a third of patients (number in study = 396) regained continence with no intervention at all.

Prompted voiding

This approach has been used for patients with severe cognitive and physical ability defects. Patients are asked, at regular intervals, if they need to use the toilet. Assistance is given only with a positive answer (Hadley, 1986). Creason et al. (1989) carried out an experimental intervention on 85 female nursing home residents having low mental state scores. Positive effects of prompted voiding were noted in comparison to a socialised only group and control. Incontinence and toileting records were kept by nursing staff which can prove unreliable measures. Despite showing an improvement in continence, no diagnosis of the patients' urinary incontinence had been established nor of an individual's base line toilet habits, which could have been useful. Learning does not necessarily take place with prompted voiding, although such a regimen is intended for the cognitively impaired.

Behaviour modification

Use of reward and punishment to re-establish continent behaviour in the elderly, or to teach toileting behaviour in adults with mental handicap, have produced encouraging results (Whitehead et al., 1984). Operant conditioning is used to modify behaviour. Psychomotor skills such as toileting may be achieved but cognitive or affective learning does not take place. A small replication study (number in study = 7) of behaviour modification for toileting and incontinence, as carried out by Foxx and Azrin (1973), has been reported (cited in Heller et al., 1989). Seven elderly patients (71–95 years) living in the community with either cognitive or mobility impairment were included. A comprehensive description of teaching methods has been provided with detailed patient characteristics, pretraining information and two-week follow-up. The intensive behaviour modification programme over a two-week period resulted in improved continence and toileting. The teaching methods used are both complex but explicit. However, due to the small sample size it is not possible to identify which elements of teaching were most important to the treatment outcome.

There is a wealth of research that has investigated treatment outcomes in relation to behavioural strategies for the promotion of continence. Invariably they have not used control groups, similar diagnoses, defined the type of incontinence suffered and have combined a number of independent variables, e.g. bladder training and drug therapy, which makes comparison impossible. The research designs, despite using teaching methods, do not rigorously document what was carried out or evaluate the methods used. The emphasis is usually upon treatment outcome of incontinence rather than combined with an evaluation of the success of teaching. A wide range of teaching methods exist and it can only be ascertained whether the most appropriate method is being used by including some form of evaluation in the research design. Another consideration which would affect outcome would be spontaneous remission of incontinence (Yarnell and St Leger, 1979). All of these issues and considerations offer an exciting challenge to the research of the future.

Teaching for appliance management of incontinence

Where behavioural approaches have not been successful in promoting continence, then the patients' incontinence will need to be managed. There are many aids and appliances available for the management of incontinence: containment – pads and pants; conduction – male urinals, penile sheaths, catheters, drainage bags; and occlusion devices – penile clamps, vaginal acclusion devices (Norton, 1986; Ryan-Wooley, 1987; ACA, 1988). Designs and materials have continued to be developed and improved in recent years with increasing emphasis on client comfort. Continence advisers are unanimous that when selecting and supplying an aid it is essential that patients and carers are taught how to use them and the correct application (Norton, 1986). This has not always been the case in practice as continence advisers cannot see all clients, and nurses in practice lack knowledge of the correct application of certain aids or what is available. A detailed account of these appliances has already been presented in Chapters 6, 7 and 8. The purpose of this section is to review research literature that has specifically looked at patient teaching in relation to these aids and appliances.

Pads and pants

To date, no research has been undertaken that has investigated patient teaching on the management of pads and pants. Recommendations have been largely in relation to application, removal and disposal (Norton, 1986). Manufacturers are largely relied upon to teach nursing staff the correct application of their own particular brand of pads.

Male urinals and penile sheaths

Male urinals are still predominantly fitted by surgical fitters, either with a manufacturer or for a wholesaler. It is not known what teaching or instruction clients receive. Penile sheaths are mainly fitted by nursing staff, and clients and carers are taught how to manage them. The main focus of research has related to evaluation of products (Watson, 1987) rather than teaching patients and carers how to manage them efficiently and safely. Recommendations and instructions given have been based largely upon common sense rather than tested practice.

Intermittent self-catheterisation

Lapides *et al.* (1975) and Hunt *et al.* (1984) have established a method of using a clean technique when carrying out intermittent self-catheterisation, with a lower prevalence of urinary tract infection being present than with indwelling urethral catheters (see Chapter 7, Intermittent self-catheterisation). However, their teaching methods have not been explicitly described, nor were they a variable tested as all patients implemented a clean technique. Nurses are largely responsible for teaching patients and carers how to intermittently self-catheterise. Norton (1986) has provided a detailed stepwise account of how this is done, using written information, consistent policy, detailed explanation and demonstration. However, this is prescriptive rather than on the basis of comparative evidence. Written information booklets may be obtained from manufacturers but have generally not been compiled on the basis of research evidence.

Indwelling urethral catheters and drainage bags

It is only recently that teaching patients and carers about catheter management has been recognised (Slade and Gillespie, 1985; Norton, 1986; Roe, 1989a). As the profile of incontinence has been raised and continence advisers have become more prevalent, the needs of patients with indwelling urethral catheters are coming to the forefront. As these patients form small numbers in medical specialities (Crow *et al.*, 1986) and the community (Roe, 1989b), they have been largely missed. Little information and initial explanation has been received by patients (Roe and Brocklehurst, 1987; Cummings *et al.*, 1982) with advice and information not always being consistent or based upon good practices (Crummy, 1989; Roe, 1989c; 1989d). An experimental study has tested the effects of an education programme on patients' knowledge and acceptance of their catheters and management of urine drainage systems (Roe, 1990a; 1990b). Forty-five new and established catheter users were included in a controlled trial and were visited on three occasions: pretest, posttest, and follow-up at five months. Trial patients received the education programme which comprised a written information booklet, used as a teaching aid and developed as part of the method from a comprehensive literature review, demonstration of bag emptying and changing (according to the booklet, Roe, (1987)) and mutual questioning and answering. The control group received conventional care. Significant differences were found, with trial patients having increased knowledge of their catheter's location, function, risks associated with their use and how they may be minimised ($p < 0.05$). New users in the trial group's acceptance of their catheter was accelerated, denoted by a decreased depression score to that of the established users. This has important implications for all clients with incontinence, in that we can help them to adjust and accept their condition, aids and appliances by teaching and supporting them.

Management of the urine drainage system by patients and carers was observed on three occasions. Bag emptying and bag changing were observed and handwashing practice, the equipment used, contamination and disposal of urine and drainage bags recorded. Before and after teaching comparisons were able to be made. A significant improvement in handwashing before and after bag emptying and changing was found at the posttest visit ($p < 0.05$). However, this improved effect had disappeared by the follow-up, which may have been due to a small sample size. However, this does prove that teaching can be effective and once commenced in hospital should be continued and reinforced in the community (Roe, 1990a; 1990b). This study concluded that teaching patients about catheter care, using an information booklet as part of the educational programme, was successful in increasing patients' knowledge and acceptance of their catheter; also management of the drainage system, but to a lesser extent.

Unlike the behavioural strategies for promotion of continence, hardly any research has been carried out that has tested teaching in relation to the management of aids and appliances. Once again, this offers a challenge to nursing research. Prescriptive information is available to say how important it is to teach patients and carers about managing their appliances safely and efficiently using the words 'explain' and 'instruct'. Literature is available from many manufacturers, although not all are based upon sound research evidence or have been tested for their effectiveness. The next stage would be to test the effects of teaching and evaluate patients' management of their appliances using the research designs described by Campbell and Stanley (1963).

Summary

This chapter has presented the theories of teaching and factors which can affect learning, a description of the teaching methods available, their suitability, advantages and disadvantages. It has also looked at the role of the nurse in patient teaching generally, and continence specifically. A review of the research evidence for teaching behavioural strategies for continence promotion and management of aids and appliances has also been described and discussed. Patient teaching has now developed as a subject in its own right within nursing research. The body of knowledge, lines of enquiry, research and critical thinking have developed and continue to do so (Wilson-Barnett, 1988; 1989; Luker and Caress, 1989). Research in relation to behavioural strategies for the promotion of continence have predominantly focused on medical treatment outcomes and have not evaluated or rigorously documented the teaching methods used. Comparison of the findings of these studies is not always possible due to inherent design differences. Such research requires expertise in urodynamics, medicine, nursing, behavioural sciences and research methods. Collaboration therefore could lead to substantial progress in the promotion of continence. Despite the importance of nursing practice in relation to the management of aids and appliances for incontinence, little research has been carried out in relation to patient teaching. This offers a great challenge to nursing research, in particular clinical nursing practice related to the promotion and management of continence.

References

ACA (1988), *Directory of Continence and Toileting Aids*, London: Disabled Living Foundation.

Anderson, R. (1987), 'The unremitting burden on carers', *British Medical Journal*, 294: 73–4.

Bloom, B.S. (ed.) (1956), *Taxonomy of educational objectives, Handbook 1: Cognitive domain*, New York: David McKay.

Boore, J.R.P. (1978), *Prescription for Recovery*, London: Royal College of Nursing.

Burgio, K.L., Whitehead, W.E. and Engel, B.T. (1985), 'Urinary Incontinence in the Elderly', *Annals of Internal Medicine*, 104: 507–15.

Campbell, D.T. and Stanley, J.C. (1963), *Experimental and quasi experimental designs for research*, Boston: Houghton Mifflin.

Cardozo, L.D., Abrams, P.D., Stanton, S.L. and Feneley, R.C.L. (1978), 'Idiopathic bladder instability treated by biofeedback', *British Journal of Urology*, 50: 521–3.

Carter, E. (1981), 'Ready for home?', *Nursing Times*, 7 May: 826–9.

Castleden, C.M., Duffin, H.M. and Mitchell, E.P. (1984), 'The effect of physiotherapy on stress incontinence', *Age and Ageing*, 13: 235–7.

Castleden, C.M., Duffin, H.M., Asher, K.J. and Yeomanson, C.W. (1985), 'Factors influencing outcome in elderly patients with urinary incontinence and detrusor instability', *Age and Ageing*, 14: 303–7.

Close, A. (1988), 'Patient education: a literature review', *Journal of Advanced Nursing*, 13: 203–13.

Cohen, S.A. (1981), 'Patient education: a review of the literature', *Journal of Advanced Nursing*, 6: 11–18.

Coutts, L.C. and Hardy, L.K. (1985), *Teaching for Health*, Edinburgh: Churchill Livingstone.

Creason, N.S., Grybowski, J.A., Burgener, S., Whippo, C., Yeo, S. and Richardson, B. (1989), 'Prompted voiding therapy for urinary incontinence in aged female nursing home residents', *Journal of Advanced Nursing*, 14: 120–6.

Crow, R.A., Chapman, R.G., Roe, B.H. and Wilson, J.A. (1986), 'A study of patients with an indwelling urethral catheter and related nursing practice', Nursing Practice Research Unit, University of Surrey.

Crummy, V. (1989), 'Ignorance can hurt', *Nursing Times*, 85(21): 66–70.

Culbert, P.A. and Kos, B.A. (1971), 'Ageing: considerations for health teaching', *Nursing Clinics of North America*, 6(4): 605–14.

Cummings, K.M., Becker, M.H., Kirscht, J.P. and Levin, N.W. (1982), 'Psychosocial factors affecting adherence to medical regimens in a group of haemiodialysis patients', *Medical Care*, 20(6): 567–80.

Dougall, D.S. (1985), 'The effects of interferential therapy on incontinence and frequency of micturition', *Physiotherapy*, 71(3): 135–6.

Frazer, M.I., Haylen, B.T. and Sutherst, J.R. (1989), 'The severity of incontinence in women', *British Journal of Urology*, 63: 14–15.

Frewen, W.K. (1978), 'An objective assessment of the unstable bladder of psychosomatic origin', *British Journal of Urology*, 50: 246–9.

Frewen, W.K. (1980), 'The management of urgency and frequency of micturition', *British Journal of Urology*, 52: 367–9.

Goodman, C. (1986), 'Research on the informal carer: a selected literature review', *Journal of Advanced Nursing*, 11: 705–12.

Gordon, H. and Logue, M. (1985), 'Perineal muscle function after childbirth', *The Lancet*, 20 July: 123–5.

Gregor, F.M. (1981), 'Teaching the patient with ischaemic heart disease: a systematic approach to instructional design', *Patient Counselling and Health Education*, 3: 57–62.

Hadley, E.C. (1986), 'Bladder training and related therapies for urinary incontinence in older people', *Journal of the American Medical Association*, 256(3): 372–9.

Haynes, R.B., Gibson, E.S., Hackett, B.C., Johnson, A.L., Sackett, D.L., Taylor, D.W. and Roberts, R.S. (1976), 'Improvement of medication compliance in uncontrolled hypertension', *The Lancet*, 1 (June): 1265–8.

Hayward, J. (1975), *Information – A prescription against pain* (1st edn), London: Royal College of Nursing.

Heller, B.R., Whitehead, W.E. and Johnson, L.D. (1989), 'Incontinence', *Journal of Gerontological Nursing*, 15(5): 16–23.

Hunt, G., Whitaker, R.H. and Doyle, P.T. (1984), 'Intermittent self catheterisation in adults', *British Medical Journal*, 289: 467–8.

Jarvis, G.J. (1981), 'Controlled trial of bladder drill and drug therapy in the management of detrusor instability', *British Journal of Urology*, 53: 565–6.

Kegel, A.H. (1948), 'Progressive resistance exercise in the functional restoration of the perineal muscles', *American Journal of Obstetrics and Gynecology*, 56(2): 238–48.

Kelly, M.P. (1987), 'Managing radical surgery: notes from the patient's viewpoint', *Gut*, 28(1): 81–7.

Krathwohl, D.K., Bloom, B.S. and Masia, B.B. (1965), *Taxonomy of educational objectives, Handbook II, Affective domain*, New York: David McKay.

Lafferty, G. and Salter, B. (1987), 'Health education as carried out by district nurses and health visitors', Health Care Research Associates, Dept of Educational Studies, University of Surrey.

Lapides, J., Diokono, A.C., Gould, F.R. and Lowe, B.S. (1975), 'Further observations on self catheterisation', *Transactions of the American Association of Genito Urinary Surgeons*, 67: 15–17.

Laycock, J. (1987), 'Graded exercises for the pelvic floor muscle in the treatment of urinary incontinence', *Physiotherapy*, 73(7): 371–3.

Laycock, J. (1989), 'Physiotherapy in the treatment of incontinence', Geriatric Workshop on Incontinence, Manchester. *Geriatric Medicine*, February: 28–9.

Luker, K.A. and Box, D. (1986), 'The response of nurses towards the management and teaching of patients on continuous ambulatory peritoneal dialysis', *International Journal of Nursing Studies*, 23(1): 51–9.

Luker, K.A. and Caress, A. (1989), 'Rethinking patient education', *Journal of Advanced Nursing*, 14(9): 711–18.

Luker, K.A. and Perkins, E.S. (1987), 'The elderly at home: service needs and provision', *Journal of the Royal College of General Practitioners*, 37: 248-50.

Mandelstam, D. (1984), 'Incontinence: re-education of the pelvic floor', *Nursing*, 29: 867–8.

Meyhoff, H.H., Gerstenberg, T.C. and Nordling, J. (1983), 'Placebo: the drug of choice in female motor urge incontinence', *British Journal of Urology*, 55: 34–7.

Norton, C. (1983), 'Teaching for urinary incontinence', in Wilson-Barnett, J. (ed.), *Patient Teaching*, Edinburgh: Churchill Livingstone.

Norton, C. (1986), *Nursing for Continence*, Beaconsfield: Beaconsfield Publishers.

Pender, N.J. (1974), 'Patient identification of health information received during hospitalisation', *Nursing Research*, 23(3): 262–7.

Pengelly, A.W. and Booth, C.M. (1980), 'A prospective trial of bladder training as treatment for detrusor instability', *British Journal of Urology*, 52: 463–6.

Plevnik, S. (1985), 'New methods for testing and strengthening the pelvic floor muscles', *Proceedings of the International Continence Society*, London: 267–8.

Plevnik S., Jarez, J., Vrtacnik, P., Trsinar, B. and Vodusek, D.B. (1986), 'Short term electrical stimulation: home treatment for urinary incontinence', *World Journal of Urology*, 4: 24–6.

Pohl, H.L. (1965), 'Teaching activities of the nursing practitioner', *Nursing Research*, 14(1): 4–11.

Redman, B.K. (1984), *The Process of Patient Education* (5th edn), St Louis: C.V. Mosby.

Roe, B.H. (1987), *Catheter Care: A Guide for Users and their Carers*, Colchester: H.G. Wallace.

Roe, B.H. (1989a), 'Catheter care and patient teaching', Unpublished PhD thesis, University of Manchester.

Roe, B.H. (1989b), 'Catheters in the community', *Nursing Times*, 85(36): 43.

Roe, B.H. (1989c), 'Use of bladder washouts: a study of nurses' recommendations', *Journal of Advanced Nursing*, 14: 494–500.

Roe, B.H. (1989d), 'Study of information given by nurses for catheter care to patients', *Journal of Advanced Nursing*, 14(3): 203–11.

Roe, B.H. (1990a), 'Study of the effects of education on patients' knowledge and acceptance of their indwelling urethral catheters', *Journal of Advanced Nursing*, I5(2): 223–31.

Roe, B.H. (1990b), 'Study of the effects of education on the management of urine drainage systems by patients and carers', *Journal of Advanced Nursing*, 15(5): 517–24.

Roe, B.H. and Brocklehurst, J.C. (1987), 'Study of patients with indwelling catheters', *Journal of Advanced Nursing*, 12: 713–18.

Rooney, V. (1989), 'Bladder re-education and timed voiding programmes', Geriatric Workshop on Incontinence, Manchester', *Geriatric Medicine*, February: 26–7.

Ryan-Wooley, B. (1987), *Aids for the Management of Incontinence*, London: King's Fund.

Shepherd, A.M. and Montgomery, E. (1983), 'Treatment of genuine stress incontinence with a new perineometer', *Physiotherapy*, 69(4): 113.

Slade, N. and Gillespie, W.A. (1985), *The urinary tract and the catheter: infection and other problems*, Chichester: Wiley.

Svigos, J.M. and Matthews, C.D. (1977), 'Assessment and treatment of female urinary incontinence by cystometrogram and bladder retraining programs', *Obstetrics and Gynaecology*, 50(1): 9–12.

Swaffield, L. (1981), 'Attitudes to incontinence', *Nursing Times, Community Outlook*, February: 51.

Syred, M.E.J. (1981), 'The abdication of the role of health education by hospital nurses', *Journal of Advanced Nursing*, 6: 27–33.

Tirrel, B.E. and Hart, L.K. (1980), 'The relationship of health beliefs and knowledge to exercise compliance in patients after coronary bypass', *Heart and Lung*, 9: 481–93.

Visser, A. Ph. (1980), 'Effects of an information booklet on well being of hospital patients', *Patient Counselling and Health Education*, 2: 51–64.

Waters, K.R. (1987), 'Discharge planning: an exploratory study of the process of discharge planning on geriatric wards', *Journal of Advanced Nursing*, 12: 71–83.

Watson, R. (1987), *An Investigation in the use of External Continuous Urine Collecting Systems for the Management of Incontinence in Elderly Male Hospitalised Patients*, Cardiff: Simpla Plastics Ltd.

Webb, C. (1983), 'Teaching for recovery from surgery', in Wilson-Barnett, J. (ed.), *Patient Teaching*, Edinburgh: Churchill Livingstone.

Wells, T.J. (1984), 'Social and psychological implications of incontinence', in Brocklehurst, J.C. (ed.), *Urology in the Elderly*, Edinburgh: Churchill Livingstone.

White, C.W., Lemon, D.K. and Albanese, M.A. (1980), 'Efficacy of health education efforts in hospitalised patients with serious cardiovascular illness: can teaching succeed?', *Patient Counselling and Health Education*, 2: 189–96.

Whitehead, W.E., Burgio, K.L. and Engel, B.T. (1984), 'Behavioural methods in the assessment and treatment of urinary incontinence', in Brocklehurst, J.C. (ed.), *Urology in the Elderly*, Edinburgh: Churchill Livingstone.

Wilson, E.H. and Desruisseaux, B. (1983), 'Stoma care and patient teaching', in Wilson Barnett, J. (ed.), *Patient Teaching*, Edinburgh: Churchill Livingstone.

Wilson-Barnett, J. (1978), 'Patients' emotional responses to barium X-rays', *Journal of Advanced Nursing*, 3: 37–46.

Wilson-Barnett, J. (1981), 'Assessment of recovery: with special reference to a study with post operative cardiac patients', *Journal of Advanced Nursing*, 6: 435–45.

Wilson-Barnett, J. (1983), *Patient Teaching*, Edinburgh: Churchill Livingstone.

Wilson-Barnett, J. (1988), 'Patient teaching or patient counselling', *Journal of Advanced Nursing*, 13: 215–22.

Wilson-Barnett, J. (1989), 'Patient teaching', in Macleod Clark, J. and Hockey, L. (eds), *Further Research for Nursing*, London: Scutari Press.

Winslow, E.H. (1976), 'The role of the nurse in patient education', *Nursing Clinics of North America*, 11: 213–22.

Wong, J. and Wong, S. (1985), 'A randomized controlled trial of a new approach to preoperative teaching and patient compliance', *International Journal of Nursing Studies*, 22(2): 105–15.

Yarnell, J.W.G. and St Leger, A.S. (1979), 'The prevalence, severity and factors associated with urinary incontinence in a random sample of the elderly', *Age and Ageing*, 8: 81–5.

Youssef, F.A. (1983), 'Compliance with therapeutic regimens: a follow-up study for patients with affective disorders', *Journal of Advanced Nursing*, 8: 513–17.

Index